gōkay fitness

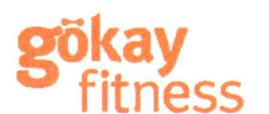

GOKAY
KURTULDUM

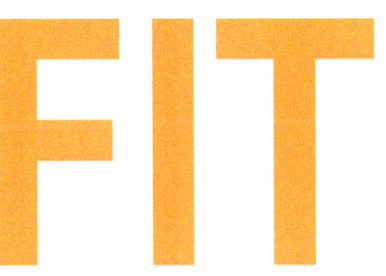

GET
FIT STAY
FIT

For Men Over 40

Get Fit, Stay Fit

Copyright © 2020 Gokay Kurtuldum

All rights reserved.

ISBN: 978-1-8380050-0-9

No parts of this publication may be reproduced, stored in a retrieval system, or transmitted in any form or by any means, electronic, mechanical, photocopying, recording, or otherwise, without the prior written permission of the copyright owner.

This book is sold subject to the condition that it shall not, by way of trade or otherwise, be lent, resold, hired out, or otherwise circulated without the publisher's prior consent in any form of binding or cover other than that in which it is published and without a similar condition including this condition being imposed on the subsequent purchaser. Under no circumstances may any part of this book be photocopied for resale.

Cover and interior design by Jessica Bell

DISCLAIMER

Gokay Kurtuldum strongly recommends that you consult your doctor and get medical approval before beginning any fitness and/or exercise programme and always consult your GP, registered dietician or nutritionist before making any significant changes to your diet, particularly if you have a medical condition.

You are voluntarily choosing to participate in a physical exercise programme. You agree that any information, instruction or advice obtained from Gokay Kurtuldum must NOT be used as a substitute for your doctor's advice or treatment. You agree that any information, instruction or advice obtained from Gokay Kurtuldum will be used at your own risk. You agree to release and discharge Gokay Kurtuldum from any and all responsibilities or liabilities from injury arising from your participation in any exercise programme.

Whilst Gokay's training programmes help most people lose weight and get fit, they have not been specifically designed for you and individual results will vary.

In the recipes, where calorie and macronutrient information is provided, it is calculated using common databases. Exact values might vary depending on the product quality and the brand.

Additional note: all client names have been changed in this book.

CONTENTS

Prologue: How I Found My Mission 11

Part One

Chapter 1: The Why and the How 14
    1.1 Is this you? 14
    1.2 Why should you care? 16
    1.3 The promise 18
    1.4 The route-map 18

Chapter 2: Time for a Wake-up Call 20
    2.1 The Slippery Slope 20
    2.2 Muscle and metabolism 21
    2.3 Optimise your life-expectancy 22
    2.4 So what's getting in your way? 22
        #1: The Knowledge Problem 23
        #2: The Accountability Problem 23
        #3: The Motivation Problem 24

Chapter 3: Trust Me, I'm a Trainer 25
    3.1 Client and coach make a team 25
    3.2 My AIMBEST method 27
    3.3 AIMBEST: the 7 steps 28
    3.4 The mind-trap minefield 35

Part Two

Chapter 4: Get Ready to Get Fit (1): Mindset Mastery 42
    4.1 Is it all or nothing - or something in between? 42
    4.2 What's your type? 43
    4.3 The obstacle course 45
    4.4 Repurpose your business skills 52
    4.5 Focus on the vision 53
    4.6 Don't lose sight of your achievements 55

Chapter 5: Get Ready to Get Fit (2): Foundations for Success 58
    5.1 Meet Alexander and Pete 58
    5.2 Heading trouble off at the pass 60
    5.3 Incentives and markers of success 64
    5.4 Define your weight goals 65
    5.5 Specific goal-setting and timetabling 66
    5.6 Planning your new improved diet 69
    5.7 Self-assessment questions 70
    5.8 Be brave, go public! 71
    5.9 Positive competitiveness 73

Part Three
Chapter 6: Fuel Your Fitness 76
    6.1 Excuses, excuses 76
    6.2 The calorie equation 77
    6.3 Why diets don't work for some people 79
    6.4 Your body is equipped with speed cameras 83
    6.5 Scales and apps: tracking your weight and the food you consume 84
        Visiting the scales 84
        Weighing yourself – when is best? 86
        Do we really weigh less in the mornings? 87
        How to stay on track with the MyFitnessPal App 87
    6.6 Your diet composition formula 89
    6.7 Macros 90
    6.8 Protein 91
    6.9 Amino acids 96
    6.10 Let fibre fill you up 98
    6.11 Carbohydrates 100
    6.12 Good Fat and Bad Fat 105
    6.13 Alcohol 106
    6.14 Secret saboteurs 107
    6.15 Temptations 107
    6.16 Fasting 108
    6.17 Eating before and after your workout 109

Part Four

Chapter 7: Get Ready to Get Fit (3): Exercise Safely 111

    7.1 Take the long view.. 111

    7.2 Let's start with a tour 112

    7.3 Where are you going to exercise?...112

    7.4 Why a gym is a great location.. 114

    7.5 Types of gym equipment.. 115

    7.6 Cardio or weights? 116

    7.7 How and when do you gain muscle mass?..117

    7.8 When is it best to exercise? 118

    7.9 How often should I exercise?.. 119

    7.10 The importance of posture 120

    7.11 Why you should monitor your heart rate 120

    7.12 Why should you use a workout app? 123

    7.13 Before and after: the importance of warming up and cooling down.......123

    7.14 Thomas becomes an addict.. 124

Chapter 8: Your 8 Week Get Fit Programme 126

    8.1 Introduction... 126

    8.2 Your Week-by-Week Exercise Programme Summary 127

    8.3 Day-by-day home workout and weight training programme exercise content.. 129

    8.4 WEEK 1 programme and journal pages...137

    8.5 WEEK 2 programme and journal pages...150

    8.6 WEEK 3 programme and journal pages.. 165

    8.7 WEEK 4 programme and journal pages 180

    8.8 WEEK 5 programme and journal pages... 191

    8.9 WEEK 6 programme and journal pages.. 207

    8.10 WEEK 7 programme and journal pages... 220

    8.11 WEEK 8 programme and journal pages...236

Part Five

Chapter 9: Optimise Your Exercise **251**

    9.1 Switch it up: different types of training methods.. 251

    9.2 Body mobility: 5 stretches you should be doing on a daily basis............. 255

    9.3 Body harmony through sleep 257

Chapter 10: You've Got Fit – Now Stay Fit **260**

    10.1 Monitor and maintain for sustained fitness success 260

    10.2 The three paths..260

    10.3 Reassess for Success...262

    10.4 Final tips to keep you on-track 263

    10.5 The end – and the beginning!... 265

Part Six

Chapter 11: Resources **268**

    11.1 Instructions for the exercises in the weight training programmes.............. 268

    11.2 Instructions for the exercises in the home workouts 280

    11.3 The recipe collection: easy, healthy and nutritious dishes......................... 298

Acknowledgements **328**

HOW I FOUND MY MISSION

The sweet runny sauce in the middle of my massive slice of chocolate cake was giving me great pleasure. But it was also making me wonder why, aged nine, I was in our local patisserie with my mum, while my sister stayed at home because she was on a diet. Throughout our childhood, I was athletic and sporty and my sister struggled with her weight. I could eat almost anything I wanted and not worry that I would put on weight; my sister, meanwhile, visited the best dieticians and professors in the Turkish city of Izmir to help her lose weight. Nothing worked.

Why was she not able to come down to a normal healthy weight even though she was on a permanent diet? Was she doing something wrong or was she meant to be obese and we just needed to accept it?

At the age of eight or nine, when most of my friends were discussing their favourite Atari computer game, this family situation was making me think about the reasons why people are overweight and the psychology behind the issue. Growing up in a family with a sister who was the polar opposite to me gave me a tremendous opportunity to observe, make comparisons, test and study weight loss, fitness and wellbeing. It also made me very empathetic.

After my mum died of a heart attack when I was thirteen, my gorgeous sister effectively became my mum and we became even closer. All I wanted was to help her solve her big problem. As the years passed, I realised that it's not so easy to give professional help to a family member.

When I was sixteen, I joined my local gym and became a regular customer, working out five or six days a week. The community at the gym was so supportive that within three years, I found myself on stage representing Turkey in an international bodybuilding contest; I became a national sportsman and 'Mr Turkey'. Fitness had become a big part of my life and I knew that I wanted to help people to get fit, lose weight and be healthy.

While preparing for bodybuilding contests, when you push yourself to your limits for 10-12 weeks even for a weekend-long competition, during the course of which you lose a massive amount of body fat, you learn so much about your body and eating habits and you discover many effective training methods. You not only read articles and books about this, but you apply these methods to your own body.

When I joined the Turkish Air Force, alongside my technical role as a communication sergeant, I trained pilots in how to improve their fitness, stamina and endurance, which helped them during flights where they endured huge G-force pressures in their F16 or F4 fighter jets.

At the age of 22, I lost my dad as well, due to his very unhealthy lifestyle, which involved excessive drinking and a bad diet. This was the final straw, telling me that fitness and wellbeing had to be my way of life. Helping other people needed to be my number one priority, so I chose this rewarding profession.

In 2010 I moved to the UK and qualified as a personal trainer. My professional fitness career had started. Since 2010, the people I've helped have collectively lost over 1,000kg body fat, plus they've gained strength, resilience and confidence. That's my personal reward: to see the transformation people can bring about in their lives, thanks to my help.

The methods you are going to learn in this book are not crash diets or magic wand fitness programmes, but true, proven techniques with lifelong beneficial effects. You will follow step-by-step methods and you'll be spoon-fed with bite-sized advice, so that everything feels easy and doable. With my help, you can get back the fitness and health you thought you'd lost forever.

PART ONE

CHAPTER 1: THE WHY AND THE HOW

1.1 IS THIS YOU?

Since you left your 20s behind, your life's path may have been conventional. Along the way you've certainly made the effort to be as successful as you can be. You may have followed the expectations of your family, making sure you had a good education; you may have taken time out to travel the world; you have settled into employment, got married, had beautiful kids. You have a roof over your head and decent food and drink. You have plans for a kitchen extension or to convert the loft. Your social life is lively and your career path may have had its ups and downs but on the whole, life is pretty good. You're in your 40s now and you're benefiting from all the hard work you put into your career. You're incredibly busy and you're committed to achieving more in your business than ever before.

And yet ...

You've started to realise amongst all this that you've lost control of something else, something crucial, even though you tried so hard to keep a grip on it. You're accustomed to controlling everything else in life. Yet your level of fitness keeps sinking.

The signals are all there and they've been there for a while, even though you've tried so hard to ignore them. Your partner makes polite – and sometimes not so polite – comments about the physical change in you. You have a belly and your face looks chubby. When you meet an old school friend at the annual beer party, you wonder how on earth he manages to look ten years younger than everyone else.

In your 20s, you used to drink seven or eight beers followed by some spirits on a weekday and you'd get up the next day and go to work as if nothing had happened the previous night. You can't do that sort of thing these days.

You are doing well in your career. However, the weight you've gained over the past decade is more significant than your salary increase and you know deep down that you need to do something about it. All those new year resolutions you make start well but still you lose traction, as you have neither a role model nor any guidance on your journey.

You lie awake feeling frustrated about feeling fat or unhealthy or having zero energy or being judged or the fact your jeans don't fit any more. I know even guys do that. Guys ask themselves questions like:

'What if I have a heart attack because I'm so unfit?'

'How can I have more energy so I can enjoy time with my partner and kids?'

'Did my boss notice me getting out of puff when we walked back from that meeting?'

'What if I go to my school reunion and they all laugh at me?'

'Why do I struggle to be as active as I should be to play with my kids?'

'What if no one ever wants to date me again because of my belly?'

You have a few colleagues you go out drinking with sometimes and they're like you, so it feels normal to eat that heavy meal and drink pint after pint in their company.

You can also afford it now as you work hard, and you want to play hard. You have been buying that expensive bottle of wine for the weekend as you can afford it and you deserve it. What's the job worth if you can't have some little perks?

You definitely don't want to go to the gym on your own. You know you should cut down on your wine and take-aways. Even everyday tasks can be challenging for you as it requires a certain level of fitness to do the gardening or play with the kids in the park.

Yes, nobody expects you to be an athlete but is this how you should be feeling at this age?

Though you know you should be taking care of yourself, you keep putting off committing yourself to action. You know you need proper guidance that resonates with your current problem. Something that takes you out of that unhealthy phase and gives you your old self back. But still you've delayed.

Until now.

Whatever has triggered your concerns, you are on the right track already.

Why do I say that?

Because you are reading this book. This means something. This shows you are prepared to make some changes and do your best to get your health and fitness back. Feeling and looking how you used to in your 20s is only a couple of months away.

If you

- struggle to lose weight
- notice how your unhealthy lifestyle impacts on your everyday life
- lack energy
- sleep badly and wake up tired
- find climbing one or two flights of stairs feels like a workout
- make poor eating choices

and if you want to improve all these aspects, just read on.

1.2   WHY SHOULD YOU CARE?

Maybe this book was a present to you from your partner and you felt obliged to read it!

Or maybe you saw it on a bookshelf and immediately grabbed it, as getting fit and healthy has been in your mind recently.

However you came to it, the first thing I want you to understand is that this book requires *action*. The actions you take will bring you tremendous benefits.

According to the NHS, there are many benefits of exercise. Let's explore some of them.

It can reduce your risk of major illnesses, such as heart disease, stroke, Type 2 diabetes and cancer by up to 50% and lower your risk of early death by up to 30%.

These numbers are absolutely unbelievable, aren't they? 50% reduction in the risk of cancer and 30% prevention of early death? Who wouldn't take action for that?

On the other hand, there are serious health risks when you don't take regular exercise.

Research shows strong evidence that physical inactivity increases the risk of many major adverse health conditions including:

- coronary heart disease
- high blood pressure

- stroke
- metabolic syndrome (including obesity and abnormal blood cholesterol levels)
- Type 2 diabetes
- breast and colon cancer
- depression

Most people working in an office sit for hours every day. After work, you go home and sit in front of the TV. You probably sit more than you walk. You might be struggling to achieve the NHS recommendation of 10,000 daily steps. You're scarcely exerting yourself physically at all. This lack of exercise, along with increasing consumption of unhealthy foods, leads to obesity, diabetes, cardiovascular disease and even depression.

Doing 15-30 minutes of moderate exercise a day will help you tremendously. According to the NHS, people who do regular physical activity have:

- up to 35% lower risk of coronary heart disease and stroke
- up to 50% lower risk of Type 2 diabetes
- up to 50% lower risk of colon cancer
- up to 20% lower risk of breast cancer
- 30% lower risk of early death
- up to 83% lower risk of osteoarthritis
- up to 68% lower risk of hip fracture
- 30% lower risk of falls (amongst older adults)
- up to 30% lower risk of depression
- up to 30% lower risk of dementia

Although you've heard often enough that we all need to do plenty of exercise, somehow you just can't seem to find the time. To be more productive, creative, energised, relaxed and happy, you need to get into the habit of incorporating a balanced and realistic exercise programme into your daily/weekly routine.

But you start with the excuses and the delaying tactics ...

You say things like:

'I don't want to be awkward.'

'I haven't got 60 minutes to spare for exercise.'

'I'm tired; it's easier to just eat what's given to me.'

'I feel fat, ill and old.'

1.3 THE PROMISE

This is a book designed to talk to men over 40, men just like you, with busy lives, who want to get back in shape; men who have been ignoring their fitness, health and wellbeing for a long time. It contains step-by-step guidance on exercise and nutrition. It is full of tips and hints, dealing with major concepts as well as minor aspects, like how to avoid poor eating habits, how to motivate yourself and keep going.

Cleverly-chosen exercise programmes will give you the opportunity to get your body back into shape, even if you are travelling a lot for work, or you have limited time or you've owned a set of dumbbells since the 1990s and you *still* don't know what to do with them. The programme will give you compelling reasons for visiting the local gym and it will give you confidence and knowledge so that you don't feel like a fool when you are on your own, exercising. (However, I will be recommending that you choose a gym if you can because of the great range of equipment you'll have access to and because of supervision – plus, if you walk to the gym, you're giving yourself another way of improving your fitness!)

I appreciate that you don't have the free time that you may have had in your 20s. So, taking your limited time into consideration, the guidance in this book will take you to a new level in just 8 weeks. From that point you will maintain and improve on this on a week-by-week basis.

From day one, the programme I've designed for you will walk you through all the necessary steps you should be taking. I'll offer clear guidance, plus there are journal sections in the programme so you can record how you are getting on and take stock of your achievements. You are a work in progress. By the time you finish the book, if you're applying my methods, you will be fitter, lighter, happier and healthier.

1.4 THE ROUTE-MAP

This book will accompany you on your journey to renewed fitness, so here's a quick summary of what lies ahead.

- Here in Part One, you're recognising your current situation and why it's so important to do something about it. You'll also learn about how I can help you take that action and how to avoid the mind-traps opening up to waylay you.

- In Part Two you'll lay down the foundations for success, both mentally and practically.
- In Part Three we'll look at what a crucial part nutrition plays both for weight-loss and increased fitness.
- In Part Four you'll learn how to exercise safely, before using your week-by-week, day-by-day programme guide, which comes with journal pages so that you can record your progress.
- Part Five shows you ways of optimising your exercise practice and how to maintain the fitness you'll have achieved by then.
- Part Six is your reference guide: here you will find the detailed instructions for each workout and weight training sequence, plus there will be a selection of delicious recipes for you to try.

CHAPTER 2: TIME FOR A WAKE-UP CALL

2.1 THE SLIPPERY SLOPE

Training hundreds of people over the years has made me realise, there is a pattern in our lives. Obviously, there might be some exceptions but the usual pattern is this:

You are born, grow up and generally during your secondary school or university years, you are at your peak in terms of fitness, health and wellbeing.

Then you graduate and you find a job.

The problems start to appear from now on. You work, find a partner, maybe have some kids and in your mid-30s to mid-40s you're focused on your career. It all sounds good so far, doesn't it? But what you don't realise at the time is that your super busy life with your family and your job, plus your unsatisfactory work/life balance, are turning you into an overweight and unhealthy person.

Then you run into the problem of time. Time to take care of yourself seems in short supply when you feel you're taking care of everyone else first.

When you hit 40, you may well have reached a good level in your career. You may have gained financial freedom. But the cost of this financial freedom might be lack of time as you work ever harder and longer. All those hours at the office, all that staying late – that's very laudable in one way, but not so much when your physical condition doesn't get a look-in.

Secondly, you might also have a family, taking up the free time that you used to spend on yourself. Less time to exercise, less time to chill, less time to muck about.

At first it is easier to give up and surrender, because after all, middle-aged spread is normal, isn't it? We accept that after being slim and active in our 20s a kind of slow ambush takes place, increasing our weight and decreasing our fitness.

All the same, you may occasionally try to take action, without much success. These attempts occur generally in the first months of the new year or in September after your summer holiday. But before you know it, you are back to your old habits, drinking and eating whatever you like. Back to square one.

It is easy to sink into defeatism. But the message of this book is this: if you establish the right mindset and work on optimising the conditions around you, can thrive again. You can become the best version of yourself - possibly even better than when you were a 20 year-old.

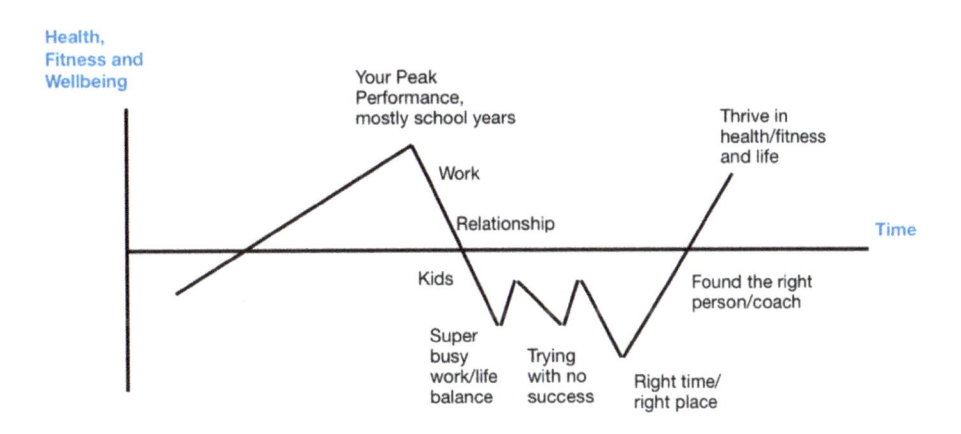

2.2 MUSCLE AND METABOLISM

Something you may have been noticing is that it takes longer to recover from any injuries. Many of my clients who are over 40 have back pain, tennis elbow, knee, hip or rotator cuff injuries. Plus, it's easier to sustain those injuries. You might hurt yourself making some banal move such as emptying the bin or getting up off the sofa. These injuries happen for two main reasons: either you are sitting down too much, which creates bad posture and weak muscles, or you delude yourself into thinking you are still 20 and can spring into action the way you used to. Whatever the reason, the fear of injury can put you off starting an exercise programme.

This is why looking after your muscle tone really matters. After you hit 40, your metabolism slows down. This is due to loss of muscle mass. The more lean muscle you have, the more calories you burn. Sarcopenia - this loss of muscle - is an inevitable part of the ageing process but with a healthy lifestyle you can turn this around. Having a good body composition with lean muscle and a healthy body fat ratio will help.

Imagine two men of the same age. One has 10 lbs (around 4.5kg) more muscle mass than the other one. If they are both inactive all day, the one with more muscle mass burns 500 calories that day, even though his body is just idling. Isn't that absolutely incredible? You therefore have to gain muscle mass if you want to lose that body fat!

GET FIT, STAY FIT | 21

Research carried out by E. Todd Schroeder, PhD, MS, CSCS, FACSM, Associate Professor of Clinical Physical Therapy at the University of Southern California's Clinical Research Centre, shows that resistance training increases your testosterone level, which is not only crucial for muscle-building but also for tissue repair and decreasing your levels of inflammation. (See https://pt.usc.edu/about-usc-biokinesiology-and-physical-therapy/faculty-directory-n-z/e-todd-schroeder-phd/)

After you turn 40, your testosterone level decreases; it might decline by around 1-2% each year. This results in low sex drive, less lean muscle mass, low bone density and loss of strength. Your mood is affected by this and you might feel low energy. The cure is exercise, eating a balanced diet, managing your stress. Research shows that strength training keeps your testosterone level high. The normal testosterone range in men is above 400-600 ng/dL (www.medicinenet.com).

I bet you can't wait to start your strength training workouts now!

2.3 OPTIMISE YOUR LIFE-EXPECTANCY

In the November 2012 issue of the peer-reviewed medical journal Public Library of Science Medicine, researchers described how people who exercise 2.5 hours a week at moderate intensity or 1 hour 15 minutes at high intensity added 3.4 years to their life-expectancy compared to the ones who were inactive. (See also: https://www.livescience.com/36723-exercise-life-expectancy-overweight-obese.html)

In addition, people who were twice as active as above, added 4.2 years.

The research also revealed that people who were active but moderately obese could still expect to live about 3 years longer than those who were inactive.

The worst outcome, however, occurred when combining inactivity and obesity. Obesity is linked to a shorter lifespan. People who were inactive and obese shortened their lifespan by about 5-7 years compared to those who were moderately active and whose weight was within the normal range.

See also https://www.nih.gov/news-events/nih-research-matters/little-exercise-might-lengthen-life.

2.4 SO WHAT'S GETTING IN YOUR WAY?

Let's start with three issues I see over and over again.

#1: THE KNOWLEDGE PROBLEM

People often genuinely don't know what they should be doing when it comes to fitness. They want to take action but they're confused. This is not the same as being in a position where they lack information: both social media and the internet as a whole are saturated with fitness information. This has partly addressed the problem in that we now have access to loads of fitness videos, recipes etc. However, that information is frequently contradictory: result, confusion! One source says 'Dieting is essential', the next says 'Do not count your calories' or 'Eat fat to lose weight'. One resource might say HIIT (High Intensity Interval Training) is the best way to get fit, the next may recommend small changes to maximise benefits.

People are confused about which fitness path to follow. Many are aware of potential 'scams' and don't want to fall into the social media trap. People ask me many questions as a result of this: 'Shall I do cardio?', 'How much cardio?', 'What is the best cardio?', 'Would strength training make me lose weight?', 'How heavy/how often, how many sets (cycles of the repetitions)/how many reps (repetitions)/how many days a week give the best results?' The questions go on and on!

If you type any of these typical questions into Google, you will get page after page of answers. But, which one should you follow?

#2: THE ACCOUNTABILITY PROBLEM

If you don't feel 100% accountable, you won't be able to lose the excess weight that's bothering you.

We are grown-ups. Unless you have a bossy partner or a friend, nobody keeps you accountable when it comes to getting fit and healthy. When you buy that delicious bottle of wine on a Thursday evening, order a take-away on a Friday evening or don't bother exercising for days/weeks, nobody keeps you accountable. It's just down to you.

You might already have a personal trainer you see weekly. The convention here is that you are buying their time to train you for that specific booked time. That's it. The rest of the time you are literally on your own. You are responsible for your own healthy eating, your own additional exercises in between sessions, if needed, and for your healthy decisions.

If a lack of accountability is affecting you, what you need are daily check-ins and regular communication. This is so essential. So if you don't have this additional service from your trainer, find a buddy, a colleague, partner or friend, so you can keep each other accountable. You might not get the kind of professional service that you get from a fitness coach, but remember if your accountability is to a friend, then it's free and it is better than not having anyone to answer to at all!

#3: THE MOTIVATION PROBLEM

Individuals have different levels of motivation. Some people are super pumped-up and full of enthusiasm throughout, and some are very reluctant to keep up to date with their exercise and healthy-eating regimes.

We all need to be motivated and a fitness coach needs the skill to realise when someone needs that extra motivational encouragement.

My highly-motivated clients have each had a specific reason for getting fit and healthy. For example, someone who came to me two years ago lost over 10 kilos in 10-12 weeks because he had his son's wedding coming up and he wanted to look better and feel healthier by the time it arrived. Someone else was going to be a father in seven months so he wanted to be in his best shape when his daughter was born. What is your reason for becoming fit and healthy? And what is your timeline for it? Pinning down the reason and knowing it's a strong one for you personally will really help, as will setting a time-goal for its completion.

Other than specific deadlines like these, I personally find it motivating to look at someone's workout video on YouTube or on social media. It gives me that buzz to get up and go! It could be something as simple as a good, upbeat playlist that motivates you.

Imagine being, let's say, 5 kilos lighter. How good would you feel? You would not only look better but also have so much more energy. Your sleep would improve, you wouldn't be out of breath when you climb up a couple of flights of stairs and as a result of all this, you'd feel so much happier.

Find out your big **why** and remember, you will always feel better after a workout.

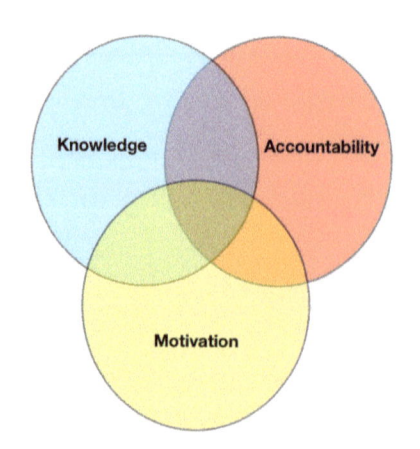

CHAPTER 3:
TRUST ME, I'M A TRAINER

3.1 CLIENT AND COACH MAKE A TEAM

When I was seven or eight, my mum ordered a piece of sit-up equipment called the 'Covvy Sit-Up Pull Spring Tension' so she could do some exercise at home. The gadget's simple concept was this: you would put your feet in the foot pedals, hold the handles on the other side of the spring and lie on your back to perform sit-ups. The tension in the spring would help to you sit up.

As was usual for her, after a few weeks of owning this piece of equipment, my mother stopped using it. Instead, I started using it in secret, thinking that using this every day would make me fit and strong even though I didn't have a clue how it worked. Eventually it dawned on me that it was just a tool to help people do sit-ups and that any piece of equipment only works when the person using it shows commitment to the process.

Fast forward twelve years and my own commitment had led to me being on stage in an international bodybuilding competition, representing Turkey in the 80kg men's bodybuilding category.

In 2010, having moved to the UK, I created Gokay Fitness from scratch and within the first few years, while many personal trainers in my area were struggling to find clients, I had not only managed to fill my diary, but had to stop accepting new clients during peak times, as I was doing up to ten sessions a day, each an hour long. This has been incredibly rewarding work and I never tire of witnessing the transformations brought about when trainer and client team up with the mutual aim of improving the client's life through fitness. I get results for my clients first by working with them as they clarify their big why. Secondly, I tailor a specific plan for them. It's gratifying when I build long-term client-coach relationships and know that I have contributed to something so important to them. No coach can do this unless they can instil a sense of trust. No client will trust a coach unless they believe in his or her knowledge and expertise.

I personally use the exercise techniques and nutrition principles in this book to keep myself fit on a daily basis. The methods you will learn here will not only help you reach your targets but keep you on track. You will learn the underlying formulae of calorie counting and macronutrient control. You will be able to use technology to help you: it is all much easier now we have smartphones, which didn't even exist when I was winning medals years ago in bodybuilding contests. I wish I had had that kind of technology back then.

Maybe you're afraid of the term 'bodybuilder'. Maybe you think I'll turn you into a 'muscle head', someone who's obsessed with growing giant muscles – and nothing else. But I assure you, this process is about so much more than that. You're reading these words because you're ready to make a change in your life and I respect that. I understand what your goals and needs are. I know how frustrated you feel and I'll use the strategies I've learned over the past decade and more to help you get much further than you ever could on your own. I'll help you avoid the pitfalls and the inclination to give up, by giving you a practical, fully-designed 8-week programme.

I'll also help you winnow out the truth from all the water-cooler wisdom that leads to the kind of discussion I occasionally have with my clients. They may pick up a fitness magazine or the exercise section of a newspaper and read a blog written by person X at the weekend. What happens is that they're inclined to believe everything in that article and it is almost impossible to convince them it might not be true. It is like trying to convince someone who is an atheist that God exists or the other way round, trying to convince a very religious person that there is no real divinity. It is *that* strong.

Discussion topics are generally on things like:

Carbs are really bad: we shouldn't eat any carbs.

Calorie counting is useless; we shouldn't count the calories and just eat healthily.

Protein powders are drugs and we should never touch them.

If I do weight training, I will bulk up and look like Arnold Schwarzenegger...

The list goes on.

Here's an example of how easy it is to be swayed and led off-track by rumour and misguided beliefs. An industry-leading high-flier wanting a healthier lifestyle may decide to hire me, a fitness coach, to help him get fit and to lose that excess body mass. Soon after working together with my 7 step methodology, he gets there. He's fitter, healthier, more energetic. As a result, he's a happy client.

That's when the difficulty starts. His friend or colleague questions him and when his colleague finds out that this guy's personal trainer (me), allows him to eat rice or red meat on a Saturday evening and have a workout-free weekend, his colleague gets annoyed as this sounds completely the opposite of what he read in that recent article in his Sunday newspaper. I must be wrong or giving the wrong advice to his friend.

I then spend ten minutes explaining the reasoning, scientific research and case studies behind my decisions, so that my client understands why we did this or that and why it was absolutely OK to do it. Because my client had created a 3000 calorie deficit over that week through my workouts and healthy eating plan, his mood and happiness also needed to be fed after consecutive weeks of hard work and discipline. His colleague obviously missed that bit!

This book is not about the latest buzz topic or alarm. This book is grounded in established, tried-and-tested practice. If you apply its advice to your life, you'll not only be the best you can be in terms of your health and fitness, but you'll also gain some great habits that will last you a lifetime.

As you progress through the programme, you'll gain the confidence to take action and you'll see a clear vision of your future, with my step-by-step guidance to becoming a new, healthy and fit you.

You'll get many compliments from your loved ones, your colleagues and even from your neighbours, about how wonderful you look and how impressed they are that you found the energy and motivation to change your life so quickly and successfully. You will connect with yourself and believe me, that connection, that feeling good about yourself, is addictive. The journal you'll keep during the programme is going to help you with that connection and this will be the best and the least harmful addiction you've ever had.

3.2 MY AIMBEST METHOD

You're about to embark on the Get Fit, Stay Fit 8-week programme, so let's give you a quick overview of what's involved.

- There are key areas we will cover – these are the 'pillars' of my programme and success relies on using all of them. Just building muscle isn't enough on its own, for instance. We are going to go through these key strategies and you'll see how they interact with one another in a holistic way.
- How this works: you'll be invited to make changes in these key areas, so that you will become leaner, stronger, more flexible, more resilient; more positive,

calmer, sleeping better. You'll start by assessing where you are now, and you'll have a weekly journal section to fill in where you record your progress and how you are feeling about that progress. I'll recommend apps and tools to help you along the way too. Week by week you'll see the evidence, recorded not just in your journal but when you look in the mirror, step on the scales, or even just get up off the sofa!

I admit, making changes and creating new habits can be hard. To make this easier, you need to follow a process. A process that is thought through, clear and easy to follow and also trackable. You need to know the changes you've made have helped you and by how much, so that you can adapt your practices as you go if you need to.

Let me stress this message: simply *wanting* something is not enough: you need action steps. You need a process. We follow processes every single day. You don't put 8 ingredients into a saucepan and expect to produce a delicious bowl of bolognese!

In health and fitness, we need to apply exactly the same principles. Over the years, I've worked out a clear 7-step process for my clients, with the kind of proven results I've been describing to you.

Welcome to **AIMBEST** - the 7 core elements of my process:

1. Assess and plan (measurements, weighing, food planning, diary clearing for workouts)

2. Initial mindset

3. Meticulous and time efficient workouts

4. Better eating

5. Essential relaxation and stretching

6. Survey, evaluate and revise (measurements and weighing, adjusting accordingly)

7. Total maintenance (knowing how to keep going)

3.3　AIMBEST: THE 7 STEPS

Let's take each of the AIMBEST steps in turn, exploring how they can help you meet your key fitness challenges.

1) **A**SSESS AND PLAN (MEASUREMENTS, WEIGHING, FOOD PLANNING, DIARY CLEARING FOR WORKOUTS)

If you had a start-up business, you would expect to do due diligence. It's very unlikely that someone can jump into a business and succeed straightaway without making plans, assessing the current situation, where they want to be in the next 3, 6, 12, 36 months' time etc.

We need to apply exactly the same principles to planning for fitness success.

Your first action should be to take some body measurements. I'll be advising you later to weigh yourself and use a tape measure to measure different areas of your body such as your waist, hips, chest, arms etc. You'll be writing all these figures down and dating them. I'll invite you to use the journal pages in the programme or you may want to keep a separate special notebook or chart for the figures you're going to record during the 8 week process.

Don't make the mistake of saying 'I will measure myself after I lose some weight'. You'll be missing the opportunity to see your most significant progress which tends to happen most dramatically in the initial stages and can be enormously encouraging and motivating.

Plan your meals in advance. I don't mean create three-course menu plans for every single meal. But you need to know what you are eating for dinner or next day's lunch in advance, even if only roughly, so that you are not grabbing the first appealing food when you are so hungry without considering whether it's healthy or not. We all know what happens when we're hungry and haven't planned what to eat! We visit the supermarket or café and pick up something we fancy there and then. And what we're likely to fancy, when we're starving and in a rush, is probably going to be something full of fat, salt or sugar, for that quick hit of energy and pleasure we crave.

So don't forget: your willpower is much weaker when you are hungry. As I write this, I know I'm eating chicken salad for lunch tomorrow. I've got salad ingredients and two pieces of chicken breast in the fridge and I'm going to prepare the salad this evening after my coaching sessions. So, it's sorted out in my head and that leaves no space for poor choices when that hungry time hits, midway through tomorrow morning!

Another useful technique is diary clearing for your workouts. Instead of a vague intention to have a couple of workouts each week, think more strategically.

During the programme I'll be planning for you on a daily basis, but afterwards you'll want to factor in at least 20, 30 or 60 minutes a couple of times a week. Plan how often per week and on which days you're going to exercise. Try to stick to this. You're making an appointment with your future self, the way you'd make an appointment with a client. Don't let yourself down!

2) INITIAL MINDSET

Every weight loss and fitness strategy has its pros and cons. What makes one work and another not work often comes down to an individual's mindset.

Everyone has their own excuses. When trying to improve lifestyle and diet, most people do fine until something unexpected happens — it could be work pressure or family issues, or something else. When you make up your mind, your healthy choices should be non-negotiable.

I was testing myself with a thirty-three hour fast a few weeks ago to detox and clear out my digestive system. I had made up my mind. I met with a friend in a pub. She had a lovely club sandwich in front of her and I just had a soda water. And you know what, I swear I didn't want to eat the sandwich although I was hungry. That's because I had made a deal with myself and I was sticking to it.

I'll tell you about my 9 strategies for dealing with temptations like this in section 6.15 of Chapter 6. I acknowledge that this is my choice rather than a sacrifice.

3) METICULOUS AND TIME-EFFICIENT WORKOUTS

Again, looking beyond the initial 8 week programme, most people think, when they commit to regular exercising, they have to find five spare hours a week. The reality is quite different from this. You could become really fit and healthy by devoting 20 minutes a day to it, 4-5 times a week. Of course it depends on how well you spend those 20 minutes, but my point is that you don't have to sleep at the gym to lose that weight.

My barber asked me the other day how often I trained. I said I had been training only twice a week lately. He laughed!

I admit, I trained very hard when I was in my late teens and early 20s. Currently I train no more than a few times a week and I spend around 30-60 minutes on the workouts each time.

If you haven't got much time available for a particular session, after a quick warm-up you could do strength-training exercises with some cardio in between.

For example, you could do a set of squats followed by 50-100 skips and move to lunges, or you could do super sets such as bench press followed by lat pull down. (If you are not familiar with these terms, by the way, don't worry: I'll be explaining them later on.)

If you are training on your own, you don't have to do all the muscle groups in one day. You should in fact split them into a sequence of 3-4 days and keep each targeted session short.

Rather than spending 50 minutes on a boring treadmill, do 15 minute sprint and jogging intervals, which could be 30 second sprints and 1 minute slow pace jogging for 15 minutes overall. Then you could work two muscle groups such as your shoulders and triceps for 10 minutes with short breaks. Within 25 minutes, your workout is over and the benefits are awesome.

4) BETTER EATING

I am pretty sure that most of us, especially in the UK, know what is good and what is bad for us when it comes to meals and snacks, thanks to increasing public awareness in the media and via the internet.

You can eat and drink whatever you want but don't expect to look lean with poor eating habits. There are tons of diet plans all over the internet; most diets work as long as you stick to them.

This is the question you should ask yourself: 'Can I stick to a certain type of eating plan and how long for? And what happens after I stop following it in two months?'

As a general guideline, we know that strength training helps you gain muscle, and lean muscle mass helps you burn more calories. To be able to gain lean muscle mass, you need to eat lean. Other than your genes, being lean relies on your consumption of fat, protein and carbohydrates: the food elements known as 'macros' or 'macronutrients'. The most important macro, I'm sure you already know, is protein. You will not gain lean muscle mass without sufficient protein in your diet. Your main calories should come from protein.

You have 2 options:

Option 1 is slow and steady weight loss. If you think you can be patient, then make small changes in your diet and be consistent for a significant amount of time (such as six months). You will see the results with this option but you can't expect fast results. For example, you may stop drinking on weekdays and swap your unhealthy snacks for vegetables or a piece of fruit rather than biscuits. If everything else is the same in your diet (portion size, some bad choices in your dinners etc.) then making these small changes will still bring you results, but not immediately.

Option 2 is a more aggressive approach, such as being very strict for 6 to 8 weeks. You could lose around 5 to 8 kilos during this time. The advantage of this approach is that getting the result you want quickly will motivate you. The disadvantage is that afterwards, you can't go back to how you used to eat, as all that weight will come back. So you need to think of a maintenance programme.

5) **E**SSENTIAL RELAXATION AND STRETCHING

This is something we ignore most of the time. Ideally you need to stretch after every single workout. You should hold that static stretching position for at least 30 seconds. Tight muscles can cause injuries. They get tight from sitting too long or after a workout.

Stretching will improve your flexibility and your range of movement. It improves your posture and your circulation and it can even help relax your mind.

Relaxation is equally important. You can't make healthy decisions when you are wired up, coping with tons of stress day after day. That's why practising some mindfulness, yoga, or meditation can help you reduce your blood pressure, lower your heart rate and improve your positive thinking.

I suggest you schedule in some meditation at least once a week. I know experts recommend daily practice. This is something I need to improve on in my life too! Our to-do list never stops. There is always something to do every single day and unless you take some time off, even for twenty minutes, to calm your mind, anxiety and stress will cause a variety of health problems.

6) **S**URVEY, EVALUATE AND REVISE (MEASUREMENTS AND WEIGHING, ADJUSTING ACCORDINGLY)

This is something people very rarely do. If you *do* already have a workout regime, when did you last take stock of and revise it?

We need to reflect and make some adjustments to our workouts and our eating habits on a regular basis. Do you weigh yourself regularly? Maybe you've put on 3 kilos during the last 5-6 weeks thanks to some work trips. Caught up in your many daily tasks, you don't notice your weight creeping up unless you keep an eye on it.

Do you time yourself when running, for example? If you include running as part of your programme or already enjoy going on runs (even short ones) for the cardio benefits, you need to get into the habit of timing yourself because unless you do, you can't know if you are making any improvements. If you're not monitoring your times, how can you make those improvements?

I had a text from a client of mine an hour ago as I was writing this section. He said that although he has been training regularly and trying to watch what he eats, he hasn't lost any weight or dropped his waist-size in the last 2.5 weeks. (He still carries around 9-10kg that he wants to lose.) We made a plan to carefully monitor his diet for a week by using the MyFitnessPal app on his phone (I'll be discussing this useful app in Chapter 6, Fuel your Fitness), just to figure out where he is going wrong. Too many carbs? Late meals? More calories consumed than he burns? Evaluating and taking action will restart progress within a week. I know this as I've experienced it many times with other clients.

7) TOTAL MAINTENANCE (HOW TO KEEP GOING)

So, you visualise reaching your targets. Imagine you've got there and it's a very good place to be. But what then? You develop a process of evaluating and monitoring your progress, linked to what we've discussed in Step 6 above. Because once you reach your targets you want to stay in that good place!

The key factor, then, is reassessing yourself regularly. Before you know it, this kind of monitoring will become part of your lifestyle. This is actually how many fitness experts live, including me. We all have a life. We are all invited to parties. The more you practise keeping an eye on where you are, the better you get at it.

When you've reached where you want to be in terms of fitness and wellbeing, but things go off-track due to work trips, big lunches or client entertainment, all you need to do is to go back to Step 6 and reassess yourself before it is too late, so that you can restore your maintenance mode again. If you realise you've put 2 kilos on, don't let another 2 kilos pile on top, as losing that initial 2 kilos will only take you a week or so. If you don't take action promptly and the weight accumulates, you may find you've lost that willpower to take charge again.

So, in Step 7, maintenance is an ongoing process, but if things get out of hand, you need to go back to Step 6 to re-evaluate, sort things out and get back into maintenance mode again.

As we get ready to embark on the Get Fit, Stay Fit programme, here are three reminders of why it may be that you couldn't achieve a healthy lifestyle and good physique before now:

1. You didn't know what to do and how to do it

2. You weren't accountable. There were no instant consequences for being inactive or having a bad diet.

3. More importantly, even if you had access to the knowledge via a personal trainer (PT) or books, videos, and online trainings, you most likely lacked willpower. You hadn't sorted out your big WHY so it was not strong enough to give you the outcome that you wished for.

How did I manage to become a gold medal winning bodybuilder? I had access to knowledge (it wasn't up to today's standards but it was enough) and I had a big why. I agreed at my local gym that I would take part in the national bodybuilding contest. I told my colleagues at work and also didn't want to embarrass myself in front of thousands in the audience on the day of the contest! (We'll be exploring the usefulness of going public in Chapter 5, Foundations for Success).

In the Get Fit programme, you'll see that monitoring progress is a key aspect of success; it is extremely important to know how you are doing as you go along and learn how to use technology to help you.

I will show you how to take control of what you eat and how to track your calories and macros; how to use a heart rate monitor efficiently and how to sync it with some great fitness apps to monitor your progress, set your own goals and also help you get accurate results.

So, we've been discussing my experience with exercise and diet and why I have the credentials to be able to help you. At the start of the book I invited you to take stock of your position, with regard to your health. I've shown you the highlights of the AIMBEST approach and I've made you the promise that I can help you.

But wait. There's something really important you need to factor in.

Your own attitude.

Time to face up to some of the get-out clauses you've been relying on!

3.4 THE MIND-TRAP MINEFIELD

Let's spend a little time examining some typical objections people make to the whole concept of a programme like Get Fit, Stay Fit. We can fall into mind-traps which seem logical and sensible to us but which lead us to take misguided actions – or worse, no action at all. Here are twelve typical attitudes and how they take you off-course or get in the way of you fully benefiting from your new regime. Do you recognise any of these get-out clauses in your own thinking?

MIND-TRAP #1

You think you have a demanding job and very busy life so there's no space for either exercise or a healthy diet. You think that your high-powered job with its overloaded schedule will give you no time or opportunity to get your health and fitness back.

So you won't take action as it doesn't seem possible for you to do anything right now. You don't invest in your health and you start to put on weight over a period of time, which makes you end up tired, feeling mentally low and weak.

MIND-TRAP #2

You think all these men with good physiques in magazines (or at the gym) were born like that. You think it is too hard to try to change, to emulate them.

You can't be bothered, because it's pointless even to try. As a consequence, you suffer from ill health.

MIND-TRAP #3

*You think you should either be doing everything or nothing. You think you risk either being like a robot doing everything to the extreme, such as crash-dieting or over-training, or you just won't do **any** of it.*

You let everything go and end up living on take-away dinners and loads of alcohol. You think working hard gives you the best excuse to treat yourself to that double whisky or an expensive bottle of wine, so you do; then you get fatter and more inactive with every passing year.

MIND-TRAP #4

You think of everything else in your business as a process. You are happy with baby steps in one part of your business development as you know the results will be rewarding in the longer term.

But when it comes to your health and fitness, baby steps in the right direction are never enough. This makes you frustrated as you want the scales to show a big drop every time you stand on them. You want an immediate return on investment: you put in a tiny amount of effort and expect a huge amount of progress. If you don't see that, you're inclined to give up.

MIND-TRAP #5

You think a daily 30 minute workout will not do you any good. It's not worth the sweat. Or you think you can draft that presentation during that time instead and that would be a better use of half an hour.

Skipping 30 minutes a day like this, you miss the opportunity of putting in 8 hours' training a month in total (3-4 times a week, 30 minutes each). This could equate to a deficit of more than 6000 calories per month, a faster metabolism and a happier mood. The benefits of an active lifestyle are amazing, equivalent to your company giving you a bonus like a car allowance or private healthcare.

Accept that taking small regular actions works. You will get back what you put in. The more exercise you do, the better your diet is, the better quality sleep you have, the healthier and fitter you will be. As a result, you will look great and feel awesome.

MIND-TRAP #6

You think that if you lose weight too quickly, you'll gain it back. So you won't even bother trying to lose weight in the first place.

Why are you worrying about something that is absolutely not a problem right now? For example, I might think that if I were to become a billionaire, I might get more money than I can spend and I might get into bad ways and even become a cocaine addict as I would be able to afford it and I'd be socialising with those types of people. I don't want that, so it's better that I don't even aim to become rich. This kind of 'what if' thinking isn't helpful!

Albert is the marketing director of an international company. His lifestyle and poor work-life balance made him gain over 10 kilograms of body fat over the last 10 years. He was not happy with it but his concern was that if he lost this weight, he might gain it back so he hadn't even tried to lose this body fat in the first place. In long conversations between our training sessions, I explained to him that he was worrying about something that was not a problem right then. I told him to deal with his future problems only when they actually became *real* and immediate. So he followed my guidance for 8 to 10 weeks and lost over 9 kilograms. This was over two years ago and he has still managed to keep his weight down.

MIND-TRAP #7

You think that your life and job won't allow you to be healthy and fit: no time, too many social events. So, once again, you don't even try to make the accommodation.

Refusing to try might make you feel better about yourself as you convince yourself you don't need to feel guilty but deep down, you know you can do better than this.

Harry is a business owner whose many client meetings take place over a lunch or boozy dinner. In his mid-forties, he started thinking his lifestyle wasn't designed to help him be fit and healthy. He had been inactive, with an alcohol-filled unhealthy diet for about fifteen years. He was worried that he couldn't go on running a successful business while trying to get fit because attending the necessary social events, with their unhealthy choices built in, would no longer be possible if he changed his lifestyle.

I persuaded him a few years ago that most of his clients were facing exactly the same issue. Meeting him for lunch, his client might also be keen to order the healthy lunch option with either limited alcohol or no alcohol at all, but they might both have been thinking it would be impolite to say 'I'll stick to the water' or 'I'll have fish and some greens'. Instead they would be ordering bottles of wine, servings of chips and many other high calorie sides. After we talked about how similar he and his clients were in terms of them both wanting to do something about their wellbeing, I asked him to mention to his clients something about his new lifestyle or the spin class he joined the other day or what his fitness goals were in the next few months.

He did exactly what I asked during the chit-chatting part of his lunches or dinners. He realised that most of his clients agreed with him and they all wanted to get healthier and fitter but they didn't want to look like an outsider or a boring person. This was a game-changer for Harry. Now, when he meets a client, he talks about what he is up to, turning the subject to health and wellbeing. This clarifies things to such an extent that most of the time, his clients join him in his healthy eating choices and they also admire him because of his motivation and the results he has achieved.

MIND-TRAP #8

You think that if you consume high levels of protein or shakes, you will bulk up, so you choose not to eat protein.

You will not build lean muscle mass unless you consume the required amount of protein, period.

After a few years of weight training, Joseph, who is a finance director of a London-based company, was frustrated because he couldn't gain all that much muscle and his body composition wasn't changing that much either. He was starting to think his genes or his metabolism might be to blame. He didn't pay attention to my nutritional advice at the beginning of his fitness journey.

After I showed him the before and after pictures of another client of mine, who'd achieved an improved body composition of 6% body fat in one tenth of the time that Joseph had been training with me, he realised his diet definitely needed to improve massively. He took my advice on board and increased his daily protein intake. In 7 or 8 weeks, he couldn't believe how much lean muscle he'd gained and also how much body fat he'd lost. He didn't bulk up; instead, he toned up amazingly.

MIND-TRAP #9

You think that if you do weights you'll build so much muscle you'll look bulky, so you don't do weights.

A dozen clients all had the same idea in their heads when they first started training with me. They said, 'Well I don't mind doing a bit of weights but I don't want to be a muscle head'. And I said to them if you read two articles about chemical reactions, would you suddenly turn into a chemical engineer? Gaining lean muscle mass will only happen through consistently following the right training programmes, getting optimum nutrition and enough rest.

It is not that hard if you really pay attention to all of these aspects for a reasonable length of time but you will not wake up one day to find you've magically turned into a mountain of muscle.

MIND-TRAP #10

You tell yourself, 'I was good all day, so it's OK to eat this treat now, even though it's s**t in nutritional terms.'

You need to commit yourself to healthy eating for a significant amount of time before you can allow yourself those treats.

Gavin is a relatively new client of mine. He works from home and feels he needs unhealthy snacks throughout the day, just to keep him going. He originally thought that coming to me twice a week would be the solution for all his weight and fitness problems and that having booked ten sessions, that would be enough to sort everything out within a few months. Then, he believed he would be able to eat anything he wanted. He tried to be healthy for a few days and he was so proud of himself, he treated himself to a nice expensive bottle of wine on a Friday evening. He was also doing some additional cycling classes on a Saturday, and that gave him the justification, he thought, to eat a take-away on a Saturday evening. He was telling himself, 'I've been good; I deserve this.' Getting virtually no tangible results over the course of three months made him realise (finally!) that he needed to do more. I chose to be very direct and firm with him one day; something clicked with him and he started to treat this fitness journey as a structured block of 8 weeks. During those weeks, he had hardly any of the unhealthy or calorific treats that he used to indulge in and he cut down on his alcohol dramatically as well. Fast forward 8 weeks: he lost 9 kg, his waist was three belt-holes smaller and his arms looked so much more toned and in shape.

MIND-TRAP #11

You think that hiring a personal trainer and working out twice a week will be enough to sort everything out; there's no need to do anything else.

A twice-weekly hour-long workout (at who knows what efficiency and intensity level) might not be enough to give you results unless you make some other changes in your lifestyle as well.

John has been seeing me twice a week for the last year. During the first three months, he got stronger, fitter and happier. However, he couldn't shift his weight and that had been the main reason he wanted to train with me in the first place. I showed him the progress he'd actually made and compared that with the progress he *could* have made if he'd taken on board all the different kinds of advice I'd given him during those three months.

Sometimes people need to experience things by themselves: that's how it was with John. He followed my guidelines with three additional workout days on his own and one group class. His additional workouts were only 25 minutes each; this didn't eat up as much time as he'd expected. He was amazed after a few months that his metabolism had speeded up, plus he lost a gratifying amount of weight within two months. He is now an exercise addict; he also finds it very useful for his mental health as he feels so much more focused in his job, making him more productive and efficient.

MIND-TRAP #12

You believe that as you run and cycle a great deal, there is no need for you to do any specific exercises for your legs.

Cycling and running are both amazing exercises. You are likely to be outdoors, and if you're cycling, your heart is pumping while you're sitting down and the fact that it is a low-impact form of exercise makes it a good choice for people with knee or hip injuries. Having said that, cycling is a repetitive movement and it is very different from strength training. It won't make you build the kind of muscle that you need to burn calories when you are resting. The biggest muscles in your body have the potential to burn the greatest number of calories, so strengthening and building lean muscle in your legs will be very beneficial for your cycling and running efficiency. They are complementary exercises, not substitutes.

I have a bunch of male clients who either play tennis, football or cycle. They all try to convince me that they have very strong legs so doing squats and lunges is a waste of time. Hugo was one of them. He only wanted to do upper body workouts and he also wanted to look toned and athletic. Introducing leg workouts gave him so much muscle tone throughout his body, *including* his upper body. He can now hit the ball much more easily when he plays tennis as doing all those lunges has given him a tremendous amount of endurance and strength – the kind he needed for his tennis games.

PART TWO

CHAPTER 4:
GET READY TO GET FIT (1): MINDSET MASTERY

You're on the launch-pad now. You understand your why and you're a lot more aware of the excuses you make for delay. You're not out of the woods yet, though! In this section we'll look at more of the sneaky get-out clauses you rely on to justify delay or inaction. I'll invite you to check what default attitude you bring to the notion of your fitness and we'll start the process of ensuring a positive mindset that will see you all the way through the programme. I'll show you how to turn around some of the potentially negative ways you have of seeing things: it's all about mastering your mindset.

4.1 IS IT ALL OR NOTHING - OR SOMETHING IN BETWEEN?

OK. Do you want to get fit and lose unwanted body weight?

Sure, exercise more and lower your calorie intake! Is it that simple? Maybe it is.

But I challenge you to take on board that most people who achieve their goals in health and fitness do it by changing their lifestyle and incorporating an exercise regime in their daily life and by eating healthily on a regular basis. So you are not alone or expected to do something very unusual.

I don't expect you to go crazy and die from hunger to lose that weight. I won't promise that you can eat all you want and achieve this either. We men are, unlike women, all or nothing types. I hear a lot from my female clients about their partners or husbands, regarding healthy eating, drinking alcohol or exercising. They either drink almost every evening or stop drinking and never touch it for a period of time, rather than reducing the amount or the number of days per week when they consume it. It's the same with exercise: they either never exercise at all or go crazy and do more than they can manage, which results in lapsing later on. However, we don't have to be like that. In fact we *shouldn't* be like that if we want sustainable results.

Imagine you want to be an airline pilot. You enrol for the training but you decide to do the reading part only and not participate in any of the practical aspects. How likely is it that you could gain the competence and confidence to fly an Airbus A380?

Similarly, if you decide to read this book but not apply its techniques and recommendations, it's unlikely you will succeed. So my message throughout this book will be 'Now *do* it, don't just read about it,' which is going to remind you to choose your approach: actively invest in your success or passively hope that reading alone will somehow do the trick!

I always hear people saying, 'I will start tomorrow'. What makes you think that you will magically have the kind of bulletproof willpower tomorrow that you are clearly lacking today?

It is very unlikely that overnight you will magically gain willpower that kicks in the moment you wake up and lasts all day. So the lesson is this: do not let yourself off today, as you never know, tomorrow you might do the same and the day after. Before you know it, the week is over and guess what. No results.

Having said that, I am not against you patting yourself on the back every now and then. We need to strike a balance in most aspects of our lives. If you are a really determined and hardworking person, it is OK to take it easy, lie on the sofa, watch TV and eat comfort food without feeling guilty about it. You need that occasional lazy afternoon sometimes.

4.2 WHAT'S YOUR TYPE?

Over the years I've observed that there are 7 types of people when it comes to approaches to health and fitness: which category do you think you fit into?

Set in their Ways: These people have been unhealthy almost all their lives. They might be aware of being unhealthy, yet they carry on with their inactive lifestyle and daily junk food habits. Or they might not even notice how unhealthy they are, which is even more dangerous. These people are generally surrounded with likeminded people who are also unhealthy and overweight. That makes things look pretty normal to them.

Of course it's possible for a 'set in their ways' type to make up his mind to reform one day, but be aware – those ingrained habits will be hard to shift.

Irregulars: Most of the UK population is in this category. These people either don't exercise or do minimal exercise now and then, irregularly. They eat convenience food, from pies to fast food. They are relatively active but don't necessarily do workouts. They might go on walks, they might go out to work, and grabbing a Tesco sandwich for lunch happens quite often.

Self-deceivers: To take an example, a city like London is densely populated, and both income and expenditure are high. Life is fast-paced. And London is full of complacent city-dwellers, fitness Self-deceivers who may well exercise once or twice a week but still drink excessively and eat rich, calorific food too often. Compared to the rest of the planet, they are healthier and more active and also much more aware of health and fitness. But they're a way off where they should be and where they deceive themselves they already are.

Lucky Ones: These people may be lucky genetically, their bodies programmed towards health, which they reinforce with healthy eating and exercise. They are lucky as when they were young they were fit and healthy and their current activity levels and healthy eating make them look great with no effort. Their colleagues and friends around them are similar in terms of their lifestyle so the results almost come naturally.

They meet with their friends during or after something like a tennis match, rather than at the pub like Irregulars or Set in their Ways people. However, if Lucky Ones change their lifestyles, stop being active and start eating unhealthy and high calorie food for a long time, they will turn into Irregulars or Set in their Ways types.

Boomerangs: People in the Set in their Ways or Irregulars categories may decide they've had enough one day and they find the willpower to improve their eating and increase their levels of regular exercise. They lose some weight and get into the healthy range. They're proud of themselves as everything gets much easier due to their being fitter and healthier, but after a while they stop taking care of themselves and gradually they put the weight back on. Before long, they're nearly back to their previous unhealthy state.

Consistent Action-takers: These people do exactly what Boomerangs do except they manage to *maintain* their fit and healthy lifestyle. So they stay fit for life. My whole focus is on helping you to be a Consistent Action-taker and not a Boomerang!

High Achievers: These people are either professional athletes or fitness professionals. A fit healthy lifestyle is a norm for them but the danger is that as soon as they stop leading this lifestyle they may become really overweight and depressed. Some examples of this are ex-professional football players after retirement.

4.3 THE OBSTACLE COURSE

When you accept that you need to make some changes in your life to become a better version of yourself, you have actually taken the hardest and biggest step on this journey. But there are many steps to come and at times you will feel like you are your own obstacle course. I'm going to mention a few of the objections that may come to you and I'm sure some will resonate. Recognising them is the first stage in dealing with them and I'm here to help you work on overcoming them.

Taking the necessary steps to get you results might not be effortless. And it's at this point that 'comparisonitis' may kick in. Comparisonitis happens when we compare ourselves to others and find ourselves wanting. Most of the time, it may feel like your colleague or neighbour does this fitness thing effortlessly – unlike you. The truth is, it is not effortless for *anybody*. I know so many people who are very healthy and they exercise regularly, but going for that 25 minute jog after a long day is a chore for them too. Somehow, though, they do it, and so can you!

I'm not going to ignore the fact that fit people might find it easier to do certain exercises or keep going without feeling exhausted, due to their stamina. You are not there yet, so it may feel hard to begin with because you run out of steam, but believe me, you will be surprised how fast that will change as long as you stick to the plan.

Imagine a stationary car. When does it burn the most petrol? Yes, in the first few seconds of acceleration, which is the hardest bit. Overcoming inertia is always hard. Once you get some momentum, you will flow easily and it will be awesome!

Many of my female clients are up against the burning issue that although their husbands are generally high achievers in their careers, and are great partners and hosts, they are however rubbish when it comes to health and exercise. I must admit, men are harder to convince to exercise or get fit. And once we are convinced then we may turn into creatures of extremes, as I mentioned earlier: we're all or nothing types.

We are so lucky that our metabolisms are faster than women's, due to the natural muscle mass we have in our bodies, plus we use more calories just fuelling our resting state, but we abuse this benefit. If we only pay attention to cutting back our snacks, we may lose a few kilos instantly and this is a very annoying thing for our partners, if they're female, as those poor women work their butts off and are only be able to lose half a kilo a week. Perhaps that's why most men can't be bothered to pay attention to their diet and exercise: we *know* we can do it (just not yet!) This is unfortunately not enough, especially after 40! Remember, the rules of the game change after 40 and what you could get away with before you won't be able to get away with now.

Let's take a look at some typical objections men may have to the very notion of taking action to get fit.

OBJECTION 1: I DON'T HAVE TIME TO EXERCISE

Tim Cook is the CEO of Apple; he runs a company worth more than $1 billion. He exercises every day.

Richard Branson, the founder of Virgin Group (who has a net worth of $5 billion) exercises every day. He either plays tennis or goes for a run or rides his bicycle.

Sir Alan Sugar used to keep himself fit by playing tennis. Now, due to groin injuries he has switched to road cycling. He's still exercising.

If these three incredibly successful people (I can count many more) can find time to exercise, tell me what your excuse is. Working too much and not finding time? You are good at everything else, and believe me you will be twice as good, as soon as you incorporate an exercise regime in your life. So we need to work on your productivity to allocate the time needed.

You think you don't have time, but think of this: every single human being on this planet has the same amount of time available to them each day. Everything depends on what you choose to do with that time.

The beauty of exercising every day is that it gives you the luxury of leaving some exercises for other days. For example, if you do strength training to tone up today, you can do your running tomorrow and abs workout the day after. Because it is happening every day (or 5 days a week), you can afford to do short workouts and you will still benefit from this 100%. That's why High Intensity Interval Training (HIIT) has become so popular recently.

In Chapter 8, the exercise-programme section of this book, we will have a look at this in detail.

What I need you to do right now is to open your calendar and imagine you have a very important task to complete with a deadline and with many people in your company or your customers relying on this work. What would you do? You would squeeze a few things together and reallocate the time needed for this important work according to the deadline. You must do the same for your exercise schedule. The good news is that it doesn't have to be an hour of workout. You must start filling in your calendar with *you* as the priority. Any meetings, deadlines, projects should come after. Believe me, you will still complete them all. We human beings are so adaptable.

When I go to the gym or do an outdoor workout, within 15 minutes I feel very satisfied and doing another 5-10 minutes would definitely tick the box for that day (so 20-25 minutes workout in total). It depends what you do in that workout and how you do it. Some days, I might do a 60 minute workout if I have time. But not exercising because I don't have an hour is absolutely not an excuse. High intensity workouts take only 15-20 minutes to complete.

Examples of time-efficient workouts:

- HIIT
- commuting to work by bicycle
- commuting to work by brisk walk or running (all or some part of the journey)
- 20 minutes whole body exercises as soon as you wake up in the morning
- booking a 30 minute class for your lunch break
- superset workouts (more details in Chapter 9, the Optimise your Exercise section)
- major muscles combined exercises

OBJECTION 2: I FEEL OK, I LOOK OK AND I HAVEN'T BEEN SUFFERING ANY MAJOR HEALTH ISSUES. WHY SHOULD I TORTURE MYSELF WITH EXERCISE AND DIETING?

This is something my female clients tell me their husbands say. It's a bit worrying as this is very dangerous. It's like someone says 'I'm absolutely fine with drink driving as I have never had an accident and my concentration is still 100% when I drive with a glass or two inside me.'

This is a risky attitude. We first need to convince the person concerned that what they are thinking is wrong and then work towards the goals. We men know that unless *we* want to make the change, nobody *else* can make us. This arrogant behaviour is unfortunately not working for us but against us. Everyone who cares about us wants us to be around for a long time and this is only achievable when we take personal responsibility for leading a healthy lifestyle.

I need to stress that exercising shouldn't be torture. Getting fit and losing body fat can be the bonus side-effects of our exercise regime. What I mean is, if you enjoy playing basketball as it is fun, you hang out with your mates and engage the competitive side of yourself, so this is far from torture: you will sweat, get rid of your negative thoughts and feel great afterwards. You will burn loads of calories and get fit while you are enjoying yourself.

So let me repeat, if you are new to fitness, do not make the mistake of thinking exercise = torture.

Having said that, some exercises are not team games and when you decide to get fit by doing some strength and conditioning workouts in your front room 4-5 days a week, it could take a few weeks for you to start enjoying that muscle burn. The satisfaction you get from strength training may be different from what you get playing football as you don't feel the kind of buzz you get from scoring a goal on the field with your mates. But there's another, better buzz waiting for you.

Spending that time on yourself gives you benefits you can't get with anything else. It's almost like resetting your entire system and starting afresh.

OBJECTION 3: IT'S TOO MUCH OF A COMMITMENT AND I DON'T HAVE THE WILLPOWER

Commitment? Yes, you do need to make some sort of commitment but it is not as hard as you think. Nobody expects you to lose 12 kilos (2 stone) in two weeks. And nobody expects you to win the Wimbledon tennis tournament if you've only just picked up a racquet for the first time.

We will talk about this aspect in more detail in Chapter 5, in my goal-setting section.

For now, you must know that you need only take one step at a time. Your willpower is there, waiting for instructions. You just need the right mindset.

OBJECTION 4: I'M SELF-CONSCIOUS ABOUT EXERCISING

Even top celebrities are self-conscious. We are all human. Once you stop worrying about what other people will think about you, you are on the right track. It's nobody's business to judge you or comment on your new exercise regime. People you think might look down on you may not be that brilliant themselves anyway! Having said that, I am not suggesting you become one of the Irregulars we mentioned earlier.

Imagine you decide to run a few times a week in your new workout regime. You can hardly run one kilometre without feeling exhausted and you have a colleague you think might make fun of you as he's completed several 5 and 10k runs. So in your eyes, he is a super-fit athlete. Now compare him with Mo Farah, a British double Olympic champion. The difference between you and your colleague is so small compared to that between your colleague and Mo Farah.

Mo Farah would probably think both of you are beginners! It's all relative! So forget about what people will think about you and focus on your personal goals. Before long, you will achieve so much that self-consciousness will be replaced by pride and triumph.

To start with, you could start working out at home or in a quiet part of your local park before you use more public spaces. Go to the gym at off-peak hours and go with a friend. Buy gym gear that you feel comfortable wearing. Don't look in mirrors too much and if you are following some fit-looking people on Instagram or Facebook, be selective and bear in mind that social media images can be fake, overwhelming and depressing. All too often they encourage us to compare ourselves with images of unattainable perfection and we feel we fall short. Our old friend comparisonitis returns!

OBJECTION 5: I DON'T WANT TO INJURE MYSELF

It's a fact that when we get older, we are more likely to injure ourselves and it also takes longer for us to recover. It's realistic to be concerned about this, but it should not stop you from working out.

What I suggest is that you pace yourself, taking small steps forward, regularly and consistently.

For example, you don't want to start a workout regime and schedule a 1.5 hour tennis match for the next day. Look out for beginners' classes and don't forget you will only be a beginner for a short period of time as long as you do the work consistently. In Chapter 7 of this book, I will be talking in detail about how to exercise safely.

OBJECTION 6: I'VE TRIED TO EXERCISE BEFORE AND FAILED

Do you know how many times Edison tried to invent the light bulb? 1000 times. These were not unsuccessful attempts, though. They were all part of a learning curve, taking him towards his successful breakthrough.

You might have failed to keep up with your exercise regime in the past. It definitely doesn't mean you will fail again. Every unsuccessful attempt is a learning point for us. Clearly you didn't have the right mindset at the time. Maybe you didn't have enough support or didn't know where to start or it was the wrong time of the year for you during a busy period at work which overwhelmed you, so you stopped.

Think about what made you fail. Write your reasons down in the space below. And write down what you think you can do to make things turn out better this time.

Problem _____

Potential Solution _____

_____

Problem _____

Potential Solution _____

_____

Problem _____

Potential Solution _____

_____

Problem _____

Potential Solution _____

_____

OBJECTION 7: I'M TOO LAZY TO EXERCISE

You are not alone. It's good to hear this, isn't it? There are so many people in the UK who think they are too lazy to exercise as well.

I really admire these people as they literally acknowledge the problem. Not only that but they are taking responsibility for it rather than blaming other people. These people are easier to work with than people who think they are OK without exercising at all. People who think they are lazy when it comes to exercise are one step ahead of the ones who think they are absolutely fine without making the effort to lead a healthy lifestyle.

How can you overcome your laziness?

Try to remember how you felt last time after exercising. It's always so much better afterwards, isn't it? When we exercise, our brains release serotonin, dopamine and norepinephrine, which are the hormones regulating our mood and happiness. Exercise lifts our mood as well as tightening our flab!

Here are a few hints if you still feel you'll be fighting laziness:

- ☐ Prepare your workout gear the night before, so all you need to do is put it on and go for it as soon as you wake up, if you're a morning exerciser.
- ☐ If you are planning on exercising after work, take your gym gear with you. Even if you choose to walk back home from your work (or some part of the journey), take your comfortable trainers with you so that you have no excuse.
- ☐ Schedule a workout with a friend. It's always easier to turn yourself down, but harder if you have a commitment to a friend or a colleague.
- ☐ Book some personal training or group classes (if you can afford it).
- ☐ Search YouTube for 'gokayfitness' workouts. They range from 10 to 26 minutes long.
- ☐ Do TABATA Workouts at home. YouTube 'TABATA': 4-minute workouts which are not only time-efficient, but also highly effective. Bear in mind, some exercises on YouTube may be intense, so please be selective so that you don't injure yourself.
- ☐ Buy good quality earphones for your workouts. Create your favourite playlist. When you choose an upbeat song, the rhythm of the music sets your rhythm of exercise and keeps the momentum going. Good music – whatever good music is for you – not only helps your endurance but boosts your mood dramatically, which in turn boosts your efficiency as you work out. I do this all the time. I have a few good pairs of earphones/headphones. I search iTunes for nice albums and create a playlist for myself, using it as motivation for those days when I don't want to exercise. Yes, even I can feel like that sometimes!
- ☐ Don't force yourself to do something you hate. If running is your least favourite exercise, go for a swim. If you hate the gym floor, go to your local park and use the bench there to do your press-ups.

You may have heard this when you were a kid: pick your friends carefully as you may find you come to embody the characteristics of the people you surround yourself with. The more lazy people there are around you, the more lazy you may get; the more unhealthy people there are around you, the more unhealthy you may become.

Remember when you were at school, how it felt permissible not to do your homework when your mates Martin and Ross didn't do theirs either? You started being conditioned to think that if you did your homework, they'd think you were a weirdo.

It's exactly the same now. You're reluctant to draw the attention of the people around you, in case they make fun of you. 'Oh look at his lunch, he is eating salad now like a girl...' or 'Are you trying to be fit now? Come on, have another pint!' or 'Come on, play Xbox with us, homework is for keenos!' Is this ringing bells? Peer pressure is very real and it's typical of humans to want to conform to the norms of their group.

4.4 REPURPOSE YOUR BUSINESS SKILLS

You may think 'I have a demanding job and a very busy life with no space for either exercise or a healthy diet. So I won't take action as it's not possible for me to do anything right now.'

People think that a high-powered job with an overloaded schedule doesn't leave them enough time to get their health and fitness back. They don't invest in their health and gradually start to put on weight, which makes them end up tired, mentally low and weak.

They think all these men with good physiques that they see in magazines (or at their gym) were born like that. They think it's too hard to make lifestyle changes, so they don't bother. As a consequence, they suffer from ill health.

They think they should be doing all or nothing. They think they will either be like a robot taking their fitness regime to an extreme, involving crash dieting or over-training, or they let everything go and end up with too many take-away dinners and lots of alcohol. They think working hard gives them the best excuse to treat themselves to a double whisky or an expensive bottle of wine, so they do and get fatter and more inactive every year.

Patrick is a very successful businessman with an incredibly busy schedule. Over the years, as he found himself gaining over 12 kilos, he felt unfit and unhappy about himself. It played on his mind for years.

He has now changed his lifestyle, with regular exercise, a healthy diet as far as possible and lots of activity at every opportunity. He started using his mobile phone for his daily step count; did workouts four times a week and went for long walks at weekends, listening to podcasts through his earphones. He has lost a big chunk of his belly, his posture has improved a lot, he has a broad chest and back, and his toned arms and legs are getting compliments from his colleagues. He feels more productive and admits that saying 'too busy, no time for exercise' was the biggest lie he used to tell himself.

So, my advice to you is to review your work-practices and consider how many of these can be transferred into your new fitness world. Use technology. Set goals (we'll be talking about that soon), think about results and timelines for those results, as you would for work-schedules. Think about exercise in terms of ROI: return on investment – what you put in will more than pay off and justify the time and effort.

Think also about how you motivate yourself. How you turn up for the day-job and show self-discipline and commitment. Think about how you encourage others in the work-force and start encouraging yourself! Think about how sometimes you need to pull someone up for laziness and letting the side down. You are a team of one: be your own team-player and coach.

4.5 FOCUS ON THE VISION

I can't stress enough that unless you are prepared to change your mindset and see this as an 8 week plan with no excuses or pauses throughout, you won't make it. In the course of these 8 weeks, you will gain some brilliant habits and this will continue afterwards to keep you going.

You won't make it if you're a part-time player; if you think you will be fine for three days of the week, then you stop watching your diet and macros as you had guests on Saturday and you had to entertain them and your colleague invited you for lunch so you had to eat that 600 calorie starter followed by... If it is so easy for you to sabotage yourself it may be that you simply haven't figured out your why.

At this point, you could opt to rethink your why and come back with a stronger one. Or you could just throw this book away or give it to someone else who might benefit from it. You can choose to go on living the way you have been living, which might be absolutely adequate for you. But you won't get toned and healthy.

OK, I've done my tough love bit. And actually, having said all that, I do want to reassure you that the programme is easier than it sounds. All I ask is that you're prepared for those rocky patches and that your overall vision of what you can be, plus your trust in the method I offer, will see you through them.

If you are my ideal reader, then it is most likely you have a good but demanding job/profession/career. That means meeting deadlines and working under relatively stressful circumstances are your norm. What happens when you have a very very busy day and a new task you have to complete appears? Plus, it's got a very strict deadline? You do it, don't you? You're even more likely to get it done than if you had no time pressure. I'm sure you've experienced times when having a deadline means you produce better results.

So why not use this concept in your health and fitness?

Your new deadline is this 8 week programme. Fill in the blanks in the lines below – do it now. Put your intentions into words rather than have a vague notion of what you want to do.

YOUR INTENTION STATEMENT

At the end of this programme, the outcome I want is:

(Examples: My ideal outcome is ...

Feeling more energetic

Losing 5 kilos)

Now fill in *yours*:

My ideal outcome is _____

_____

CREATE THE VISION

If your aim is to have a better physique and look good, to achieve your goals, you need to know who you want to look like at the end of your challenge. Some descriptions are basically not enough. For example, saying 'I want a six-pack' won't trigger that willpower of yours as you can't see the whole picture.

You've probably heard how effective it is to create a vision board for your future desires. For example, cutting out an image of a summer-house and sticking it to your board in your study is going to make you focus twice as much on that desire to build one in your garden. The visual reminder will keep the goal at a high level in your consciousness, making it more likely that you will be able to spot the opportunities to achieve what you want in the end.

Three years ago, I added two images to my personal vision board. One was of a convertible BMW car and the other one was of a villa with an infinity pool and an amazing sea view. One year later, I've achieved the first one! The second one hasn't come true yet but I know I will have it one day. These were the materialistic aspects of my vision board. I also have Richard Branson's image on the lifestyle side of my vision board as a high-achieving positive can-do role-model.

What I need you to do is to create a vision board now. I need you to either search online or get a fitness magazine and find a few images of men who have the kind of body that you would like to have. Cut out those images and stick them on your vision board. I always say this is a journey because you are going from A to B. Right now we are at A, and B is that person on your wall. Your aim is to get there as directly as possible.

Imagine you want to go to Vienna by car. You are in the UK right now. What do you do? You cross the Channel. Drive through France a bit and towards Germany afterwards and head to Vienna. Do you visit Bilbao in Spain on your way there? You could, but that would delay everything! Before you know it, you'd be tired, lose concentration and willpower and want to come back home. Waste of effort.

Let's go to our destination with as few diversions as possible. With those images on your vision board, you now know exactly who you want to be when you achieve your goals. It's time to make the necessary changes to get there. It's time to increase your activity, work on the quality of your sleep, cut all the crap in your diet and replace it with healthy and nutritious food.

4.6 DON'T LOSE SIGHT OF YOUR ACHIEVEMENTS

There may be times when you will lose faith in your ability to stick to your intentions so instead of looking forward, you could try looking back.

Take some paper and write down some of your previous achievements. For example: became a manager in your company, raised/raising a lovely child, bought a house, attended a cycling event and finished it without fainting, gave a great dinner party where everyone loved the food you cooked, finished a book on holiday.

I know these are random examples but my point is that every single person has achieved something important in their life, no matter how big or small and they did it despite life's ups and downs.

When the going gets tough, it really helps to remind yourself of what you have managed to achieve in life so far, so please list 3 things you have achieved in the past that you're most proud of.

1. _____

2. _____

3. _____

Now, what are your intentions for the next two months? Not a crazy aim like losing 30kg in 8 weeks but something achievable. Think about how you would *really* like to look and feel in 8 weeks' time.

How can you maximise your chances of succeeding? You may have to play some mind-games with yourself. As a trainer, I have found this really works when I am encouraging people to stretch themselves and go for targets they don't at first believe they can hit. Here's an example:

Running can be a hard exercise for some people, so I conducted a mini-experiment with more than 30 of my clients. Every single time, I got this remarkable result.

During my personal training sessions, I often ask my clients to run about 100 metres to a post and run back, in between doing other exercises. If I am training someone new or a relatively unfit person, they run to the post, getting so out of breath that they pause there for 10-15 seconds before they run back. Many of these individuals stop on the way back and walk the last 20-30 metres.

Now, this is the interesting bit. I may set a target linked to a penalty, such as 'If you pause more than 3 seconds when you arrive at the post or if you stop running either way, I will ask you to repeat this exercise and run again.' Guess what happens! Yes, every single individual completes the task perfectly without fail.

Another interesting experiment involves skipping. In my personal training session, a part of my client's cardio workout could be to do 100 skips, just to raise their heart rate in between some weight exercises. Again people who stop or trip over by mistake a few times during these 100 skips, magically improve when I say 'If you stop (by mistake or as you get tired), I will ask you to start again or we will add 20 skips each time you stop.' They all seem to be brilliant after this mini-challenge!

The answer, it seems, is to bargain with yourself or issue challenges to yourself that you rise to meet – and then you feel extra satisfaction, if not triumph.

ENJOY YOURSELF

Whatever you do, have fun. Things you don't like doing might feel like chores, but they can also be fun as long as you change your mindset.

Remember, nobody is forcing you to do something that you don't really want to do. If you choose to become healthy, by going to the gym or doing a workout at home for twenty minutes, it should not feel like a chore as this is your private time between you and your own self. It should feel good because you are investing in you and you should feel free to feel selfish. It's your time and you can do whatever you want to do with it.

CHAPTER 5: GET READY TO GET FIT (2): FOUNDATIONS FOR SUCCESS

5.1 MEET ALEXANDER AND PETE

We've talked about mindset and in a way, mindset is something you will always have to bear in ... er, mind. In this section, though, we are looking at the interface between mindset and action, where you translate your will and your intentions into actual doable plans. You're at a crossroads. You can keep reading and *thinking* about taking action, or you can actually take that action! Action is the only way you'll take charge of your health and fitness: no amount of advice or detailed exercise structures can help you if you stay passive or eternally procrastinate. It's decision time!

We're going to start with a preliminary exercise because for the programme to work you need to set it up to work. In earlier sections we looked at the ways you may self-sabotage, the kinds of *internal* excuses and delaying tactics you may come up with. Now, we are going to look at some of the *external* sabotages that may affect you. But before we do, let's meet Alexander and Pete. Both in their 40s, they wanted to lose weight and become fitter. Both seemed really keen and motivated but, when they came to me, one met the challenges rather better than the other. I wonder which of them you'll be most like? Will you be Alexander? Or will you be Pete?

Why did Alexander manage to get fit and lose about 5-6% of his body fat in just 10 weeks and Pete made almost no progress whatsoever for weeks on end?

I have been studying these people for a while so I know the reasons: I'd love to share them with you.

First of all, no one can *make* you do something unless you want to. If I had the best French teacher in the world and had his/her unlimited attention and time for a year, could I be fluent at the end of the year? Only if I wanted to enough.

Here are the reasons I observed for their relative success or failure:

Goal Setting:

Alexander came to me with a time limit in mind. He said, 'I'd like to lose 10 kg. Can I do this in 10 weeks? Pete said, 'I think I'd better lose some weight and get fit. Maybe about 10 kg. I am not bothered about how long it takes.' I did explain to him about the importance of time in setting goals that are SMART. SMART stands for:

- S – Specific. You need to have a specified goal, such as 'I'd like to lose 6 kg.'
- M – Measurable. You need some way of measuring your achievement of the goal, such as dropping a clothing size.
- A – Achievable. The goal needs to be something you can reasonably achieve, so not something like losing 12 kg in 7 days ...
- R – Relevant. The goal needs to resonate with you. You need to know the reason behind it.
- T – Time-based. You need a deadline, such as losing 8 cm round your waist in 8 weeks.

Alexander wanted to know exactly what else he could do outside of his Personal Training (PT) sessions. So I gave him a detailed workout plan via my online app and he also followed a strict healthy eating plan (without starving himself).

Pete not only ignored me when I said he needed to do some additional activities in his own time but also tried to persuade me that one hour a week of training would be enough as he was very busy.

Mindset:

Alexander had already made up his mind before he booked his appointment with me that he wanted to be fit and healthy.

Pete hadn't. He was magically expecting to be convinced to do that, as if I were to enrol at Dulwich College (a top private school in South East London) and expect the headmaster to convince me I could be a brain surgeon.

Alexander planned his weeks in advance in terms of his nutrition as well as his workouts. He travels to a few countries a week for seminars, so you can imagine how hard that is, but he still did it.

After a few weeks, Pete thought losing 10 kg was too much to achieve as he hadn't broken his goal down into bite-sized achievable pieces.

Alexander had a great reason. He had his son's wedding coming up so he felt he had to be fit and healthy in time for that.

Pete had no real reason other than his reaction to some peer pressure.

Alexander saw this as a cumulative weekly progress so this helped him not to feel overwhelmed during the difficult times.

Pete thought he could just take it easy and see how he felt.

Alexander put on his earphones, put on his gym gear and got on with his workouts at the gym (doing the homework exercises I designed for him), without feeling self-conscious as he had his main reason in his mind all the time.

Pete found it difficult to complete his exercises as he compared himself with those super-fit guys in the weights room and forgot why he was there in the first place.

Creating Support:

Alexander had fantastic support from his wife and kids and his colleagues.

Pete didn't even mention to his wife that he had set some goals for himself. So nobody knew about his weight loss goal other than that he had booked some PT sessions.

Now we have compared them I hope you'll choose to be like Alexander rather than Pete!

5.2 HEADING TROUBLE OFF AT THE PASS

In your fitness journey, you are bound to meet obstacles and hurdles. For example, there may be some dinner parties that you absolutely have to attend, with the kind of high calorie food and drink you may find difficult to turn down. Or you might have a few business trips coming up, also pretty compulsory, which may result in eating hotel breakfasts as well as unhealthy business lunches. You'll also be short of time for the workouts you need to be completing in this programme. I get it, it's life.

In order to head all this off at the pass, your first task is to look ahead. Pre-emptive action will save you a lot of trouble later on. First, take a look at your diary and list all the birthday celebrations you need to attend, all the possible trips, all the weekend parties – all the *social interruptions* you're going to face in the coming 8 weeks. I am perfectly aware that life goes on and it can be very hard or impossible to say no to all these events in your diary in the next 8 weeks.

What we are going to do now is to plan ahead and address how to minimise the damage these events create when we attend them.

For example, if you're going abroad on a business trip for five days, write it in the list below and come up with ways you could handle it better. It might be 'Pick a hotel that has a decent gym' or 'Pick a hotel that is two miles from the daily meetings, so I can walk there and back to increase my activity on those days'. I know your circumstances might be different but this gives you an idea.

My point is that this is like making a business plan. Everything is arbitrary. Who knows how many sales you will make next year or within the next five years or what percentage of the market you will be able to gain? You can't know for sure but still you make a business plan to have a broad impression at least of what is ahead of you and how you can eliminate or mitigate any upcoming risks.

This programme is like that business plan. Have you ever watched *Dragon's Den* on TV? Entrepreneurs pitch their business ideas to a board of (pretty scary) multimillionaire businessmen and women. Have you ever seen any of them come in and say, 'Hey, I have this business idea. But I haven't got a business plan. I'm waiting to see how I feel. Of course I want to make a profit but you know, life is always in the way: I have kids; weekends I get wasted sometimes'. They would hardly be able to secure investment funds if they sounded as flakey and ill-prepared as that!

So, here at the start of the programme I want you to plan ahead, maximizing your chance of the best outcome. Here is a table of the coming eight weeks. Write down the issues you're expecting may sabotage you – and also write down the strategies you'll put in place to address them.

WEEK 1

Which days are tricky? _____

How will I deal with this? _____

WEEK 2

Which days are tricky? _____

_____

How will I deal with this? _____

_____

_____

WEEK 3

Which days are tricky? _____

_____

How will I deal with this? _____

_____

_____

WEEK 4

Which days are tricky? _____

_____

How will I deal with this? _____

_____

_____

WEEK 5

Which days are tricky? _____

_____

How will I deal with this? _____

_____

WEEK 6

Which days are tricky? _____

_____

How will I deal with this? _____

_____

WEEK 7

Which days are tricky? _____

_____

How will I deal with this? _____

_____

WEEK 8

Which days are tricky? _____

_____

How will I deal with this? _____

_____

_____

5.3 INCENTIVES AND MARKERS OF SUCCESS

Returning to the notion we covered earlier, of the inner mind-games you may need to play with yourself, think of them in terms of public visibility and accountability. As we mentioned, one way of getting the results you want is to book a *public* event, such as a 10k race, a mini-triathlon, a cycling weekend aiming for 150k in two days etc.

You could create a different type of deadline by setting up a challenge in your office or with a mate. Who is going to lose more body fat by the end of eight weeks or gain more strength or do more press-ups (the loser pays £100 or you name it). Competition is a great spur to achievement!

Scales: these are our close friends when we start losing weight, but they can also be our worst enemy if we are not making progress or if we are actually gaining fat! I will be talking about this in 'Visiting the Scales' in Chapter 6.

Waist: all you need is a tape measure. Measure around your waist, just over your belly button. You won't go wrong. Numbers will tell! There is no way you can say 'Agh, I must have put on muscle mass because I've gained three pounds over the last week!', as measuring your waistline is more or less a true indicator of whether or not you are losing body fat.

Comments: do not ignore nice comments you get from the people around you. In England, people are so polite that nobody likes to say anything if they think you're putting weight on. However, if you are hearing comments such as, 'You look healthier'; 'You look like you've lost some weight'; 'Are you exercising as your shape has changed so much recently?', then accept these compliments and use them to motivate you further.

Mirror: some days we look in the mirror and have to face up to the fact that we're not as toned as we'd like to be or our belly is sticking out a bit and so on. However, when you lose weight, when that magical time comes, you definitely notice that change either in the circumference of your arm or around your waist, or in the contours of your face. If you stare hard at yourself in the mirror every single day, you're more likely see the difference. When you do see it, it's a fabulous feeling!

Clothes: losing weight could be an expensive experience but it's all worth it. I have some clients who have changed their entire wardrobe as they lost a considerable amount of weight: their torso, shoulders and arms are much larger, due to the muscle mass gain, while their waist and hips are smaller. When you start feeling your trousers are getting loose or your shirt is slightly tight around your chest, you will be over the moon!

Mood, sleep and energy: once you change your lifestyle by exercising regularly and eating healthily, your mood will improve, you will sleep better and your energy levels will be much higher. So this is another great indicator that you are on the right track my friend.

5.4 DEFINE YOUR WEIGHT GOALS

You can't know if you've succeeded in any project in life unless you first set out what it is you want to achieve, so let's write down your weight goals. First of all, I need you to take two basic measurements.

1. Weigh yourself with a scale that you have access to regularly.

2. Measure your waist by using a tape measure (I do it on top of my belly button as a reference).

Record these numbers – your current weight and current waist-size.

Be aware that when you set anything more than a 7-8 kilo weight-loss goal in 8 weeks that might be too much too soon unless you already have 25 kilos or more of body fat. You might gain it back afterwards or lose muscle mass, which is not what we want. So if you need to lose more weight you should feel free to carry on longer than the initial 8 weeks to achieve your goal in a healthy way.

Now I need you to write down how much you want to lose:

_____ (kg/stone/lb)

Does this target look daunting to you? Maybe your healthy weight should be 10 kg less than your current weight but you're just too scared to write it down as losing even 3 kg seems an impossible task for you right now.

How much, then, do you realistically want to lose during this time period? Remember that setting a moderate goal can be better than an over-ambitious one. Make it enough to spur you on, not to daunt you.

My weight loss target during the programme is: _____ (kg/stone/lb)

Your weight loss goal might be over 12 kg and let's say with the right guidance, support and motivation you are able to lose 8 kg in 8 weeks. Can you imagine how wonderful you will look and feel being 8 kg lighter? (Remember what we said about having a vision, in the previous section?) Losing the remaining 4 kg will only take another 3-4 weeks. You can actually achieve your goal in 11-12 weeks. So if you start this task on September the 1st, for example, before Christmas you will be the person you dreamt of being!

Think about all the praise you'll get from friends and family. They will all ask you how you did it. Your kids will be proud of you and believe me, you will get a completely different level of attention from your partner!

Now let's take things further.

5.5 SPECIFIC GOAL-SETTING AND TIMETABLING

OK, let's go back to the notion of goal-setting. Not only goal-setting but being aware of the timescale of your goals. If you don't set precise time-goals, the risk is you will drift rather aimlessly, full of good intentions but little else. How did I become a gold medallist in bodybuilding? I had access to the knowledge (it wasn't up to today's standards but it was enough), certainly, but do you know what was the most important factor in my success? *I had my big 'why'.* My big why helped me tremendously. In addition, though, every time I lacked willpower or felt too lazy for that workout after eight or nine hours of solid work in the Air Force, I reminded myself that I had a *deadline*. So, let's get clear on yours. You may find my scorecard app helpful https://www.gokayfitness.com/scorecard.

1. Write down your 8 week weight loss goal.

2. Now divide that number by 2 (your monthly weight loss goal).

3. Add 1kg to the result from answer 2. This is your goal for the first month. You

will most likely lose more in the early stages of your challenge. (This is why faddy diets are so appealing. But remember, you are in this for the long haul and you're going to aim for a steady loss over time, not a quick crash and rebound.)

4. Now divide this answer by 4 to find out your weekly weight loss goal for the first month.

5. Do the same thing for the second month but this time subtract 1 from the half of your weight loss goal. And divide it by 4 to find out your weekly goal for the second month.

Next, write down the activities you will start taking part in.

The first one is going to be a regular weekly exercise routine, such as joining a circuit class/spinning class twice a week etc. The frequency is for you to choose: I appreciate everyone's needs are different.

The second one is something you will incorporate into the routine of your everyday life, such as walking to work, jogging/running (for part of your journey perhaps). It needs to be an activity that you are not already doing.

The third one is a fun activity that you will enjoy. No restrictions here. Join a swimming class, take your kid to a park for a ride, hire a bike to discover your local town or local parks or the countryside, play badminton. There are activities you can engage in with friends or with your kids. If you are alone, then Google activities or groups that you can join locally.

Activities I can aim to take part in:

1. _____

2. _____

3. _____

Involvement in these activities is going to carry on for at least 8 weeks but my aim is you'll continue with them afterwards, so that they become a lifestyle change rather than a quick temporary fix.

Now you need to set yourself weekly goals. Complete the following statement:

At the end of Week 1, I will have achieved _____

(E.g. 1kg weight loss/worked out 5 times a week/walked 70 minutes longer than usual using a suitable app such as MapMyWalk, Record, Strava/ consumed _____ calories on average.)

MY GOAL PLANNER

My Starting Weight: _____

My Starting Waist Measurement: _____

Week 1 Goals: _____

Week 2 Goals: _____

Week 3 Goals: _____

Week 4 Goals: _____

Week 5 Goals: _____

Week 6 Goals: _____

Week 7 Goals: _____

Week 8 Goals: _____

5.6 PLANNING YOUR NEW IMPROVED DIET

Diet. The word itself sounds harsh so 'healthy eating' is how I tend to refer to it. We'll be exploring this in a lot more detail in Chapter 6 but right now you can start to plan for optimizing your relationship with food.

Download the MyFitnessPal app, which is free, and use it for at least 3 days to analyse what you are currently eating and what your current calorie consumption is. The longer you use it, the better it works!

You can visit my sample healthy food shopping list page on my website if you need guidance: https://www.gokayfitness.com/healthyfoodshoppinglist.

Write down what you will cut out or reduce consumption of in the next 8 weeks. (Examples might be beer, wine, cakes, crisps, second portions.)

1. _____

2. _____

3. _____

Now write down what you will replace these with.

1. _____

2. _____

_____

3. _____

_____

As with exercise, it helps to make a plan rather than stumble haphazardly through the 8 week challenge with no clear notion of how nutrition will help you. Knowing what to do helps you to focus, keep motivated and aids success. You'll find more guidance and advice in the next chapter.

5.7   SELF-ASSESSMENT QUESTIONS

Any process in business or in the routine of your day-job needs evaluation. Things are no different here, so at the end of each week I encourage you to review your progress. Here are the kinds of questions you can ask yourself in a notebook you keep for the purpose.

WEEK _____

What were my goals for the week?

How many did I achieve?

How many did I get close to achieving?

How does it feel?

Were there any I didn't achieve?

What stopped me?

Was it family commitments, too much work, no time, not motivated enough? Can I define exactly what hindered my progress? Can I take action on that next week?

What were my wins

I've achieved _____ (e.g. weight loss, mileage run etc.)

Or I was very close to achieving _____ Next week, I will nail it.

Next week, I am going to do _____ to make sure I achieve this or I am closer to achieving this.

Note: to help you with this, I have also created journal pages for you to fill in each week during the programme: they can be found at the end of each week's programme in Chapter 8.

5.8 BE BRAVE, GO PUBLIC!

Now, it's all well and good to make a private pact with yourself, setting your intentions or creating a vision board as we've discussed. These techniques do work. But another way to encourage yourself to see things through is to go public. I know! Scary thought! If we have an intention and we fall short of achieving it, and we told nobody in the first place, then nobody need know we failed. Going public is nailing your colours to the mast. When other people know, when they have expectations, when they show you encouragement, then you may be more likely to deliver. You want to please or impress them. You don't want to let them down or shame yourself in front of them.

I proved this technique works when I made that agreement at my local gym so many years ago, that I was going to take part in the national bodybuilding contest. I'd told my colleagues at work, so I felt accountable to them. I also didn't want to embarrass myself in front of thousands on the day of the contest!

You'll find it really useful to sign up for an event: a 5 or 10k run, mini Iron Man, half marathon, regional fitness competition or even your kid's end of the year parents' fitness competition! Whatever it is, just pick something that suits you best, then see what happens. You will not only just turn up for your preparatory workouts, but also try really hard during each one, because you know there's an overall purpose to it.

If running is not your thing, sign up for something like the London to Brighton Bike Ride or an event like it in your region. Believe me, you don't need to be super fit. You will manage it, just as many other people have managed it in the past; there's no reason you should be any different.

Last year, I had a client called Andrew who started training with me. He'd not done any running since he was in Year 5 at school! He was overweight (obese according to the UK fat percentage chart), and very unfit. His diet was absolutely appalling. He drank alcohol most days of the week. Plus he had a dodgy knee that had been bothering him.

On the other hand, Andrew was successful in his career and was bringing in nearly half a million a year. He was super-smart, witty and fun to be around. He didn't have much free time for exercise as he was travelling a lot with his job and what time he had left over was spent with his family.

We first sat down and discussed why he wanted to work with me. What was he expecting from my expertise and how keen was he to *actually* take action? We then created space in his diary and set short and mid-term goals.

After we made the initial plan, I signed him up for a 10k run. He was unfit, overweight and had a knee injury so you might think that to sign him up for a run of that length, only five months away, was a bit unrealistic…

We set to work. I arranged physiotherapy treatments for his knee and after four or five treatments, plus work to increase the flexibility of his hamstring and strengthen his quads and gluteus, his knee started to feel better. The physio gave the green light for him to start running and by that time we had been working all the muscles around without aggravating his knee. Within a month, he'd lost about 4.5-5kg (around 10lbs). The 10K run was by then four months away.

Andrew's mindset had shifted from a vague 'I might take part in this running event in a few months' time'. The run was now part of his daily conversation with his colleagues, family and even with himself.

I'm an ex-bodybuilder, not a running expert. So I signed him up with his local running club to get him additional help. By the time the 10k run was about a month away, he was able to run 7-8k. I helped him gain lean muscle and lose around 14-15 kilos (around 30lbs). I changed his mindset so much he was already thinking about signing up for a cycling event six months off.

As all this was going on, the main benefits started to appear. His energy level rose, his sleep improved tremendously, his stress level came down and his mood was elevated. All in a mere five months.

When Andrew travels overseas now, instead of trying to locate the nearest bar, he is checking out where the nearest gym is. When booking his hotel, his PA only picks hotels with either a swimming pool or a decent gym (or both!) He now chooses healthier options at that business lunch and sticks with water or a non-alcoholic drink, or at worst he stops after one drink.

5.9 POSITIVE COMPETITIVENESS

I acknowledge that everyone is different. Therefore, what motivates you or what keeps you going might be completely different from what motivates someone else. This applies even to brothers or sisters or close friends.

You might be the type of person who works best on your own; someone else might prefer to be involved in teamwork and thrives on other people's presence and input.

You might be very focused and determined and don't need any extra motivation to help you succeed but in my experience everyone has some degree of competitiveness in them. You must know at least a handful of people around you who turn into monsters when you give them a task and ask them to compete against their friend or colleague.

That's why sales teams do great when you give them a target and mention how well the other team is performing.

That's why GCSE exam pass marks are published after everyone sits the exams and all the students' exam papers are marked so that you get compared to the rest of the attendees. If the majority of students haven't done all that well, the pass mark goes down or vice versa. We are all affected by what our peer group is doing. We all sit somewhere within a spectrum of achievement.

In today's society as everyone knows, comparison and trying to keep up with the Joneses is not very healthy mentally as it does bring you down and make you doubt yourself. You may feel unhappy even if you have all you need in your life.

The downside of this is that you may be comparing yourself financially with other people around you or you are only looking at the materialistic side of things. Yes, you will try to find opportunities to compete with that neighbour to make more money so that you don't feel inferior; however, that will continue to make you unhappy as nothing will be ever be enough, even if your achievements are tremendous. It will block you from seeing how incredibly you performed and stop you from acknowledging and celebrating your achievements.

The upside is that competition might give you the motivation to work more on your goals and keep you on track as long as you keep it all in proportion. So we need to ignite your competitive side. Believe it or not, you can potentially double the speed of your success, if not more.

Let me explain. When clients come to me to get fit, lose weight or get lean - whatever the goal is, if they are not focused and determined, they may not get where they want to be. Life has a tendency of getting in the way of us achieving our goals, so some weeks they may not be doing all that well. I appreciate that. If this carries on week after week, then we revisit what they really want to achieve. In addition, I came up with a competition idea that has helped so many of them.

It works like this: I pair up two men or women with similar lifestyles, who are of similar size and activity level and fitness. Each of them wants to get fit, lose some weight and gain some lean muscle.

I speak to them individually and we set a goal to be achieved within the next four to six weeks. It could be weight loss or a fitness level goal. I weigh them at the beginning and give each one the same goal, such as, for example, losing 5% of their body fat in five weeks. Every week I weigh them again and the person who loses more that week is paid a pre-arranged sum of money, generally around £20, by the loser. At the end of the overall four to six week period, the overall winner gets paid £50 or £100 by the loser. You won't believe how competitive and determined people get when I apply this method. They both lose more weight than they would have on their own and even the loser of the game actually loses a big chunk of his/her body fat.

That's what I would like you to do. Think about people around you. Colleagues, friends - whoever is similar to you in terms of weight, fitness and lifestyle. Dare them to join this challenge with you.

You could set your own rules: the competition could be for 8 weeks, it could be a condition that if someone pulls out of the programme prematurely, they need to pay £100 or do 200 burpees etc. You've got the point. You set a start date, decide when you will be weighing yourself and when it will end. If you don't live close to one another, you could send screen shots of the readings on your scales.

By doing this, you're working with a competitive version of the accountability strategy we looked at earlier in the book. Every time you're close to succumbing to food temptation you'll think of your competitor sending a screenshot of the scales showing their weight-loss, and you'll stand firm rather than let them beat you!

PART THREE

CHAPTER 6: FUEL YOUR FITNESS

6.1 EXCUSES, EXCUSES

In this section we're concentrating on how a good diet can really help you as you proceed with your exercise programme. It's crucial to pay attention to this: the fuel you put in the tank helps that vehicle, your body, to function well!

But first, a bit of straight talking.

I hear this from many clients on a regular basis: 'Oh my diet is very healthy, I eat lots of vegetables and no junk food'. But this type of person's visceral fat (the fat around the internal organs) could be at a quite high level and they may not actually be that healthy, in spite of their outward appearance.

Healthy means avoiding illness, being in good shape, having high energy levels and being strong. If you are 10kg over the recommended weight (due to excessive fat tissue not muscle mass) you might not suffer from any illnesses but you are also not healthy. Over the course of 8 weeks with this programme, you can lower your visceral fat by a significant amount and be much healthier, fitter and more likely to live longer.

So the lesson is, don't deceive yourself! You need to pay attention to the hidden levels of fat there may be within your body and you need to be honest with yourself when it comes to just how varied your diet is and how many servings of fruit and vegetables you consume each day. Don't forget the form those servings take! You don't need to tell me that raw or steamed vegetables are better for you than fried ones.

If you need help and inspiration, I'm including a selection of delicious recipes you can access in Chapter 11's Resources section at the back of this book.

6.2 THE CALORIE EQUATION

Right, now let's accentuate the positive as we dive in to one of the most important contributing factors to health and wellbeing. I'll give you the calorie-count and recommended protein intakes for you to get optimum results. Bear in mind, though, that these numbers are only guidelines. It can be very hard to hit those targets every single day.

Bear this in mind as well: I don't expect you to eat exactly the same quantities of calories, vitamins and macros on a daily basis, as life often gets in the way of our intentions. The key is to try to be as consistent as possible during these 8 weeks at least.

We don't sleep exactly the same number of hours every single night, we don't walk exactly the same number of steps every day, we don't move around the same amount, so I appreciate that we are not robots.

When it comes to weight loss or weight gain, calories in versus calories out is a law. Accept it or not, this a law. It is like Newton's Three Laws of Motion, the Archimedes Eureka principle or Galileo's discoveries in astronomy.

What I mean by that is you can argue against it by following other fancy and commercial trends. You could try eating only during a six-hour window each day (intermittent fasting), or calling your treat a sin (Slimming World) or only eating the kind of 'stone age' food hunter-gatherers would have eaten in ancient times (Paleo Diet) or collect points for each food you eat and have a specified allowance of daily points (Weight Watchers). All you are doing by following different trendy diets is restricting your calorie intake in some way or other.

Calories in, Calories out.

I cannot stress this enough.

You will not lose weight magically with a high fat low carb diet if your total daily calorie intake is more than you burn.

You will not lose weight by separating your carbs and protein into different meals if your daily calories total comes to more than you burn.

Research conducted by the American Physiological Society in 2017 established that you will definitely not lose weight if you starve yourself for 15 hours a day and consume 4500 calories in the remaining 9 hours unless you burn more than 4500 calories a day in the first place.

These days there are so many differing opinions around diets with all sorts of fancy names. Almost every year, we hear of a new popular diet being advocated amongst gym freaks or even at the office. All of this makes it difficult to know where to start.

The key thing is that you find a food plan that is *sustainable* and does not make you feel miserable as you are starving day after day. Food should be enjoyed: making, sharing and consuming food is a social event. My healthy eating recipes and guidance will provide you with an easy sustainable way to enjoy your food, one that fits in with your lifestyle.

One of the most common mistakes we make in our nutrition is to allow our blood sugar levels to rise and fall dramatically during the day. Missing meals causes our blood sugar to fall too low. Then to compensate, we eat high GI food (sweet and simple carbohydrates, such as white pasta, bread and pastries), and this raises blood sugar levels significantly. The result is an unhealthy roller-coaster of highs and lows. However, if you are following a fasting diet, your blood sugar still goes down during the fasting period. Then your body uses its own fat stores to replace the missing blood sugar until you eat once more. This is more controlled than irregular instant highs and lows.

CALORIE DEFICIT VERSUS WEIGHT LOSS

I'd like to talk about how many calories you need to burn to lose a pound (half a kilo) a week.

As you probably know by now, I love numbers and maths, but I have to admit that weight loss doesn't always follow a linear graph. If you reduce the amount of calories you consume or increase your activity (or both) to create a calorie deficit, you start losing weight. However, once you start losing weight, your body will be spending less energy to do the same work, as it doesn't need to fuel the same body size as before. Therefore, you need to adjust your diet and exercise accordingly. There are many factors you need to consider: your sex, age, basal metabolic rate, even your genes.

In the late 1950s, some research showed that if you were to create a 500 calorie deficit per day, it would come to a total 3500 calorie deficit a week, which is equal to losing a pound per week. This is a rough guideline. You could create this deficit by eating less or exercising more (even walking more daily counts) or doing both at the same time to speed the process up.

A rough sample calculation: you are in your mid-40s and are about a stone heavier than you should be. Let's say from Monday onwards, every single day, you were to consume 200 fewer calories (equivalent to 175ml of wine) and also exercised and burnt 300 calories (an hour of walking/30 mins jogging/30 mins swimming) on a daily basis. If every other factor in your diet and activity stayed the same, at the end of the week you would see around a pound of weight loss.

And consuming 200 fewer calories is absolutely doable: for example, eat no starters, cut down one daily naughty snack – even a pint of beer has over 200 calories! In three months, you'd be a stone lighter. And this is without killing yourself with starvation and effort! The key thing here is being *consistent*.

6.3 WHY DIETS DON'T WORK FOR SOME PEOPLE

I haven't met anyone who doesn't want to look good. I don't mean everyone wants to be pumped up or have a six-pack. It could be your hair, your clothing or your physical appearance that matters to you. Some people can put in more effort than others; some just can't be bothered. It doesn't change the fact that deep inside everyone wants to look good.

Here, in the western world, we are used to thinking that we can eat whatever we want and as much as we want. People can die of starvation during a famine but in developed countries these days they are more likely to perish because of obesity-related diseases, such as Type 2 diabetes or heart disease. We live to eat, rather than eating to live.

The level of obesity within the UK population has gone up from 10% to 30% in only forty years, according to the World Health Organisation. The number of calories we consume every day is absolutely ridiculous. On top of that our daily activity is nowhere near what it used to be even fifty years ago. We walk less, robots or machinery have taken the place of human labour; in cities, Uber is two minutes away so everything is more convenient. All of this comes at a cost. In 1975 you would have seen one in ten people as obese, and in 2016 almost one in every three people was obese. Scary, isn't it?

From the late 1970s to the mid-2000s, average calorie consumption per person went up by about 570 calories a day as food got cheaper and more accessible. Fast food and calorific food is much cheaper than wholesome and healthy nutrition.

One of the reasons for the increase in obesity-levels has been the consumption of processed food. Human beings have always subjected foodstuffs to processes, of course, to make the foods more palatable and long-lasting. But we are seeing this on an industrial scale and, more worryingly, we are taking foods a long way from their original nutritional functions and values. Simple processes which do not mess with foods too much include drying, freezing, baking and canning. But nowadays when you look at the ingredients list on the side of the product you're considering buying you will see a whole range of additives. Processed food is homogenized, made all too easy to eat (smooth, sappy, not involving too much chewing) and has added sugars (in a dizzying array of forms), salt, trans fats, emulsifiers and preservatives.

DIET FADS AND FASHIONS

This rise in obesity has sustained the market for powders/pills, diet plans, bestselling diet books and global companies, all promising to reveal the secret of weight loss. It looks like we still haven't found it yet! Most people use these special diets to lose a little bit of weight but once they stop they put back on more weight than they lost originally. So they start to diet again ...

We now have lots of diet options to choose from. Almost every year, a new diet comes up and some of them are more or less the same as earlier ones.

In the 1960s, there was a popular diet called 'Sleeping Beauty'. It was literally based on you taking some sedatives in order to sleep for 20 hours. No need for me to comment further on this ridiculous idea, I hope! (Although, worryingly, this diet has reappeared in connection with anorexia websites, as a way for anorexics to control their intake.)

In 1963, the Weight Watchers organisation was founded. Starting locally, a bit like Facebook, it was initially a small group of people gathering together to discuss their dietary challenges and successes. It eventually became huge with 1.1 million members, including celebrities like Oprah Winfrey.

In the 1970s, there was the grapefruit diet that required people to eat grapefruit at every meal in the belief that it contained some special enzyme which burns fat. The main reason why people lost weight on the grapefruit diet was not that it had special enzymes, but because people consumed fewer calories.

In the 1980s, the cabbage soup diet became incredibly popular. You would eat cabbage soup for 7-10 days in a row; some people lost around 4-5 kilos. Cabbage has very few calories and almost no protein. Most of the dieters' weight loss was water and muscle mass, unfortunately.

In the 1990s, meal replacement products were a phenomenon. For example, Slim-Fast required people to replace two of their meals with SlimFast products and have one sensible third meal of their choice. People who followed this diet lost weight because they were restricted to around 1200 calories a day.

The low-fat diet was extremely popular in the 90s as well. Ironically, low-fat products often have more carbs and even more calories in them.

Then there was the 'Blood Type Diet' with its claims that eating according to your blood type would help people absorb food with better efficiency and lose weight. A study by the University of Toronto of 1455 participants disproves that and actually says it prevents people eating various essential nutrients.

Another popular diet was the Atkins Diet, promulgated by Dr Robert J. Atkins in 1972 and remaining popular in spite of controversy until his death in 2003. He claimed that if you kept to a high fat, low carb diet you would still lose weight. This went against all received wisdom about the dangers of animal fat, and studies by the *American Journal of Clinical Nutrition* disprove Atkins' theory.

Around the time of Dr Atkins' death the South Beach diet, similar to the Atkins in its emphasis on high fat, low carb foods, became popular. Criticism of the diet arose because it encouraged people to consume processed vegetable oils which we now know are not healthy.

In the 2000s, the Dukan Diet, created by Pierre Dukan in the 1970s, encouraged people to eat high protein foods and very limited amounts of carbohydrate. Due to such limited calorie consumption and tough restrictions, people, including many celebrities, lost a lot of weight following this. However, no solid evidence was found that it works or that it can be sustainable after initial weight-loss.

In the mid-2010s, juicing became popular. People who juiced rather than ate their vegetables and followed this for 7-10 days, lost lots and lots of weight. This was a no-brainer, as the number of calories consumed daily was so minimal. People who lost weight also lost some muscle mass as they couldn't consume necessary proteins when consuming vegetables in juiced form. And we know muscles are your friend when it comes to weight loss as they need energy.

The gluten-free diet of the early 2010s emerged because of increasing awareness of coeliac disease. Although avoiding gluten products didn't initially start for slimming reasons, avoiding bread, pasta and some common carbs led to it being considered as a diet. Coeliac disease is a genetic autoimmune disorder which affects people's small intestines. It occurs in 1 in 100 people. Thinking gluten-free equals weight loss was also a big mistake as gluten-free products contain as many calories as their gluten-filled equivalents.

The Paleo (Low Carb) Diet came along in the mid-2010s. It says we should eat only what our hunter-gatherer ancestors used to eat. It allows mainly fruits, vegetables, meats, seafood and nuts. It basically means giving up on modern food and in this era of highly-processed food, the attraction is clear. However, eating out is nearly impossible and after a certain period of time, deficiencies of calcium and vitamin D may start to cause problems.

In the late 2010s, the Ketogenic diet became one of the trendy diets highlighted in the media. Once again, it is a high fat, low carb diet like the Atkins diet. It limits carb intake to around 50 grams a day. Consider this: one banana or apple can contain around 20-25 grams of carbs! What people consume on this diet is mainly red meat, butter, nuts, seeds, avocados and MCT* (medium-chain triglycerides found in oils such as coconut and palm, or dairy products). The limited range of fruit and vegetables on the diet can put people at risk of vitamin and mineral deficiencies. It also leads to constipation due to lack of fibre.

*MCT – an extra note: medium-chain triglycerides are found, as mentioned, in some oils such as coconut, palm and dairy products. There are several benefits of MCT oil. According to the Alzheimer Drug Discovery Foundation in April 2006, patients with dementia might find short-term benefit using MCTs. Another study in Japan in 2009, 'Effect of Medium-chain Triacylglycerols on Moderate- and High-intensity Exercise in Recreational Athletes' suggests that MCT oil increases endurance time during HIIT exercising.

In 2018, Dr Christopher D. Gardner of Stanford University conducted a twelve-month study amongst overweight adults: half of them followed a low fat diet and the other half a low carbohydrate diet. Neither group restricted calorie intake; they just focused on avoiding high fat or high carbohydrate foods according to which group they were in. It was important that people taking part weren't hungry. The results of this study were identical for both groups. Some people lost a lot of weight no matter what diet they chose, whether it was the low carbohydrate or low fat one. Some people didn't lose any weight. The bottom line is, arguably, that if people can't lose weight with a particular diet, it's because they can't stick to it for a certain period of time and once they stop it and go back to their usual eating, they regain the weight they lost.

It all comes back to this set of basic principles: eat fruit and vegetables, base your meals on high fibre wholesome foods, consume some dairy (or dairy alternatives such as soya drinks), lower your saturated fat intake (the NHS recommends a maximum of 30g a day) and cut down on sugar as much as you can, consume high quality protein such as pulses and/or meat and fish, restrict your salt intake (max 6g a day) and drink plenty of water, plus maintain a sustainable level of activity each day.

6.4 YOUR BODY IS EQUIPPED WITH SPEED CAMERAS

Although I'd like you to take an easy approach to food and dieting, with a plan you can follow without putting a lot of effort and thought into it, I would also like you to get results. Being aware of the rough macro content of the food you consume and your overall rough daily calorie consumption is very important.

For us men, it's dead easy to consume an extra 1000-1500 calories a day but imagine doing this every Saturday and Sunday! You can be super-virtuous during the week, but end up sabotaging the good you've done because cheating over the weekend will make you gain more weight than you managed to lose during those weekdays. A full English breakfast contains around 1000 calories. Imagine you decide to treat yourself to four pints of beer and a small packet of crisps at the pub on a Saturday, (an extra 1000 calories), and a full English breakfast on your beautiful Sunday morning, (another 1000 calories over and above your quota). And you do that every week ...

You know that there are lots of speed cameras all around the country. Imagine you didn't have a speedometer in your vehicle. How on earth would you decide how fast you are travelling? Perhaps by looking at other cars and adjusting your speed accordingly while passing the speed camera so that you don't get a speeding ticket. But what if there are no other cars around as it's very early in the morning or late at night? You would be overly cautious and most likely pass the speed camera way slower than you needed, to just to be on the safe side because, remember, you haven't got a speedometer.

If the speed limit is 30 mph, would you get a ticket if you were going at 35 mph? Hell yes!

If your body burns 2200 calories a day, would you gain weight if you ate 2400 calories a day (over a period of time)? Hell yes!

How would you know how much you consume each day without counting your calories at least for a few days to get an idea of the general food/calorie/macros concept?

When people say they can't be bothered counting their calories, it's like saying they can't be bothered having a speedometer in their car. They will just guess their speed. Good luck with never getting a speeding ticket!

I totally hear you. I totally understand how inconvenient it is to measure what you eat or scan the product to work out the protein/carbohydrate/fat content on a daily basis. But unless you do this for at least a short period of time, you'll have no idea what you are consuming and how many grams of protein you have in your diet. You just won't.

Losing weight consistently is similar to this speeding concept but more so. Do you know there are speed cameras that measure average speeds, especially on some motorways? Authorities place a series of cameras on sections of motorways. The first camera registers your number plate as you pass it and the second one is positioned let's say half a mile away. Doing simple maths, speed equals distance divided by time, they know that if you arrive at the second speed camera before a certain time, you've been speeding. This monitoring carries on along the 'average speed check' section of the motorway, generally 10-15 miles long.

Why am I talking about speed cameras again? Well, have you ever driven your vehicle at the required speed along the average speed camera section at, let's say 50 mph, but between the last two cameras you did 60 mph? What happens? Yes, you're sent a speeding ticket.

Do you think the authorities would say, 'Oh no, he drove so well for ten miles staying below the maximum speed limit, so let's ignore the last section where he was speeding?' They absolutely wouldn't. Your body is exactly the same. You may be virtuous with your eating for five days but if you consume way over what you should over the weekend, I'm sorry my friend, but your body won't forgive you. Occasionally falling off the wagon doesn't do long-term harm: all it does is slow your progress, but repeatedly indulging to excess every weekend will continue to undermine your efforts and negate the progress you've made.

So, treat your body as if you are driving your car in an area full of speed cameras. Your body watches you. Be good to it and you will be rewarded with high energy, a healthy heart and organs, good strength, strong bones and happiness.

6.5 SCALES AND APPS: TRACKING YOUR WEIGHT AND THE FOOD YOU CONSUME

Before we go into more detail about the types of foods and drinks I recommend you consume or limit, you're going to find it helpful if you have some way of monitoring things. The obvious first resource is your trusty set of bathroom scales!

VISITING THE SCALES

When you're trying to lose weight, one of the most exciting or demoralising times can be when you step on the scales. Many people join slimming groups where the weekly weigh-in seems to act as an incentive to help keep them on track. But whether weighing yourself in public or alone at home, there are a number of factors to consider.

How often should you weigh yourself? What do you do when you have started your new exercise regime and healthy eating plan, you stand on the scales and horror of horrors, you have not lost a single pound? AGH!

Do you think all your hard work has been in vain? As it is clearly not working do you reach for that chocolate biscuit or do you tighten your belt and go slightly mad, restricting your eating even more, hoping to lose weight even faster?

It's at these times it is important to remain focused no matter what, as there are a number of reasons why weight loss can fluctuate.

It can depend on when your last meal was, what it consisted of, your bathroom habits, the climate you live in, how often you exercise, the speed of your metabolism and how hydrated you are. I always find it strange when you think you have had a really naughty night eating-wise and yet the next morning you stand on the scales and you have lost a pound! With any lifestyle change our body weight will fluctuate while it regulates its normal functions so you must keep this in mind when choosing your weighing-in options.

I experiment with different diets for different lengths of times. I also weigh myself at different times of the day to see how my daily life affects my weight. Let me share two bizarre experiences I've had recently.

One evening I weighed myself before I went to bed and recorded my weight and body fat percentage. I didn't eat or drink anything all night. Next morning after about seven hours' sleep, I weighed about 700g more than before and I'd gained 1% body fat, which was not a true reflection of my body's condition.

Another time, when I was trying the 5:2 diet (5 days off, 2 days at 600 calories max) I weighed myself in the morning of the 600 calorie day and during that day I consumed 600 calories. No more. Next morning, I was hoping to see some weight loss. I started to laugh when I saw a 500g weight gain!

My point is that you should not be obsessed with these numbers. As long as you are consistent with your healthy diet and losing body fat over a period of time, you are on the right track.

WEIGHING YOURSELF – WHEN IS BEST?

Daily weigh-ins: there are arguments about whether you should weigh yourself on a daily basis. Personally, I like to do this so that I am in control and can understand how my weight can fluctuate depending on my daily habits. It provides me with more data over the month rather than just four readings in a month. This of course is my personal preference. You need to discover for yourself what is the best motivator for you.

Weighing in daily makes me accountable for my actions and helps me to think more about what I am eating every day. If seeing how your weight can fluctuate on a daily basis will make you more stressed and affect your mood and behaviour, then this option is not for you. A friend of mine's wife literally had to hide the scales as her husband could not cope with his daily weight fluctuations!

One really important thing to remember, is to place the scales in the same place each day and try and weigh yourself at the same time of day.

There is no point weighing yourself more than once a day. This will not do you any good mentally and it will not reflect any kind of accuracy. Unless you are conducting experiments like me!

Weekly weigh-ins: having a mathematical brain that loves statistics and figures, a week is definitely too long for me to wait to see results. However one obvious advantage of this approach is that you do get six whole days of not focusing on your weight and standing on the scales!

Some people avoid weighing themselves on a Monday for fear of what they have let slip over the weekend but I like to see what the damage is and get back into the right headspace. Sometimes you can even be pleasantly surprised!

So ideally you should weigh yourself on the same day each week and in the morning. Consider all the factors I mentioned earlier and look on this as a long-term journey.

Occasional weigh-ins: some people absolutely hate standing on the scales and will only do so at the gym quickly or when necessary at the GP. These people tend to judge their weight loss on how their clothes are fitting instead, plus the state of their mood and energy levels and performance in their exercises. This again is down to personal preference.

You know by now that I am a daily weigh-in person but I can of course identify my own signs too without using the scales. My jeans get slightly tight around the waist if I put on a few kilos, so this is a good indicator for me too!

So there is no right or wrong in this area. You have to find what works for you and then use the scales as a positive tool to aid you in your weight monitoring.

DO WE REALLY WEIGH LESS IN THE MORNINGS?

The straight answer is 'Yes' but I will explain why this might not be true on certain occasions.

We let our bodies rest for 8 hours (on average, mine is around 6!) during the night without any food or water. Let's say you ate your dinner at 8 p.m. and went to bed at 11 p.m., slept for 8 hours, hopefully undisrupted, and woke up at 7 a.m. The food you had last night is by now more or less broken down and digested, unless it is red meat which might take longer; the water or any liquid you drank last night is gone through sweating, breathing and peeing first thing (or during the night). If you tend to move your bowels in the mornings, that's around 250 grams (half a pound) and one cup of liquid (around 250 ml) weighs about 250 grams as well. Because of all these reasons, you weigh less in the mornings.

Weigh yourself before breakfast. Make sure you are wearing the same type of clothes each time; ideally when you're in your underwear or fully naked so that the extra weight of those jeans doesn't make you feel depressed in the winter.

WHY MIGHT THIS NOT BE TRUE?

Well, if you wake up in the middle of the night and hydrate yourself or even have some munchies then you are literally replacing that lost water and this might be one reason why you don't weigh any less than the night before. An accurate way to measure yourself would be to weigh yourself on an empty stomach at the same time each day.

That weight loss in the mornings doesn't necessarily mean you are losing fat unless you were running a power station in your body during the night! The true indication of fat loss is the change in your clothing size and the change of your body composition over a period of time.

HOW TO STAY ON TRACK WITH THE MYFITNESSPAL APP

Although scales, especially fancy electronic ones, can tell you a lot, including aspects of body composition, what you're looking at here is the result of your eating and exercise habits. That's the 'after' – what about the 'before'? What about your intake? One way to get results is to track your calories and your macros (protein, carbs, fat – more about this in a minute), so I'd like to recommend you use a calorie tracker app.

There are many nutrition-tracking apps out there but the one I am going to ask you to download is MyFitnessPal, as I recommended earlier.

The app has more than 3 million food products listed in its database and it is really easy to use. Best of all, it's FREE!

Here's what to do: download the app and sign up, using your email address or your Facebook account.

When you sign in, the app asks you what your goal is. You can choose losing weight, maintaining or gaining weight. Select one of these options.

Then it asks you how active you are. Choose from 'Not Very Active', 'Lightly Active', 'Active', 'Very Active'.

Enter if you are male or female, plus your birthday and country, then click the tick icon and enter your height, either in cm or inches, followed by your weight in lbs, stones, or kg. Now you enter your goal weight. How many pounds do you want to lose per week, from the options '½', '1', '1½' and '2'? I think that 2 is generally what most people want to lose and it is healthy and sustainable. Then you enter your email and password. You can click if you want updates or not. I generally click 'No'. Click 'Next' and your account will be created. You now have your calorie intake recommendation and are ready to go. Please click the box that says 'Use my phone to track my steps'. This is a great motivation for you to be active enough to reach the 10,000 steps a day goal. Skip the next pages and the premium option.

Setting your macros: I would now like you to go to the 'more' button on the bottom right and click on goals. Under the 'nutrition goals' title, click on calorie and macronutrient goals. Now you are going to alter the percentages: Carbs 30%, Protein 40% and Fat 30%.

Return to the 'More' button and now click on 'Steps'. If you have a device like a Fitbit, Apple watch, Jawbone etc., then you click on 'Add a device' and you can link the device to the app.

There are many things you can use MyFitnessPal for but you are going to be using it for food entries so that you can monitor your macronutrient intake and total calorie intake on a weekly basis.

Home screen: the home page shows you lots of interesting stories and articles which help motivate you. You can see at the top of the page your Goal, Food, Exercise and most importantly how much of your calorie allocation for the day is left.

Diary: this is where you can add your food and liquid intake each day. In Breakfast, for example click on 'ADD FOOD' and you can search for your food at the top of the page – e.g. All Bran – then enter your size serving and number of servings and click the tick at the top of the page. This will now appear in your 'Breakfast' listing with the number of calories next to it. This is also now stored in your 'Frequent foods' and 'Recent foods' and so you can quickly add from there. The dots to the right of the entry enable you to add, entering the detail yourself, save as a meal, copy to or from a date and to share. If you want to add more than one thing at a time you can click 'Multi-add' and if you press the 'Scan' icon at the top right then you simply scan the barcode on your food and it will bring up its calorie value so that you can then enter the amount you are eating.

Now let's try a recipe for dinner: choose one of my healthy recipes from the selection in Chapter 11. In 'Dinner' click on 'ADD FOOD' and click on 'Recipes' at the top of the page; now click on 'Create a recipe'. You can manually input the ingredients in the correct amounts. This recipe will now be saved in your recipes. If you choose a recipe from the internet, you can import it. Bear in mind, you will need a basic set of kitchen scales for this, to make sure that the portion weights you input are accurate.

Note that under the 'More' button, when you start losing weight you can update your goals.

You are now ready to go and can enter everything that you eat and drink on a daily basis into this app.

6.6 YOUR DIET COMPOSITION FORMULA

OK, now that you're set to monitor your weight and food, it's time to focus on designing the right balance of the nutrients you need. If you're a man who works out, you're recommended to consume around 1.8 times your body weight (in grams) of protein. That means that if you weigh 90kg: 90 x 1.8 = 162g protein a day.

It is also recommended you should consume around 130-140 grams of carbohydrate a day to have enough energy to carry out your daily activities and exercises but not so much carbohydrate that it gets stored as fat.

Your fat target is around 0.7 times your body weight, in grams. This means 90 x 0.7 = 63g.

How do we calculate our required daily calories?

Remember:

1g protein has 4 calories

1g fat has 9 calories

1g carbohydrate has 4 calories

So, the calculations look like this:

Protein: 162g x 4 = 648 calories

Fat: 63g x 9 = 567 calories

Carbohydrate: 140g x 4 = 560 calories

Total Calories: 1775 calories

Does that make sense? This is a rough calculation, but it works as long as you are consistent with your intake. This is why when you lose weight, the number of calories you should be consuming also changes because your weight is used in the formula!

6.7 MACROS

Remember, macros are macronutrients: protein, carbohydrate and fat. Counting your macros means adjusting the ratios of these 3 components within our overall calorie-intake. Counting your macros is crucial as it helps you with weight loss, gaining lean muscle or maintaining your current form. Eating enough fat, carbohydrate and protein is essential in our lives but how much of each should you aim to eat?

Firstly, fat has more calories than either protein or carbohydrate, as we saw.

- 1g fat has 9 calories
- 1g carbohydrate has 4 calories
- 1g protein has 4 calories

I always say if you are doing strength training (weight/resistance training), you need to increase your protein intake. Why do I say that?

Because, if you get your calories from protein rather than carbs, you use that protein to repair the muscles and this will help you gain lean muscle mass which will contribute to burning more calories. But if you get those calories from carbohydrates, you will obviously burn some of them to give you energy but the rest will be stored as body fat.

6.8 PROTEIN

What is protein?

Protein is an organic compound made of amino acids that is essential in our everyday life, for the growth and repair of the body and for muscle growth. However, different protein sources are made up of different sequences of amino acids.

Reducing your calorie intake to lose weight will also reduce your lean muscle mass which is catastrophic as you are getting rid of your friends in your weight loss journey. Your lean muscle is your ally when you want to increase your BMR (basal metabolic rate) and burn more calories; you can only preserve your lean muscle mass with sufficient protein intake. Therefore, reducing your calories definitely requires a higher protein intake to compensate, if you want to do this properly.

When you think of protein in your diet the first thing that usually springs to mind is chicken, chicken and more chicken! But there really are a lot of other delicious options to help you increase your protein intake, including vegetarian options.

So how much protein should we be consuming on a daily basis?

If we don't get enough from our diet then our health and body composition suffers. As we mentioned earlier, according to most official nutrition organisations the DRI (Dietary Reference Intake) is 0.8 grams of protein per kilo of body weight or 0.36 grams per pound.

This amounts to 56 grams per day for the average sedentary man and 46 grams per day for the average sedentary woman. However, the amount of protein for any one individual depends on many factors including activity, age, muscle mass, goals and current state of health.

If your aim is to get fit, gain lean muscle and tone up, then you might need to increase your protein intake: the International Society of Sports Nutrition recommends as much as around 200 grams a day for a man (and up to 135 grams a day for a woman). This is why many people in training use protein supplements to be able to top up.

If you are not eating enough protein this might be one of the reasons why you struggle to gain that lean muscle tone.

Protein helps you keep fuller for longer. It speeds up your metabolism as it helps build lean muscle.

HERE ARE SOME HIGH PROTEIN FOOD SOURCES:

Yoghurt

Supermarket yoghurt often has many additives and sugars but natural Greek or Turkish (of course my favourite!) yoghurt can have up to almost 20 grams of protein per serving. Yoghurt makes a great snack any time and a great breakfast with berries to combine your fibre and protein. If you want to add some flavour you can add a scoop of protein powder to increase your intake further (I do this for breakfast myself). Additionally a spoonful or two on the side of a nice chilli is delicious or you can make your own cucumber, mint and yoghurt dip.

Eggs

Swapping your cereal for eggs for breakfast is another alternative: hard-boiled, soft scrambled, poached or however you like them. You can add peppers, onion and mushrooms plus herbs and spices for that extra flavour without increasing your calories. A hard-boiled egg makes a great snack with around six grams of protein in each egg.

Almonds

Nuts add a lovely texture to salads or stir-fry veggies, and are also packed with protein and antioxidants. Almonds are filling too and are full of magnesium, potassium, calcium and vitamin E. Don't overdo it though, as 10 almonds contain about 70 calories!

Cottage cheese

Cottage cheese comes in a few varieties, such as with pineapple or chives etc. It is creamy in taste and high in protein, while being low in calories and fat. Believe it or not zero-fat cottage cheese actually has more carbs and calories than normal cottage cheese so read the macro labels carefully. A portion of cottage cheese will give you around 12g of protein.

Lentils

A hot favourite with me is lentils. They are an excellent addition to soups, stews, curries and salads. There are even lentil crisps now which are delicious and help you feel like you are not missing out when people are snacking on other types of crisps. Yushoi baked lentil snacks are delicious. You can add lentils to rice and noodles and they're a staple for vegetarians. Try my flavoursome lentil and cauliflower masaman curry or my traditional Turkish lentil soup. Visit Chapter 11 for the recipes.

Peanut butter

Peanut butter is rich in protein and provides 4 grams of protein per tablespoon. The only difficulty is restricting yourself to one tablespoon! I love spreading it on celery sticks and it really is very filling.

Hummus

Chickpeas are very high in protein but you have to watch the calorie intake on this. The best way I find to eat this in moderation is by using it in a sandwich instead of mayonnaise. Make sure you spread it fairly thinly though. You can still taste the flavour even with a small amount.

Tinned fish and lean meat

Fish, lean cuts of meat and skinless white poultry are all excellent sources of protein, including yes, you've guessed it, our old favourite, chicken!

Tinned tuna is a staple for my larder and so easy to throw into a salad as it's full of flavour; I particularly like John West no-drain version. However, be mindful not to consume too much tuna because of the levels of mercury it contains. Try not to consume it every day. Now go on...try my delicious minced beef with fresh runner beans, which you will find in the Recipes section, in Chapter 11.

Quorn veggie cocktail sausages

There are many Quorn options and these are always rich in protein. My favourites that I wanted to share with you are the Quorn veggie cocktail sausages which I must admit have become a bit of an addiction of mine. Eaten as they are from the packet or chopped up and mixed with eggs they are absolutely delicious.

Frozen chicken pieces

Frozen chicken pieces are also very tasty and I add them into stews or serve them with veggie casseroles.

Tahini

Tahini, made from sesame seed paste, is also very tasty and can be used to make salad dressings instead of oil. One tablespoon has three and a half grams of protein compared to olive oil which has literally no protein. You can add lemon juice, herbs and just a tiny bit of oil.

Peas

Green peas have about 5.5 grams of protein per 100 grams. You can add them to stews and soups or even blend and make dips from them. Pea and mint soup is a delicious recipe full of protein, as is pea and mint dip. Also consider pea protein, if you are looking for a plant-based protein powder. Again there are some delicious baked pea snacks and I would recommend Yushoi.

Tofu

One hundred grams of firm tofu will give you 8.2 grams of excellent, flavourless protein. Tofu can be marinated to your taste and is delicious in soups, stews and even as a thickener in smoothies.

Quinoa

Quinoa is packed with fibre. It is one of the few plant foods that have all nine essential amino acids. It's anti-inflammatory and gluten free. I have a delicious quinoa and black bean salad that I guarantee you will love, also in the Recipes section.

Beef jerky

Jerky is a meat that has no fat, has been cut into strips and dried. It is then put into portable bags and makes a great snack when you're on the move. It contains 9 grams of protein per 28 grams. Be careful, though, as some versions are high in sugar.

Dairy

Consuming yoghurt and milk is going to give you a different type of protein compared to consuming meat or chicken or beans. Each has a different structure, once broken down and absorbed by the body. Your body then uses these proteins to repair your muscles, for muscle and cell growth, as well as providing structure to your skin, bones, hair and nails, boosting immune function and hormone production. Protein is also vital for releasing two very important hormones for our muscle growth: testosterone and growth hormone.

SHOULD I TAKE PROTEIN SUPPLEMENTS?

If you are working out to build muscle and even to get toned, you need 1.4-2g of protein per kilogram of your bodyweight per day. It can be difficult to consume that amount of protein from chicken breasts, eggs and pulses. It can be expensive and it also increases your daily calories.

Protein shakes are:

- easy to make
- relatively cheap
- give you a sufficient amount of protein per serving
- save you from the temptations of a sit-down meal

Having said that, these are supplements: protein powders are not meal replacements and you will still need nutrients from proper food.

ARE THERE ANY SIDE-EFFECTS OF PROTEIN POWDERS?

There is very little evidence to support the theory that protein powders have side-effects if used properly. High doses, however, might cause nausea, thirst, bloating, cramps and reduced appetite. If you experience constipation, increase your fibre intake. I also recommend you consult your doctor before consuming any supplements.

WHEN SHOULD YOU HAVE PROTEIN SHAKES?

The best time to consume protein shakes is after your workout so that your body gets the necessary protein and amino acids without delay and can start repairing and growing your muscle tissues effectively.

WHERE CAN YOU BUY THEM?

You can buy protein powders even from big supermarkets these days. There's also Holland and Barrett, Amazon and my favourite online store at https://www.myprotein.com.

WHAT SHOULD YOU BE MINDFUL OF?

Make sure the product you choose has high protein and low sugar/calorie content. On average 70-80% (20g + per portion) protein and around 100 calories per portion is pretty good. Also some products say 20g protein per portion but their one portion could be a 1.5 scoop of powder rather than an ordinary single scoop. So it might be a good idea to have a look at not only the amount of protein per portion but also the percentage.

If you are asking the question, 'Should I take both amino acids and protein powders', then my answer would be if you really want to achieve the best results and are aiming to tone up and build lean muscle, then yes, but always consult a doctor if you have any concerns.

6.9 AMINO ACIDS

Many people think that muscle soreness is caused by the build up of lactic acid. However, recent research by Mike T. Nelson, an exercise physiologist, has found it is caused by the small-scale trauma to the muscle fibres themselves that happens during an intense training session.

I personally believe that you can help speed up the repair to these fibres by increasing your protein intake. In the gym, we see people sipping from plastic bottles filled with protein shake.

But let me start by answering some common questions I get asked about protein and amino acids.

WHAT ARE AMINO ACIDS?

Amino acids are the building blocks of protein and are thus an essential part of all living organisms. We need amino acids in our body to build and repair. Therefore, they are essential for building lean muscle.

There are 20 different types of amino acids. 9 of them are essential and the rest non-essential. Our bodies can synthesize non-essential amino acids but we need to consume essential amino acids from external sources such as meat, eggs, lentils and so on, in order to be able to function properly, as essential amino acids cannot be synthesized: they need to come from an external source.

DO I HAVE TO TAKE AMINO ACID SUPPLEMENTS?

If you are doing strength training exercises, you are creating small-scale trauma to your muscle fibres and unless you consume an enormous amount of chicken, eggs, dairy products, pulses etc., you are virtually abusing your body and not giving it enough nutrients. It's like driving your brand new car at top speed on the motorway with no oil and expecting it to run at full capacity! The advantage of using amino acid supplements is that they contain virtually no calories.

ARE THERE ANY SIDE-EFFECTS OF AMINO ACIDS?

This is a very common question! Unless you overdose on amino acid (and recommendations will be written on the packaging), no side-effects have yet been discovered, as far as I am aware, unless you are pregnant or post-operative. There are claims that too much tyrosine can cause anxiety and restlessness. But if you follow recommended levels of intake, your body will benefit. However, I'd still like to advise you to consult your doctor before consuming any supplements.

BCAA (BRANCH-CHAINED AMINO ACIDS):

L-Leucine, L-Isoleucine and L-Valine form branch-chained amino acids, which should be supplied by our diet, as our bodies cannot produce them on their own. Dairy foods, eggs, fish, poultry and meat are good sources of BCAA. The difference between BCAA and the other amino acids is that BCAA are metabolised in the muscles rather than the liver, helping to delay fatigue during workouts as the body is less likely to use its own amino acids. That means we can use them for energy and also as the most important amino acids in the manufacture, maintenance and repair of muscle tissue.

A study called 'Exercise promotes BCAA catabolism: effects of BCAA supplementation on skeletal muscle during exercise' in 2004 suggests that consuming BCAA supplementation before and after exercise helps in decreasing exercise-induced muscle damage and promoting muscle-protein synthesis.

WHEN SHOULD I TAKE AMINO ACIDS (ESPECIALLY BCAAS)?

There are different opinions on this. Taking them before your workout reduces DOMS (Delayed Onset Muscle Soreness). Taking them afterwards will help reduce the breakdown of your muscles. Remember, when you do strength training you are breaking down your muscle tissues!

So the answer in an ideal world is to take them before and after your workout. Keep in mind, that without being part of a healthy and nutritious diet, amino acid supplements on their own will be no good.

6.10 LET FIBRE FILL YOU UP

I follow a macro-controlled eating plan which means that I carefully consider my carbohydrate, fibre, sugar, protein and fat intakes. One thing that nearly all my clients are surprised to discover is that they are not eating enough fibre in their diet. Most people in the UK eat only about 18g of fibre a day, but you should actually aim to eat at least 30g.

But what does fibre bring to our diet?

There is evidence that fibre keeps your bowels healthy and can help reduce cholesterol. It has been shown to keep your digestive system running smoothly and help reduce the risk of heart disease, diabetes and certain types of cancer such as bowel cancer. Increasing your fibre can also aid in weight loss because meals containing more fibre are digested more slowly and that can help make you feel fuller longer so you're more likely to stick to your calorie limit. If you want to increase your fibre intake you must do this gradually, otherwise you might end up with cramps and constipation. You must also make sure that you drink plenty of water. Fibre needs water to create a gel-like substance during digestion so 1 or 2 litres a day will help and also reduce cramp and constipation.

TWO TYPES OF FIBRE

Soluble: this type of fibre is broken down naturally by the natural bacteria in your bowels. Foods that contain soluble fibre include oats, barley, pulses, dry beans, fruit such as apples and citrus fruits.

Insoluble: this type of fibre passes through your body mostly unchanged but it does absorb water. Foods with insoluble fibre include fruit and vegetables with skins and pips, such as cauliflower, green beans and potatoes, nuts and wholegrain cereals such as wheat, rye and rice.

Both types of fibre are beneficial to your body and most plant foods contain a mixture of both soluble and insoluble types, so my advice is to eat a wide variety of high fibre foods.

EASY WAYS TO BOOST THE FIBRE IN YOUR SNACKS AND MEALS:

Breakfast: Add some fibre to your breakfast. Choose cereals with at least 3g of fibre per serving. All-Bran or bran flakes are good options. Instead of sugary cereals, try high fibre cereals such as wholegrain wheat cereals, muesli or porridge. You can also add a handful of fibre-rich berries. I always have frozen berries in my freezer.

This will also help you to stay feeling full longer, thus reducing the urge for an unhealthy mid-morning snack.

Change white bread to wholemeal or wholegrain options. The salt content in these might be high, so be mindful of this as an adult's daily salt allowance is 6 grams.

Delicious breakfast ideas include muesli which is typically a dry cereal made from toasted whole oats, nuts, fruit and wheat flakes. You can add some sliced fruit and yoghurt for extra interest. Or natural peanut butter on wholewheat toast, or a fruit smoothie blended with yoghurt. Swap butter for natural almond butter. Almond butter is so tasty, it is easy to consume a lot of it, so be aware of the high calorie content.

Lunch and dinner: the good news is that many of the regular places that you might go for lunch now offer high fibre options. These are generally described as 'stay fuller longer' options. I particularly like the smashed beets and veggie pot from Pret a Manger. Delicious. Vegetables are an excellent source of fibre, so try swapping some of the things on your plate for more veg. Aim for at least two portions of veg on your plate at dinner. Vegetables high in fibre are beans, broccoli, Brussels sprouts, carrots, cauliflower and green peas. Again swap white rice and pasta for wholemeal options. Implementing this simple change will actually double your fibre intake. Pulses, beans, lentils and peas are delicious and there are plenty of recipes on my website for soups, casseroles, curries and dips etc.

Snacks: try the more healthy snacks containing fibre such as fruit – fresh, canned or frozen – and pure fruit snacks. The skins on fruits are a good source of fibre. Fruits high in fibre include figs, apples, berries, prunes, pears and oranges. Snack on veg sticks such as carrot, celery or cucumber sticks or a packet of sugar snap peas. I love sugar snaps and some days I take a packet to work with me and graze!

You can also enjoy these low-calorie snacks if you feel hungry in between your meals. Air-popped, plain popcorn: homemade is best, to avoid the high fat, sugar or salt content of commercial popcorn. Try baked pea and lentil crisps instead of the other varieties. Nuts, wholemeal crackers, rye crispbreads and oatcakes are all tasty snacks too.

SAMPLE GOOD SOURCES OF FIBRE:

- wholegrain and wholemeal bread
- brown rice
- wholewheat couscous

- jacket potato with skin
- peas, beans and pulses
- porridge
- bran cereals
- nuts
- dried fruit
- fresh fruit and vegetables

6.11 CARBOHYDRATES

Clients who work with me follow my high protein and low/moderate carb healthy eating plan. Cutting back on carbohydrates can have major health benefits such as weight loss, reduced hunger, better control over insulin and blood sugar and improved energy. When you enter your food in the MyFitnessPal app we are using, you can see the macro breakdown and so keep an eye on your daily carb intake.

SO WHAT ARE TYPICAL TYPES OF CARBOHYDRATE FOODS?

- bread
- cereal
- rice
- pasta
- dairy
- beans and legumes
- starchy vegetables such as potatoes and corn
- sugary sweets

There are good carbs and bad carbs. Consuming healthy carbs on a daily basis is extremely important in order to have a healthy lifestyle and also to lose weight. You cannot lose weight if you don't have the energy to exercise. Your body needs to be fuelled correctly so that it functions properly. Although this may change depending on your sex, size and activity level, to be able to lose weight and gain lean muscle mass and tone up, you should be aiming at around 130g of carbohydrates a day.

The majority of your food should come from good carbs, especially during your weight loss programme. We are of course going to have some days for treating ourselves with some bad carbs, but not too soon. In this weight loss programme, you need to lose a considerable amount of body weight to deserve some of the bad carbs as a reward.

Once you get to your ideal weight and build lean muscle, your body will be able to deal with bad carbs much more easily, as your muscles will be burning more energy than they are burning now and your metabolism will also be faster. We will however never go back to our old habits and eat bad carbs full time again. They will be treats, that's all.

Good carbs include sweet potatoes, vegetables, whole fruits, legumes and wholegrain products.

WHAT IS WHOLEGRAIN?

Wholegrain products make use of the entire seed of a plant containing three parts: bran, germ and endosperm.

WHY IS IT IMPORTANT TO CONSUME WHOLEGRAINS?

Because wholegrain products are more nutritious. For example, if you consume white rice, you are eating processed rice; its germ and its bran have been removed, yet they are the most nutritious parts.

Wholemeal products provide many B vitamins (which help prevent infections and are important for energy levels, brain function and a healthy nervous system), some protein, minerals, and healthy fats, antioxidants and fibre.

WHAT ARE WHOLEMEAL PRODUCTS?

- brown rice
- wholegrain pasta
- wholewheat bread
- quinoa
- wild rice
- whole oats
- buckwheat
- millet
- whole rye
- wholegrain barley

WHICH CARBS ARE BAD CARBS?

Sugar: this is the worst, because it offers only empty calories and has no nutritional value whatsoever. Consuming sugar regularly reduces the capacity of your taste buds and a delicious piece of peach or an apple doesn't taste as nice. Sugar doesn't fill you up and sort out your hunger. In fact, once you've eaten sugar it isn't long before your blood-sugar levels drop and you need another hit. It's almost like a drug.

Products that contain sugar are chocolate, soft drinks, sweets, juice, sports drinks, cakes, buns, pastries, ice cream, most breakfast cereals.

Also:

- white bread, pasta, rice, crisps, potatoes, chips
- beer: liquid bread!
- fruit: the very sweet types

Having said that, I am not completely against some of these treats as long as you've achieved your goals and are limiting your intake, only having them as treats.

It all depends on your goals and deadlines. Trying to lose a stone in 5-6 weeks for a special event might require you to cut down on almost all these high-carb foods, but if your goal is maintaining a healthy diet it is only possible and enjoyable if you allow yourself that odd beer or ice cream. We are not robots!

RECOMMENDED CARBS

Here are 7 carbs I recommend you eat (not all of them in one day!)

1) **Brown rice:** this should be one of the essential foods in your diet. It contains bran and several vitamins and minerals. It may help reduce cholesterol and lower the risk of stroke, heart disease, and Type 2 diabetes.

2) **Quinoa:** considered a superfood and originally from South America, quinoa has twice as much protein as brown rice with branch-chained amino acids (essential amino acids the body cannot produce itself) which help you to build and repair lean muscle. However, although I listed it in the proteins section, I don't consider quinoa as a protein source. This fills the carbs section of my plate as the protein percentage is far lower than that of a piece of chicken.

3) **Oats:** they reduce your risk of heart disease, high blood pressure and Type 2 diabetes. I prepare my oats overnight so that they are ready and waiting in the morning and they taste delicious.

4) **Granola:** a tasty breakfast or snack option especially when mixed with some dried fruit and nuts. The number of calories in a serving of commercial granola can be quite high because of the proportion of sugar, but it has a good amount of vitamins and minerals. You can of course make your own so you have better control of your calorie intake.

5) **Barley:** a great replacement if you are bored with other types of carbs. You can even consume barley for breakfast. So it's not only for soups!

6) **Bulgur wheat:** another tasty source of carbs which has minerals and fibre. It goes very well with sun-dried tomatoes, roasted peppers, garlic and onion. I LOVE bulgur wheat.

7) **Sweet potatoes:** these are considered as a super-food. I'm not saying normal potatoes are bad for you but sweet potatoes have fewer calories, fewer carbs and less starch in them compared to normal potatoes. The GI (Glycaemic Index) of sweet potatoes is also less than that of ordinary potatoes.

THE GLYCAEMIC INDEX EXPLAINED

GI stands for the 'glycaemic index' rating system for foods containing carbohydrates in terms of how quickly they convert to glucose. The food is rated out of 100. Low GI food is below 55 and includes wholewheat, oat bran, muesli, sweet potato, beans, lentils, peas and starchy vegetables, plus certain fruits.

The GI Index is also a measure of how each food affects your blood sugar level when you eat it. For example, the more mature a piece of fruit is, the higher its GI is. That's why an overripe banana tastes so much sweeter. Sometimes you need fast energy, but the price is the drop afterwards, if you've consumed high-GI food and drink. What you want to aim for as much as possible is a steady level of energy, not the sugar-spike followed by sharp slump roller-coaster of energy.

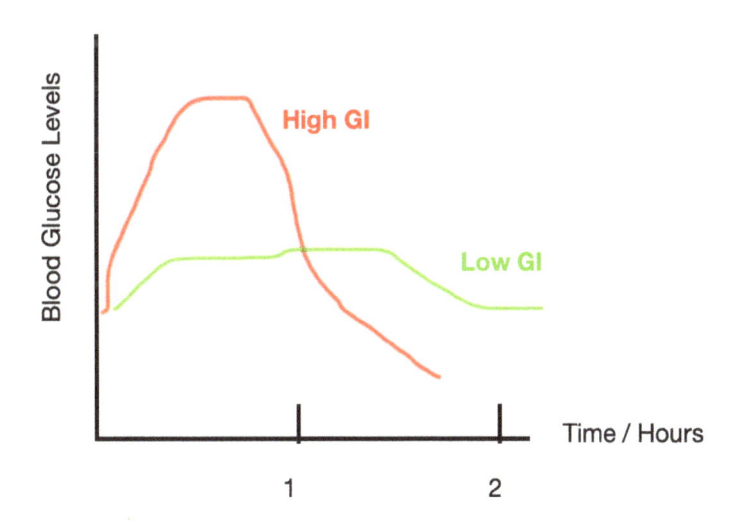

LET'S LOOK AT HOW TO CUT DOWN ON YOUR CARBOHYDRATE INTAKE

Most of your calories should come from protein, the rest from carbs and fat. In order to reduce your carbohydrate:

- ☐ Try to cook home-made more, rather than buying ready meals as you know what you put in your own recipes but you don't always know what is in your ready meals.
- ☐ Stop or reduce your bread consumption, especially white bread which is high in carbs and low in fibre.
- ☐ Try rye bread which contains about 15 grams of carbs per slice. A Warburton brand brown sandwich thin contains 19.3 grams per slice and a wholemeal pitta 29 grams per pitta.
- ☐ Swap breakfast cereals for eggs. Most of the breakfast cereals you can buy in supermarkets are very high in carbs. For example 55g of granola contains around 30 grams of carbs before you add milk. Substitute eggs when you can. They only contain 1g of carb per egg.
- ☐ Stop drinking fruit juice. In one glass of orange juice, there are about 2-4 oranges, but you're losing the fibre they contain. You wouldn't sit and eat 4 oranges in one go but it's so easy to drink a glass of orange juice and this has the effect of creating a spike in blood sugar. I know that compared to Coke, orange juice sounds virtuous but remember we are on a mission for 8 weeks and let's do our best to cut down on all unnecessary calories, while at the same time maintaining as stable a blood sugar level as possible.
- ☐ Replace cow's milk with almond or coconut milk. Cow's milk contains a type of sugar called lactose and it is fairly high in carbs. One glass of milk contains about 12-13 grams of carbs. Coconut or almond milk contain 6.5 grams of carbs. I have both cow's and coconut milk in my fridge so I can switch between them. Having said that, almond and coconut milk don't have as much protein as cow's milk. Plant milks may be fortified with calcium but don't have as much as cow's milk, so unless you have an intolerance it is worth having some cow's milk for both the protein and the calcium content.
- ☐ Choose veggies instead of potatoes. Fill your plate with extra vegetables instead of potatoes. Peppers, broccoli, greens, asparagus, cauliflower, mushrooms, courgettes, spinach, avocado, green beans, lettuce, garlic, curly kale, cucumber, Brussels sprouts, celery, tomatoes, radishes, onions, aubergines, cabbage and artichokes are all low carb. The starchy vegetables are peas, corn, potatoes, sweet potatoes, yams, parsnips, beans, carrots and squash
- ☐ Cut out sugar-sweetened drinks. Fizzy drinks are extremely unhealthy and also very high in sugar which can be linked to Type 2 diabetes. A can of Coke has as many as 40 grams of carbohydrate as it contains 10 teaspoons of sugar. Try a simple sparkling water and add a squeeze of lemon or lime or orange

if you want a tasty sugar-free fizz. I sometimes add a splash of Robinsons No Added Sugar Squash to my water.

- ☐ Use natural sweeteners instead of sugar. Honey is one option although one tablespoon represents 15 grams of carbs. Learning to enjoy the natural flavour of foods without adding any sweetener may ultimately be best.
- ☐ Stop or seriously reduce your alcohol intake. Alcohol contains an enormous amount of sugar and therefore calories. What's more, these are 'dead' calories with no nutritional value.
- ☐ Choose low-carb snacks such as nuts.

6.12 GOOD FAT AND BAD FAT

Can any fat be our friend? In this section I'd like to talk about the different types and how they can benefit or harm us, as well as where these fats can be found.

What happens if you stop consuming fat completely? Well ... you would suffer several consequences. Sounds a bit funny, doesn't it? You were probably expecting me to warn you about what happens if you eat too *much* fat, but now I'm saying the opposite: there are some risks to your health if you don't consume fats at all.

In general, the benefits of including fats in our diet are improved brain functionality, hormone regulation, and maintenance of a healthy heart. Insufficient fat causes a decrease in testosterone, which results in a low metabolic rate and decreased muscle mass, as well as depression, risk of heart disease and raised cholesterol.

TYPES OF FATS

There are two main types of fats: saturated and unsaturated.

Saturated fats: these are often referred to as bad fats. However, they benefit your immune system. They play a key role in reducing cardiovascular risks as long as we consume saturated fats in moderation. What does 'in moderation' mean? According to some studies, about 10% of our total calories, which is around 16-22g of saturated fat per day.

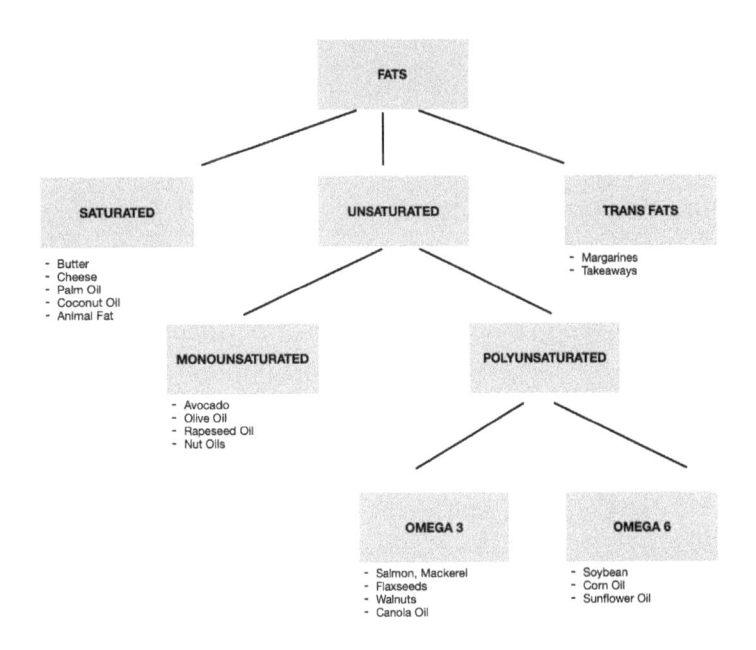

FATS
- SATURATED
  - Butter
  - Cheese
  - Palm Oil
  - Coconut Oil
  - Animal Fat
- UNSATURATED
  - MONOUNSATURATED
    - Avocado
    - Olive Oil
    - Rapeseed Oil
    - Nut Oils
  - POLYUNSATURATED
    - OMEGA 3
      - Salmon, Mackerel
      - Flaxseeds
      - Walnuts
      - Canola Oil
    - OMEGA 6
      - Soybean
      - Corn Oil
      - Sunflower Oil
- TRANS FATS
  - Margarines
  - Takeaways

Regularly consuming too much saturated fat can increase your bad cholesterol (LDL) which can clog up the arteries carrying blood around your body. This could result in heart disease and stroke.

Which foods contain saturated fats? These fats are solid at room temperature, in the form of butter, lard, palm and coconut oil. You can find them in cakes and biscuits, cheese, red meat, cured meat like salami and pepperoni, pastries, cream and chocolate.

Unsaturated fats: these are often referred to as good fats and are liquid at room temperature. They reduce bad cholesterol (LDL) and help to lessen the risk of heart disease and stroke. We split unsaturated fats into two categories: mono and polyunsaturated fats.

Monounsaturated fats help lower your bad cholesterol and also maintain the level of good cholesterol (HDL). They can be found in olive oil, rapeseed oil, avocados, and some nuts such as almonds and peanuts.

Polyunsaturated fats also lower your bad cholesterol. I promise, no more splitting these into different categories after this! There are three types of polyunsaturated fats: Omega 3, Omega 6 and trans fats. Omega 3 can be found in oily fish such as mackerel, trout, sardines, salmon and tuna. Omega 6 can be found in vegetable oil and some nuts.

However, both types of unsaturated fat contain a lot of calories. So if you consume too much, they will cause some weight gain.

Trans fat is a man-made polyunsaturated fat. It is formed by turning polyunsaturated liquid fats into solid fats using an industrial process. Trans fats are very unhealthy and are found in margarines, popcorn, fried salty snack foods, crackers, biscuits and cakes.

The bottom line is that fats have a crucial part to play in our diet and we need them. They help the body absorb Vitamin A, D and E. Without consuming enough fat, you will not be able to benefit from these vitamins either. Try to consume both saturated and unsaturated fats in moderation. If possible, replace saturated fats with unsaturated fats. Try to stay away from fast food and ready meals. Make a habit of reading the label on the food that you are buying.

6.13 ALCOHOL

A little drop or the whole bottle?

Alcohol is an important part of how we celebrate and socialise in the UK, and in moderation I suppose it is not harmful to our health or relationships. The hardest part is the judgement call. It is about knowing how much is too much and our own judgement can be variable.

Alcohol is also not a diet food: a 250 ml glass of red wine has around **170 calories** and a pint of beer around **220 calories**.

For every drink you have, you have to subtract something else from your diet or jog another mile on the treadmill; otherwise you risk weight gain and certainly won't lose if you are trying to.

Use this quick reference guide to find out how many calories are in different alcoholic drinks or MyFitnessPal, the app we referred to earlier.

https://www.nhs.uk/live-well/alcohol-support/calculating-alcohol-units/

6.14 SECRET SABOTEURS

You won't believe how quickly these secret calories add up and send your daily allowance over the limit! For example:

- one shortbread biscuit with your tea (105 calories)
- one piece of toast with butter (190 cals)
- a whole avocado instead of half (extra 120 cals)
- 2 tablespoons of olive oil (240 cals)
- 40g Cheddar cheese (166 cals)
- 30g mixed nuts (193 cals)

It is so easy to mindlessly snack or 'graze' on and off all day, racking up those calories. It might take a mere couple of minutes to eat two shortbread biscuits, or five seconds to add a splash of olive oil to a salad. But what you need to bear in mind is how dense in calories easily-consumed snacks can be. We have a habit of sidelining this sort of consumption, focusing instead on the calorie-count for our main meals. But beware! Be on your guard against those sneaky saboteurs!

6.15 TEMPTATIONS

Here's a list of the ways in which I try to avoid food temptations. I don't use all of these tactics in one go, but I mix and match according to the situation I am in.

- I drink a large cup of water. Thirst is often confused with hunger or food cravings
- I avoid getting extremely hungry in the first place
- I acknowledge that this is my choice rather than a sacrifice
- I stop and ask myself why I am craving this particular food and try to remind myself what I have already eaten that day
- I remind myself how good I felt when I resisted last time and how I don't want to disappoint myself
- I use a 'postponing tactic'! I say to myself, 'Yes, I want to eat this piece of cake but I will have it later' (e.g. 2 hours later) and then I almost always forget about it
- I visualise the saturated fat and unnecessary sugar I will ingest from that cookie floating in my system, visiting my stomach and heart
- I also visualise myself on holiday by the beach with a physique that I am happy with and how eating this temptation will divert me from achieving that look.

6.16 FASTING

We've been talking about the composition of your diet, but we also need to address a concept that you've probably noticed over the past few years, through popular books and TV programmes advocating types of fasting diets. I'd like to discuss a couple of the main ways to introduce fasting into your life, but I want to stress that this approach is something to consider carefully and with full awareness of what it entails. The very word 'fast' feels a little extreme, doesn't it? It feels all about denial and about somehow punishing your body by not giving it food. That is certainly how fasting has been used in past centuries, for religious reasons, for example. What matters here is to look at two recent types of fasting practice which are not about total denial but about a strategic approach to how much you eat and when you eat it.

The 5:2 diet: this is popular because it's easy to follow and it doesn't seem too taxing. You eat normally for 5 days a week and restrict your calorie intake to 600 calories on each of two non-consecutive days. This allows you to bring down your overall calorie intake for the week without feeling as if you're punishing yourself. Given that an overly-strict diet can lead to a rebound effect and binge-eating, you can see why this appeals.

The 16:8 diet takes place on all 7 days of the week. This time you focus on creating a window of time during the day when you're not eating. The theory is that this gives your body time to rest from digestion, burn calories and concentrate on repair and cleaning up of damaged cells (known as autophagy). You would fast for 16 hours although water, tea and coffee are allowed. Then your day's eating takes place during the remaining 8 hours. The temptation might be to cram a load of main meals and snacking into those hours but this is not likely to create a calorie deficit. What is helpful here is to work out where to place your eating window. For instance –

and most of my clients following this type of fast do this – you could eat after midday and until 8 p.m. Or you could eat your first meal at 8 a.m. and your last at 4 p.m. You adapt this to fit your personal lifestyle.

Total fasting is, as I mentioned, what we normally understand by the word 'fast'. I occasionally fast for 24 or even 36 hours, but I'm not going to suggest that you try this right now as it can be complicated and, as I just mentioned, if you're not used to this approach, you might well overeat afterwards, which doesn't exactly help you achieve your aim!

6.17 EATING BEFORE AND AFTER YOUR WORKOUT

My clients ask me what they should eat before a workout, so if you are also wondering, here are my tips. The first question is, how long before a workout? Because my answer is going to be completely different depending on how much time you have before your workout starts.

The first principle is not to exercise on a full stomach. If you have 2-3 hours before your workout, then you need to be eating low GI carbohydrates. This will help your blood sugar rise and fall, slowly, not in a sudden spike but in a way that sustains your energy level throughout your workout.

The next question may be 'What should I be eating after a workout?'

It's very important to give your body the nutrients it needs when you complete your workout. During your workout, your body uses its glycogen stores and now is the time to nourish your body with sufficient amounts of carbs and protein.

It also depends on the type of activity you were engaged in. If you went for a run or cycled (more cardio-based) then you would need more carbohydrate than protein. However, if you did some weight/resistance training then you would need more protein.

It again depends on the time of your workout. I'm not going to say eat two pieces of chicken breast if your workout was at 6.30am! So here are my favourite post-workout meals:

- a piece of protein (e.g. chicken breast, tuna, prawns, salmon or even steak – around 200g) with some complex carbs (brown rice, sweet potatoes, wholemeal pasta)
- scrambled eggs with half an avocado and a slice of brown seeded bread
- smoked salmon with half an avocado and corn on the cob
- cottage cheese and fruit
- protein shake with a piece of fruit
- bran cereal and skimmed milk (if it is a cardio session)

PART FOUR

CHAPTER 7:
GET READY TO GET FIT (3): EXERCISE SAFELY

You're about to embark on a journey of transformation as you start the 8-week Get Fit, Stay Fit programme. In this section we're going to pause to consider how best to ensure you stay safe while you exercise.

Remember, I strongly recommend that you should consult a doctor before you embark on this programme.

7.1   TAKE THE LONG VIEW

We all train for different reasons, from wanting to keep fit, to losing weight, toning up, improving our general feeling of wellbeing or for specific targets such as performing better in our careers or private lives, getting married or simply to look good for ourselves or our partners.

One thing to keep you motivated during the weeks ahead is to remember that your training, discipline, knowledge and commitment to your health is providing you with even longer term benefits. By continuously incorporating strong self-care habits into your everyday routine, you'll find it is easier to deal with and manage the things that life throws at you, things that may not be in your control.

So in reality you are also training for the complexities of life itself.

Do you see yourself having a fit and healthy lifestyle over the next six months to a year? Are you arming yourself or equipping yourself with some healthy long-term lifestyle habits or are you only aiming for a short term special event and you will let it all slip after that?

Your training equips you better to help others and helps you make decisions to the best of your ability.

With this in mind, enjoy every step of your journey and know that even when those last ten burpees are pushing you to your max, they will benefit you in so many other ways!

7.2 LET'S START WITH A TOUR

As you'll be putting your muscles to work in the workouts and weight training sequences, it does really help to know a little about the muscles and muscle groups and how they work.

We have three main types of muscle in our bodies: skeletal, cardiac and smooth muscles. What I am focusing on in this section are the skeletal muscles. They are the voluntary muscles which are attached to our bones. When we squeeze a muscle or group of muscles, we contract them, which means that they get shorter and pull on the bone. Although we do need to perform some movements that require pushing, such as press-ups or pushing a door open, muscles in fact cannot push: they can only pull. So the way the action works is this: the opposite (antagonist) muscle contracts to carry out the push movement. To be able to push a door open, you need your triceps muscle to contract, thus extending your arm.

So, the antagonist muscles are those performing opposing movements. For example, the biceps and triceps; pectoralis major (chest muscles – the 'pecs'); latissimus dorsi (the 'lats' – the back muscles); abductor and adductor muscles. The main muscles performing pulling actions are the back (latissimus dorsi), biceps and hamstrings and the ones performing the push action are the chest (pectoralis major), shoulders (the deltoids), triceps and quadriceps.

Your gluteus muscles (glutes) are the muscles in your buttocks responsible for moving your thighs and hips.

Abdominals (abs) are your stomach muscles. When you gain definition of these through exercise you're likely to refer to your abs as your six-pack. Some people imagine they don't have any abdominal muscles because they're not visible, but you wouldn't even be able to get off the sofa if you didn't have them! Reducing your padding round the middle, the fatty tissue above your abs, also helps them become visible.

7.3 WHERE ARE YOU GOING TO EXERCISE?

The most obvious answer to this question, especially if you are feeling cautious, might be 'at home'. You could be thinking of setting up gym equipment in your garage or spare room. Certainly there are advantages to working out at home: it's a familiar, low-cost environment. In the programme that follows there are workouts with certain types of exercise that you can perform at home. However, my advice is to choose a gym. It's unlikely that you would be able to incorporate the range of machines I'll be recommending in your own home, which would affect how effectively you can follow the weight-training programme. To be able to hit those muscles from different angles, you'll need to be able to use weights, cable machines, barbells, dumbbells and adjustable benches. On certain days in the 8 week programme, you can do the workouts at home as some don't need any equipment; there will be full descriptions in Chapter 11's Resources section. But to benefit properly from the entire programme I've designed for you, you also need to have access to a gym.

WHICH GYM?

First, you need to choose the right gym, so here are some questions you might like to ask:

- Which gyms are close by or accessible? If you have to take three buses just to get there, it's unlikely you'll persevere.
- Is it more useful to have the gym close to work than home? If it's near work then you could fit in exercise before you start work or at lunchtime or immediately after work. However, you might like to come home after work and go out to the gym later.
- Are the opening times convenient?
- Can you have a trial of its services? How impressed are you with the facilities and the level of cleanliness?
- What kind of fees does it charge? Is this on a contract-only basis or a rolling or per visit charge?
- Does it offer any special rates or deals?
- Does it have extra facilities attached, such as a swimming pool?
- Will there be trainers there to ensure you exercise safely?

Of course, you might already be a member of a gym or have an idea in your mind. Ask your colleagues, friends or Uncle Google!

Personally, I like to use different gyms on different days. I have a membership type that allows me to visit different branches of my gym. Although they all have similar machines and equipment, I find changing the location keeps it more interesting so I don't feel I'm at the same old gym every time. You might be more comfortable with the same location: it is a personal choice. Whatever you choose, I think going to a gym is great, taking you away from your home fridge and all its temptations. Repeated visits help you to train your mind as well as your body so that when you arrive, you are getting down to business, taking the health of your body seriously and taking consistent action.

7.4 WHY A GYM IS A GREAT LOCATION

I often come across clients who are over 40, who haven't exercised for the last decade and yet think, as soon as they start, that they are still in their 20s. It's human nature and understandable. As soon as you pick up a ball or a set of dumbbells, time winds back for you and you think nothing has significantly changed in the past 10 years. Reality is, unfortunately, different; remember what we discussed in the earlier sections. You are now probably heavier than you were, your core is weaker and you have less muscle mass.

I strongly advise you not to over-exert yourself in the beginning. Take it steady and don't become daunted if it's hard at first.

What really helps is to follow instructions to the letter. This is another reason that training at a gym is so useful: the gym instructors are there to help and guide you. So don't be frightened to ask a trainer to take you through the sequence, making sure you do the exercises safely by being in the right positions for each.

Some people may feel daunted by the gym environment if they are unfamiliar with it. This is also perfectly natural. It can be unnerving, especially around the free-weights area, to see men lifting heavy weights with ease and looking as if they know exactly what they're doing. You may, by comparison, feel your confidence has deserted you and you're sticking out like a sore thumb. Here's a secret: I feel the same occasionally when I arrive at a gym to do my workouts. Even though I hold several bodybuilding medals, I still feel the same.

You may feel uncomfortable with the notion of being seen exercising in public. You may fear being judged by others. I get it. But once you allow yourself the time to get to know the machines, interact with the instructors and make potential friends with other people attending the gym (most of whom have experienced those initial feelings of unease), you'll be surprised how quickly you settle in.

The secret is to get down to it. Once you've begun the uncertain feeling starts to evaporate. We all feel strange when entering a new environment but humans are infinitely adaptable and we soon accustom ourselves to that environment. The machines will stop feeling like mysteries and more like tools or friends. Keep the focus on getting your workout started and don't let anything stand in your way.

7.5 TYPES OF GYM EQUIPMENT

When you visit a gym, there will be a range of equipment available to you and you'll quickly become familiar with it all. There are two main categories I'd like to introduce you to: strength training equipment and cardio equipment.

CARDIO EQUIPMENT:

Many of you will already know or have used these machines. With their focus on heart-health and stamina, they include treadmills for running or walking, cross-trainers, stationary bicycles and rowing machines.

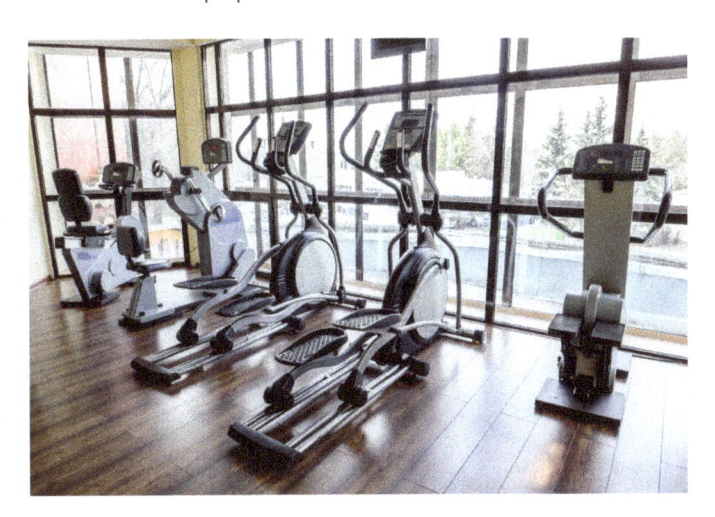

STRENGTH TRAINING EQUIPMENT:

These machines, of course, are designed to help you develop your strength. They fall into 3 main types:

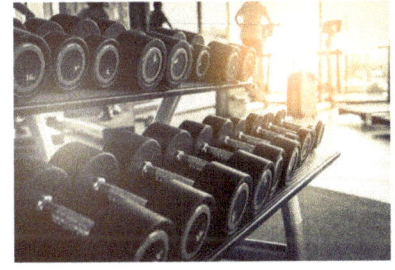

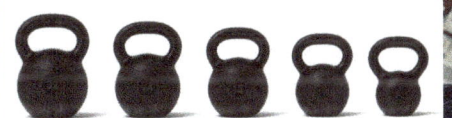

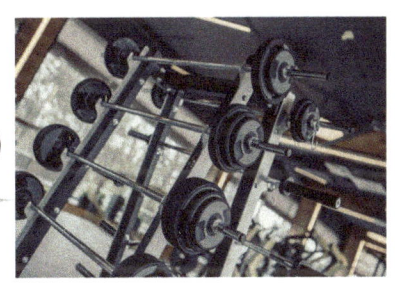

1) Free Weights: dumbbells, barbells and kettlebells. Some dumbbells and barbells are at pre-set weights or they may be single bars you load with selected weights, securing them with a clip.

2) Machines: extremely solid, stationary pieces of fitness equipment. These can be subdivided into two categories.

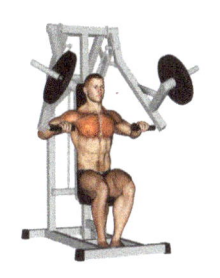

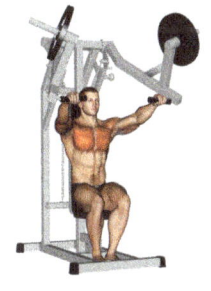

(a) Plate-loaded machines: these have no weights already loaded on them. You simply add the plate weights before using them.

GET FIT, STAY FIT | 115

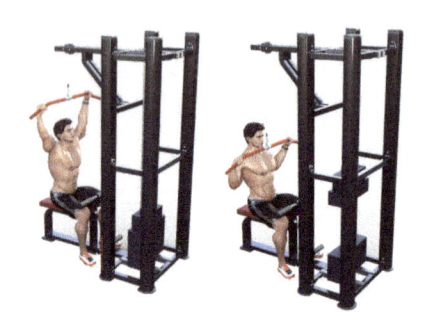

(b) Pin-adjustable plate-loaded machines. Similar to the plate-loaded machines, these are loaded with the weights and all you need to do is move the pin to set the weight*. These are generally limited in terms of weight capacity but are still very useful pieces of equipment.

*Setting the weight means choosing the weight for the exercises. It's important to choose the weight correctly. For instance, if the workout plan says 3 sets of 12 repetitions, you need to choose the weight at a level where you can perform 12 repetitions and 3 sets. If you could easily do another 2-3 repetitions, that means the weight you chose was light; if you feel you can't do more than 9-10 repetitions, it means that the weight you chose was too heavy. So set a weight appropriate for your ability to perform the repetitions and sets.

(c) Multiple-use cable machines: these are some of my favourites. You can easily adjust the weight with the pin, attach different handles with a carabiner, change the height of the handles – all this helps with using different angles for the specific exercise in question. Some of the most common handle types are small bar, V-bar, V-handle rotating bar, rope, single handle and resistance-band handle grips.

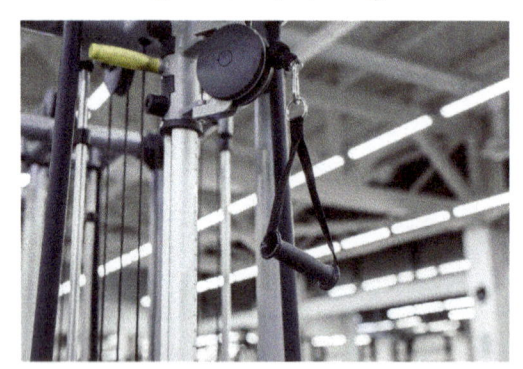

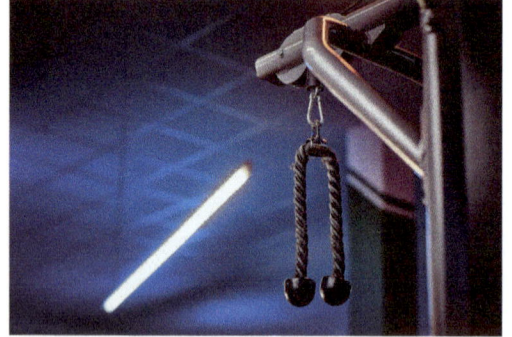

7.6 CARDIO OR WEIGHTS?

My clients ask me what they should start with when they go to the gym for their own workouts. Should they start with running on the treadmill, or use the exercise bike or start with weights and strength training first?

And I always have the same answer!

It all depends on your goal.

1) If you want to bulk up, get big and put on muscle mass, then you need to start with strength training so that you use your maximum energy in your weight session. Then whatever is left is spent on your cardio workout. (As long as they are on the same

day; sometimes you separate these workouts into different days, depending on your programme and goals).

2) If you want to tone up, gain lean muscle and lose some fat tissue, then start with cardio. However, on some days, especially leg days, it would be good to change this order by starting with weight training. Ideally you start with your cardio workout and burn as many calories as possible while you have the energy and then carry on with some weights to add a strength training element afterwards. Again this depends on your workout programme. If I wrote a high intensity, high reps with minimal rest period workout plan for you, then it would be perfectly fine to start with your weight training as your heart rate would be almost as high as during your cardio workout.

7.7 HOW AND WHEN DO YOU GAIN MUSCLE MASS?

If you have ever pumped iron (sounds a bit macho!), you must know that it makes you feel good whether you are male or female. It's a great feeling when your chest and biceps expand or you start to feel those gluteus and abs muscles burning after a workout.

Studies show that to be able to feel the difference in your physique and muscle tone, you need to carry on with your routine for at least 4-6 weeks. You will increase the blood flow in your muscles with your resistance training workout. If you feel pumped up and even feel jelly-like after training, then feed yourself with some good quality protein and carbs every day and have plenty of rest time. So what happens next? Yes, you start seeing some changes in your body. If your carbohydrate intake is not more than you are able to burn, and you have enough protein in your diet, you will really see that muscle tone develop and feel over the moon about it.

The muscles you just worked out will actually grow during your repair and rest time. Yes, you read it correctly. While you are resting, sleeping, watching TV or at your desk working, your body uses the nutrients you've given it and starts repairing those torn muscle tissues, burns the fat tissues and makes you ready for your next workout. Imagine you have a team of shift workers helping your body change! One shift helps you work out, forces your muscles to work hard and uses the energy to improve your fitness level. The next shift waits until you give them nutrients and rest so that they can then start repairing you.

What happens if you tire out those shift workers and don't feed them enough? They go on strike and you gain almost nothing after that workout. One of the most common mistakes people make is just focusing on their workouts and repetitions, not their rest periods, both in between sets and in between workouts. Resting a muscle group that is being trained is equally important in order to gain that lean muscle mass. The second mistake is not to have enough of the necessary macronutrients in your diary, thinking that doing the strength training will be enough on its own to change your body composition.

Bottom line: work hard during your workouts, follow a good quality diet, rest and repeat!

7.8 WHEN IS IT BEST TO EXERCISE?

This is the million dollar question! Unless you are an Olympic-level athlete, the simple answer is whenever it suits you.

For example, some studies say doing cardio early morning on an empty stomach will use all your glycogen stores within the first 15-20 minutes and then you will start burning fat, which is what most of us want.

However, if you are doing weight training on an empty stomach in the morning, your performance might be low as you haven't got sufficient fuel, in the form of protein and carbohydrate, in your body.

This is highlighted by two studies. First, the *British Journal of Nutrition* found when they studied a group of men exercising on an empty stomach that skipping breakfast after an overnight fast resulted in 20% more fat burn. This is so significant you might wonder why not everyone chooses to exercise after fasting overnight! However, another study carried out by Canada's McMaster University found exactly the opposite: no difference in fat loss, whether people were fasting or fed. Similar results were found by *The Journal of the International Society of Sports Nutrition*.

Some people perform so much better if they train in the late evening. Some find it more useful to go for a run mid-afternoon; they clear their minds and come back refreshed enough to work for another 3-4 hours.

THE ADVANTAGES OF WORKING OUT IN THE MORNINGS ARE:

- Your body's testosterone level is high
- Testosterone increases protein synthesis
- Protein is needed to repair damaged muscle fibre in weight training
- Exercising helps you elevate your mood, so working out in the mornings will help you enjoy a better mood throughout the day
- You've got your session out of the way and there's no need to worry about trying to find time during the day or evening

THE ADVANTAGES OF WORKING OUT IN THE AFTERNOONS ARE:

- You have consumed at least one or two meals already which helps with your performance.
- Mentally it could be a break from a stressful work environment

THE ADVANTAGES OF WORKING OUT IN THE EVENINGS ARE:

- It's less likely you will rush your workout
- You get rid of the stress of the day

However, in the evenings, your body starts producing a hormone called melatonin which prepares you for sleep. Having a hardcore session might affect your ability to wind down and have a good night's rest. Having said that, I do know a number of people who prefer an evening workout and sleep like a baby afterwards!

So as you can see, the bottom line is, it really depends on the person. I would say if you have an opportunity, try to pick different times of the day during the week and experiment with which works best for you.

7.9 HOW OFTEN SHOULD I EXERCISE?

I often get asked this and the answer is that it depends on the activities you choose and how intense they are. You may have seen on social media that many online fitness packages claim you can be super fit with no effort, spending only 5 minutes a day on workouts, while you go on eating everything you want. I'm afraid I strongly disagree! If you currently have an unhealthy lifestyle, getting fit and healthy may not prove to be effortless. To get the best out of this book and programme you need to be willing to make real changes in your life.

If you're keen to have clear guidance, my own example, and real life success stories of how I helped many people to achieve transformation, and if you are ready to take action, then please go ahead, read more...

A 5 days a week moderate intensity workout would be ideal. If you are doing strength training workouts with a high volume of repetitions for each muscle group, you definitely need to rest that particular muscle group afterwards.

For example, if you have a split weight training programme and you do a leg workout, you need to rest your leg muscles for 48 hours afterwards and for small muscles such as those in your arms, rest is needed for 24 hours at least. Otherwise, you do more harm than good.

However, if you are doing moderate intensity cardio workouts, you could do them on 5 consecutive days.

7.10 THE IMPORTANCE OF POSTURE

The key thing is posture awareness, knowing your limits and increasing the intensity gradually. You need to warm up for longer and you should also make sure you stretch when you finish your workouts.

One crucial aspect of posture is the technique of engaging your core. This means that you tighten your stomach muscles and pull your belly button in when doing certain exercises. If you are doing exercises, tightening your core often requires tilting your pelvis to engage those core muscles. If you're not familiar with the technique, ask for guidance from the gym instructor and practise until you feel in control. Soon you'll be able to activate those core muscles at will. Your main reason for learning how to engage your core is to help reduce strain on your lower back and protect it from injury. You'll also find you're 'holding' yourself better: your posture is better.

7.11 WHY YOU SHOULD MONITOR YOUR HEART RATE

I'm a numbers man. I love statistics, graphs, and results in numbers. Personally it motivates me to see that I've covered 100 metres more on an exercise bike than I did last week in the same amount of time.

Before we start, let me tell you what a heart rate (HR) monitor is: it's a device that you wear (on your chest with a strap or on your wrist) that instantly tracks your heart's beats per minute. So when you start moving faster, the number goes up simultaneously. The trick is how quick your HR comes back to normal when you stop/rest. This is one true indication of how fit you are.

WHY SHOULD YOU WEAR ONE?

All modern cardio machines and workout apps are compatible with heart rate monitors these days. For example, if you are running on a treadmill it tells you how many calories you burned at the end of the workout (and during it as well).The more data you put in the machine, e.g. your age, sex, weight, the more accurate your result will be as the machine is going to take this data into account to estimate your calories burned. Now we're talking! When the cardio machine or your workout app (as, for example when you are running outdoors or doing a weights session at the gym) knows your heart rate, it will adjust and perfect the calculation of how many calories you are burning during the exercise.

Accurate results/stats from your workouts mean accurate results for your goals.

I think you might now have two questions in your mind: 'What should my HR be during the workouts and which HR monitor should I get?'

Now what might happen is if you're like me, you'll never want to workout without a HR monitor again as once you wear it you'll be thinking that the exercises you do without one don't really count!

CALCULATING YOUR OWN RESTING AND MAXIMUM HEART RATE

What should your heart rate be during your workouts? How do you calculate your own resting and maximum heart rate? What are the benefits of working different heart rate zones?

As I just mentioned, your heart rate is the number of times your heart beats per minute (your BPM).

Your Resting Heart Rate (RHR) is the number of times your heart beats per minute at rest; sitting or lying down, for instance. It is a very good indicator of your fitness level, as the fitter you are the lower your heart rate will be. It should be somewhere between 60-100. As a guideline, a fit athlete's RHR is around 40-60 bpm.

How can you calculate your maximum heart rate (MHR)? Let's do a bit of maths (my favourite subject!) To be able to calculate your MHR, you need to find out what your RHR is. The easiest thing to do is to wear a heart rate monitor. Alternatively, you could place two of your fingers (not your thumb) on your wrist and count the beats for 15 seconds and multiply the answer by 4. Everyone's MHR can be different; even if you are the same age as someone else your RHR might be different.

Here is the formula: (MHR=220 minus your age). For instance, a 55-year-old man would have a MHR of 165. However, to be able to calculate 70%, 80%, 90% of your MHR for different training zones, you need to include your RHR in the equation. To find out 80% of your MHR: ((220-your age-RHR) x 0.8) + RHR. If you want to find out 70% of your MHR, you need to change the variable 0.8 to 0.7. So, for a 55-year-old man with a resting heart rate of 60, 80% of MHR would be (220-55-60) x 0.8 + 60 = 144 BPM.

WHAT SHOULD YOUR HEART RATE BE DURING YOUR WORKOUT?

I will say my favourite thing here ... it depends!! The most beneficial thing would be to vary your heart rate zones during your workouts.

Zone 1: 50-60% of your MHR. This is a very easy zone. It's so easy that you feel like you are not doing much and almost feel guilty! E.g. going for a casual walk: this could be dog-walking, as long as you are not running after your dog.

Zone 2: 60-70% of your MHR. This is a very low-key workout which you would have during walking or a warm up and cool down. It is beneficial for a recovery training which could be a day after you did a really hardcore workout. You can maintain a steady workout for a long time in this zone and you will see the benefits if done regularly.

Zone 3: 70-80% of your MHR. This is your fat burn zone as your body uses approximately 85% fat, 10% carbohydrates and 5% protein. If you want to benefit from this zone, you need to stay in the range between 10-40 mins. The benefit of working in this zone is your body will be able to carry more oxygen to your muscles and get rid of more waste products.

Zone 4: 80-90% of your MHR. This is the anaerobic zone which is just before you exhaust yourself. It is good for improving your athletic performance but not for fat burn. (In contrast, 'aerobic' means requiring the presence of air: at the aerobic level, you are at 70-85% of your maximum heart rate.)

Strange, isn't it? You would have thought, the more effort you put in, the more calories you burn, which results in more fat burn… Well, not on this occasion, my friend! Yes, you do burn more calories, but not from fat. This zone burns your carbohydrates and the glucose in your bloodstream. Anaerobic means 'without oxygen', usually when you're functioning at 85% of your maximum heart rate. So it is the zone where lactic acid, a by-product of muscle activity, accumulates in your muscles as you feel that burn. You hear your breathing very noticeably in this zone and you would be capable of uttering single words at a time during long runs. I personally like to come up to this zone for a short period of time (max up to 10 mins total) or as part of my interval training (HIIT) and I wouldn't advise working this hard for a long period of time every single day unless you are on a specific training regime and are accompanied by a professional fitness coach. This zone helps you increase the amount of oxygen you can consume (VO2 Max, the optimum rate at which you use oxygen during exercise). In it, you burn approximately 85% carbohydrate, 15% fat and a tiny amount of protein. The lactic acid resistance also increases in this zone.

Zone 5: 90-100% of your MHR. This is the zone where you're too out of breath to speak and should be used in your interval trainings only. If you've just started your training regime, you should not be in this zone.

7.12 WHY SHOULD YOU USE A WORKOUT APP?

I mentioned earlier that I am a numbers man, so I like statistics and charts.

Using a workout app and linking it with a heart rate monitor will keep track of all your different workouts, times, the number of calories you've burned, what your max and average heart rates were and so on. It is like a detailed profit and loss sheet but this is for your activities and workout!

Would you run a business without knowing how much money you're making, who your maximum paying client is, what your average monthly income and expenditure breakdowns are? You need all this to gauge how your business is performing and where it may be in trouble. That is why I encourage you to use a workout app for your activities, to gauge your body's performance.

One of my favourites for this purpose is the MapMyFitness App (currently owned by Under Armour).

The reasons I like this workout app are:

- you can choose your workout from many many options
- it shows your average and max heart rate during your workout
- there is a heart rate zone showing you which zone you are currently in
- you can control your music during your workout without leaving the app
- you can link your calorie tracker (MyFitnessPal) and also your sleep tracker app so that you can monitor them all in one app
- you can create online challenges and invite friends

When you get used to using a workout app, after a while you might be like me, thinking if you don't use a workout app, it feels like you haven't done that workout as it hasn't been recorded!

7.13 BEFORE AND AFTER: THE IMPORTANCE OF WARMING UP AND COOLING DOWN

Whether you're experienced or not, you probably know already that it's not a great idea to plunge into an exercise session without giving your body good warning beforehand! If you take your muscles by surprise like that, you're likely to get injured, so you need to get into the habit of warming up prior to the main exercise session and also cooling down by doing stretches afterwards, to stop things seizing up.

Some warm-ups might consist of dynamic stretching, especially if you are going to engage in cardio exercise such as running.

For strength training gym workouts, I warm up my muscles with light weights in a combination of exercises. For example, if I am working my upper body, then my warm-up routine would be a few sets of press-ups, resistance band or cable rowing, dumbbell shoulder presses and dumbbell biceps curls. Similarly, if I am doing a lower body workout, then I warm up with some hamstring and quads stretches, followed by some lunges and squats.

A HIIT (high intensity interval training) session would entail a few minutes of skipping, then some press-ups, butt kicks, arm rotations, steps up and down, lunges and light dumbbell shoulder-presses.

There is no strict rule for a warm-up, just as long as you don't over-exert yourself by starting a fast workout. The purpose of a warm-up is to get your muscles used to the range of movement and encourage your joints to secrete synovial fluid which lubricates the joint and reduces wear and tear.

Once your session is over, do some stretching to gently wind down from the intensity of what you've just done. In Chapter 9 I include 5 useful stretches you should be doing every day. Your joints and muscles will thank you for it!

7.14 THOMAS BECOMES AN ADDICT

Thomas is a 52-year-old married man from Dulwich, with three grown-up kids. He works in insurance in the city of London, so that involves quite a lot of foreign travel, plus his days are varied, with lots of client entertaining. He has been training with me since 2011 after his wife actually signed him up with me.

Back in his schooldays, he played lots of sport, swam in the swimming team three or four times a week, and was in the rugby, football and cricket teams. So sport was a big part of his life then.

Once he started working, all that structure fell away. He tried to play rugby for a club in London for while but didn't really pursue it.

Until he started training with me, he'd fallen into a cycle of joining a gym, being really keen for six months or a year, going three times a week, getting really fit, losing lots of weight ... and then something would happen: he'd get out of sync and he'd pile the weight back on. And when it comes to weight control, yo-yoing is never a good thing.

Just before he started training with me, he was going through a period of not exercising much, so his core and strength had deteriorated. His back and neck were hurting.

Back then a typical week for him involved long days, five days a week, travelling a bit, two nights out with clients and two or three business lunches a week. It was busy, full on and tough. The funny thing is, he is *still* a very busy man! What has changed is that now he gets up very early and comes to see me as opposed to getting up very early to go to the office. He's now making time for himself which still means he is tired at the end of the day but a better kind of tired than when he was going straight to the office at 7 a.m.

There are a number of factors to explain why he's now getting results. He says he used to hate seeing himself in family photos looking overweight and with lots of chins on show. He also knew that he wasn't working efficiently. And generally he was feeling tired all the time, whether at work or at home.

Now he feels fit, he works better, his concentration is much stronger. He has better ideas and home-life is better too. He asks why anyone wouldn't want to feel better and take steps to bring it about.

He tells me there's a massive difference between traditional personal training and my elite concierge personal training service. Constant communication is important for him because having someone at his shoulder nagging him daily makes him feel responsible for his actions. When I ask him 'Did you do your home workout on my fitness app?' or 'Did you do the run this morning?', it makes him feel guilty if he hasn't, but in a good way. I give him the nudge: he goes and takes action. Even when he doesn't see me on the days he is busy or travelling, our constant communication encourages him to do things that he normally wouldn't do: stay in it for the long haul, being committed and active.

He is also aware that he has the kind of metabolism that means he is liable to put on weight if he is not active and not watching his diet, so he needs to compensate for that. He basically wants to be in the world for as long as he can, by remaining healthy. There is only one way to do that: eat well, not drink too much and exercise. He gets a buzz from the exercising and he now finds it addictive, in a good way.

Now, you're reading this book. You're not in a gym or a park with me and you're not hearing me nag you in the ear. (Although you can, if you want to sign up for some personal training some time!) So why am I talking about Thomas at all? Because I am so proud of what he has achieved: he has shown the kind of lasting commitment that brings real results and that's what I want from you and *for* you. When you're reading this book, remember Thomas. See this book as your personal trainer. Imagine I am calling you to check up on you. Ask a friend or family member to do the same for you. Stop the yo-yoing and the slip-sliding in and out of good habits. Start living them.

CHAPTER 8: YOUR 8 WEEK GET FIT PROGRAMME

8.1 INTRODUCTION

Welcome to the core 8 week programme, which I have designed to take you on your journey to fitness. Every stage, every day of the programme, contains carefully tailored exercise routines, where each component is designed to work cumulatively and in a complementary manner, making sure that strength, tone and flexibility are achieved. Simply take it day by day and on that final day, you are going to be so proud of yourself. In fact, I suggest you take a photo of yourself on Day 1, then at the start of each week of the programme, rounding it all off with a photo of yourself at the finishing line. You could tag @gokayfitness on Instagram and share your photos with me, I'd love to know how you are getting on.

The programme contains both gym-based and home-based workouts. The workouts you do at home will get progressively longer, week by week. The gym workouts make use of the equipment there and these workouts are divided into two sections. Programme 1 has starter workouts, with separate upper and lower body workouts in it. Programme 2 has two categories, a and b, which again have separate upper and lower body workouts.

The Resources section in Chapter 11 at the back of the book contains the detailed instructions for each weight training programme or home workout to ensure you do the exercises safely and accurately: visit sections 11.1 and 11.2. Please refer to those instructions constantly, until you are absolutely sure you've mastered the techniques.

In the meantime, in 8.2 and 8.3 following this introduction you'll see summary lists of the day-to-day programme and of the contents of your weekly gym and home workouts, so that you can easily keep track of where you are. From 8.4 through to 8.11 you have each week's detailed programme and your journal pages where you can record your intentions for the week, followed by a summary of the progress you made and how you feel about it.

8.2 YOUR WEEK-BY-WEEK EXERCISE PROGRAMME SUMMARY

Here, for overall reference, is a summary of the programme you're embarking on. This will take you through a carefully designed process which over the course of 8 weeks will help you build your body's strength and resilience. You'll see that on each day you will either be following a workout or a specific weight training sequence, listed below. Remember, you'll find the step-by-step instructions for each in Chapter 11, sections 11.2 and 11.3, for easy access.

The time for preparation is over – the time for action is here!

DAILY LIST OF WORKOUTS AND WEIGHT-TRAINING SEQUENCES:

Week 1

Day 1	Home Workout 1
Day 2	Upper Body Weight Training P1
Day 3	Home Workout 2
Day 4	Lower Body Weight Training P1
Day 5	Home Workout 3
Day 6	Home Workout 4
Day 7	OFF

Week 2

Day 8	Home Workout 5
Day 9	Upper Body Weight Training P1
Day 10	Home Workout 6
Day 11	Lower Body Weight Training P1
Day 12	Home Workout 7
Day 13	Home Workout 8
Day 14	OFF

Week 3

Day 15	Home Workout 9
Day 16	Upper Body Weight Training P1
Day 17	Home Workout 10 (Pyramid)
Day 18	Lower Body Weight Training P1

Day 19   Home Workout 6
Day 20   Home Workout 7
Day 21   OFF

Week 4

Day 22   Upper Body Weight Training P2(a)
Day 23   Lower Body Weight Training P2(a)
Day 24   Home Workout 8
Day 25   Upper Body Weight Training P2(b)
Day 26   Lower Body Weight Training P2(b)
Day 27   OFF
Day 28   OFF

Week 5

Day 29   Home Workout 9
Day 30   Upper Body Weight Training P2(a)
Day 31   Home Workout 10 (Pyramid)
Day 32   Lower Body Weight Training P2(a)
Day 33   Home Workout 11
Day 34   Home Workout 12
Day 35   OFF

Week 6

Day 36   Upper Body Weight Training P2(b)
Day 37   Lower Body Weight Training P2(b)
Day 38   Home Workout 13
Day 39   Upper Body Weight Training P2(a)
Day 40   Lower Body Weight Training P2(a)
Day 41   Home Workout 14
Day 42   OFF

Week 7

Day 43   Home Workout 15

Day 44 Upper Body Weight Training P2(b)
Day 45 Home Workout 11
Day 46 Lower Body Weight Training P2(b)
Day 47 Home Workout 12
Day 48 Home Workout 13
Day 49 OFF

Week 8

Day 50 Upper Body Weight Training P2(a)
Day 51 Lower Body Weight Training P2(a)
Day 52 Home Workout 14
Day 53 Upper Body Weight Training P2(b)
Day 54 Lower Body Weight Training P2(b)
Day 55 OFF
Day 56 Home Workout 15

8.3 DAY-BY-DAY HOME WORKOUT AND WEIGHT TRAINING PROGRAMME EXERCISE CONTENT

Day 1
Home Workout 1
1. Squats
2. Horizontal Knees to Chest
3. Press-ups
4. High Knees

Day 2
Upper Body Weight Training Programme 1
1. Barbell Chest Press
2. Cable Fly
3. Lat Pull Down
4. Seated Rowing
5. Machine Shoulder Press
6. Barbell Biceps Curl
7. Cable V-Bar Triceps Extension
8. Plank

Day 3
Home Workout 2
1. Star Jumps
2. Alternating Backward Lunges
3. Hooks
4. Side Planks

Day 4
Lower Body Weight Training Programme 1
1. Leg Extension
2. Leg Curl
3. Leg Press

 4. Dumbbell Alternating Backward Lunges
 5. Side Plank
 6. Abs Vertical Scissors
 7. Abs Crunches with Hands on Thighs

Day 5
Home Workout 3
1. Oblique Curl Right
2. Oblique Curl Left
3. Cycling in the Air
4. Plank
5. Side Touch Shuttles

Day 6
Home Workout 4
1. Side Lunges
2. Horizontal Side Jumps
3. Heel Touches
4. Leg Kicks

Day 7 OFF

Day 8
Home Workout 5
1. Hip Extensions Right
2. Hip Extensions Left
3. Burpees
4. Leg Raises

Day 9
Upper Body Weight Training Programme 1
1. Barbell Chest Press
2. Cable Fly
3. Lat Pull Down
4. Seated Rowing
5. Machine Shoulder Press
6. Barbell Biceps Curl
7. Cable V-Bar Triceps Extension
8. Plank

Day 10
Home Workout 6
1. Squats
2. Alternating Backward Lunges
3. Upper Cuts
4. Lateral Plank Walks
5. Rhomboid Squeezes
6. Arm Circles

Day 11
Lower Body Weight Training Programme 1
1. Leg Extension
2. Leg Curl
3. Leg Press
4. Dumbbell Alternating Backward Lunges
5. Side Plank
6. Abs Vertical Scissors
7. Abs Crunches with Hands on Thighs

Day 12
Home Workout 7
1. Split Squats Right
2. Split Squats Left
3. Dead Bug
4. Press-ups and Rotate

5. Slalom Side-hops
6. Plank Step In and Out

Day 13
Home Workout 8
1. Good Morning
2. Side Touch Shuttles
3. Plank with Knee Flexion
4. Squat and Jump
5. Floor Triceps Dips
6. Spotty Dog

Day 14 OFF

Day 15
Home Workout 9
1. Clams Right
2. Clams Left
3. Bridge
4. Leg Kicks Right
5. Leg Kicks Left
6. Skydiver
7. Side Leg Kicks Right
8. Side Leg Kicks Left

Day 16
Upper Body Weight Training Programme 1
1. Barbell Chest Press
2. Cable Fly
3. Lat Pull Down
4. Seated Rowing
5. Machine Shoulder Press
6. Barbell Biceps Curl
7. Cable V-Bar Triceps Extension
8. Plank

Day 17
Home Workout 10 (Pyramid)
1. Pyramid Press-ups
2. Pyramid Abs Scissors
3. Pyramid Horizontal Side Jumps

Day 18
Lower Body Weight Training Programme 1
1. Leg Extension
2. Leg Curl
3. Leg Press
4. Dumbbell Alternating Backward Lunges
5. Side Plank
6. Abs Vertical Scissors
7. Abs Crunches with Hands on Thighs

Day 19
Home Workout 6
1. Squats
2. Alternating Backward Lunges
3. Upper Cuts
4. Lateral Plank Walks
5. Rhomboid Squeezes
6. Arm Circles

Day 20
Home Workout 7
1. Split Squats Right
2. Split Squats Left
3. Dead Bug
4. Press-ups and Rotate
5. Slalom Side-hops
6. Plank Step In and Out

Day 21 OFF

Day 22
Upper Body Weight Training Programme 2(a)
1. Inclined Barbell Bench Press
2. Dumbbells Chest Fly
3. Dumbbells Inclined Bench Press
4. Dumbbell One Arm Rowing
5. Cable Reverse Fly (Back Extension)
6. Lat Pull Down Wide Overhand Grip
7. Cable Crunches
8. Leg Raises

Day 23
Lower Body Weight Training Programme 2(a)
1. Barbell Squats
2. Side Lunges
3. Barbell Deadlift
4. Oblique (Russian) Twist
5. Plank
6. Oblique Crunches
7. Slow Release Sit-ups

Day 24
Home Workout 8
1. Good Morning
2. Side Touch Shuttles
3. Plank with Knee Flexion
4. Squat and Jump
5. Floor Triceps Dip
6. Spotty Dog

Day 25
Upper Body Weight Training Programme 2(b)
1. Barbell Shoulder Press
2. Dumbbell Side Laterals
3. Cable Front Raise
4. EZ Barbell Biceps Curl
5. Dumbbell Inclined Biceps Curl
6. Standing EZ Bar Triceps Extension
7. Dumbbell One Arm Triceps Kick
8. Cycling in the Air
9. Dead Bug

Day 26
Lower Body Weight Training Programme 2(b)
1. Leg Extension
2. TRX Squat Jumps
3. Leg Curl
4. Split Squats
5. Abdominal Crunches with Raised Arms
6. Abs Scissors Heel Taps
7. Oblique Crunches
8. Plank Weight Rotation

Day 27 OFF

Day 28 OFF

Day 29
Home Workout 9
1. Clams Right
2. Clams Left

3. Bridge
4. Leg Kicks Right
5. Leg Kicks Left
6. Skydiver
7. Side Leg Kicks Right
8. Side Leg Kicks Left

Day 30
Upper Body Weight Training Programme 2(a)
1. Inclined Barbell Bench Press
2. Dumbbells Chest Fly
3. Dumbbells Inclined Bench Press
4. Dumbbell One Arm Rowing
5. Cable Reverse Fly (Back Extension)
6. Lat Pull Down Wide Overhand Grip
7. Cable Crunches
8. Leg Raises

Day 31
Home Workout 10 (Pyramid)
1. Pyramid Press-ups
2. Pyramid Abs Scissors
3. Pyramid Horizontal Side Jumps

Day 32
Lower Body Weight Training Programme 2(a)
1. Barbell Squats
2. Side Lunges
3. Barbell Deadlift
4. Oblique (Russian) Twist
5. Plank
6. Oblique Crunches
7. Slow Release Sit-ups

Day 33
Home Workout 11
1. Lunge Back and Side
2. Squat Thrust to Sides
3. Scissors
4. Duck Squats
5. Dynamic Plank to Press-ups with a Jump
6. Knee Hits

Day 34
Home Workout 12
1. Skiing Torso Rotation
2. Squats Increasing Claps
3. Leg Kick, Tap with Opposite Hand
4. Reverse Crunches with Knee Flexion
5. Side Tap, Side Laterals
6. Burpees and Forward Lunges

Day 35 OFF

Day 36
Upper Body Weight Training Programme 2(b)
1. Barbell Shoulder Press
2. Dumbbell Side Laterals
3. Cable Front Raise
4. EZ Barbell Biceps Curl
5. Dumbbell Inclined Biceps Curl
6. Standing EZ Bar Triceps Extension
7. Dumbbell One Arm Triceps Kick
8. Cycling in the Air
9. Dead Bug

Day 37

Lower Body Weight Training Programme 2(b)

1. Leg Extension
2. TRX Squat Jumps
3. Leg Curl
4. Split Squats
5. Abdominal Crunches with Raised Arms
6. Abs Scissors Heel Taps
7. Oblique Crunches
8. Plank Weight Rotation

Day 38

Home Workout 13

1. Press-ups/Star Jumps
2. Low Kick Dance
3. Squat Side Jumps
4. Triceps Dips
5. Single Leg Hops
6. Lying Flying

Day 39

Upper Body Weight Training Programme 2(a)

1. Inclined Barbell Bench Press
2. Dumbbells Chest Fly
3. Dumbbells Inclined Bench Press
4. Dumbbell One Arm Rowing
5. Cable Reverse Fly (Back Extension)
6. Lat Pull Down Wide Overhand Grip
7. Cable Crunches
8. Leg Raises

Day 40

Lower Body Weight Training Programme 2(a)

1. Barbell Squats
2. Side Lunges
3. Barbell Deadlift
4. Oblique (Russian) Twist
5. Plank
6. Oblique Crunches
7. Slow Release Sit-ups

Day 41

Home Workout 14

1. 5 Split Squats and Jumps to Alternate Foot
2. Diagonal Toe Touch Crunches
3. Clap under Thighs/Squat Jumps
4. Plank
5. Press-ups to Sides
6. Leg Oblique Side Drops

Day 42 OFF

Day 43

Home Workout 15

1. Horizontal Side Jumps
2. Leg Raises
3. Press-ups and Diagonal Touch
4. Heel Touches
5. Jumping Lunges

Day 44

Upper Body Weight Training Programme 2(b)

1. Barbell Shoulder Press

2. Dumbbell Side Laterals
3. Cable Front Raise
4. EZ Barbell Biceps Curl
5. Dumbbell Inclined Biceps Curl
6. Standing EZ Bar Triceps Extension
7. Dumbbell One Arm Triceps Kick
8. Cycling in the Air
9. Dead Bug

Day 45
Home Workout 11
1. Lunge Back and Side
2. Squat Thrust to Sides
3. Scissors
4. Duck Squats
5. Dynamic Plank to Press-ups with a Jump
6. Knee Hits

Day 46
Lower Body Weight Training Programme 2(b)
1. Leg Extension
2. TRX Squat Jumps
3. Leg Curl
4. Split Squats
5. Abdominal Crunches with Raised Arms
6. Abs Scissors Heel Taps
7. Oblique Crunches
8. Plank Weight Rotation

Day 47
Home Workout 12
1. Skiing Torso Rotation
2. Squats Increasing Claps
3. Leg Kick, Tap with Opposite Hand
4. Reverse Crunches with Knee Flexion
5. Side Tap, Side Laterals
6. Burpees and Forward Lunges

Day 48
Home Workout 13
1. Press-ups/Star Jumps
2. Low Kick Dance
3. Squat Side Jumps
4. Triceps Dips
5. Single Leg Hops
6. Lying Flying

Day 49 OFF

Day 50
Upper Body Weight Training Programme 2(a)
1. Inclined Barbell Bench Press
2. Dumbbells Chest Fly
3. Dumbbells Inclined Bench Press
4. Dumbbell One Arm Rowing
5. Cable Reverse Fly (Back Extension)
6. Lat Pull Down Wide Overhand Grip
7. Cable Crunches
8. Leg Raises

Day 51
Lower Body Weight Training Programme 2(a)
1. Barbell Squats
2. Side Lunges

3. Barbell Deadlift
4. Oblique (Russian) Twist
5. Plank
6. Oblique Crunches
7. Slow Release Sit-ups

Day 52
Home Workout 14
1. 5 Split Squats and Jumps to Alternate Foot
2. Diagonal Toe Touch Crunches
3. Clap under Thighs/Squat Jumps
4. Plank
5. Press-ups to Sides
6. Leg Oblique Side Drops

Day 53
Upper Body Weight Training Programme 2(b)
1. Barbell Shoulder Press
2. Dumbbell Side Laterals
3. Cable Front Raise
4. EZ Barbell Biceps Curl
5. Dumbbell Inclined Biceps Curl
6. Standing EZ Bar Triceps Extension
7. Dumbbell One Arm Triceps Kick
8. Cycling in the Air
9. Dead Bug

Day 54
Lower Body Weight Training Programme 2(b)
1. Leg Extension
2. TRX Squat Jumps
3. Leg Curl
4. Split Squats
5. Abdominal Crunches with Raised Arms
6. Abs Scissors Heel Taps
7. Oblique Crunches
8. Plank Weight Rotation

Day 55 OFF

Day 56
Home Workout 15
1. Horizontal Side Jumps
2. Leg Raises
3. Press-ups and Diagonal Touch
4. Heel Touches
5. Jumping Lunges

8.4 WEEK 1 PROGRAMME AND JOURNAL PAGES

I'm very excited that we are starting our fitness journey this week. This week's workouts are basic and short, especially the home workouts, which last only 10 minutes. However, do not underestimate this as these exercises will help you get ready for the following weeks. I want to prepare you gradually, so that you don't overdo it and injure yourself, while at the same time increasing your strength, endurance and cardiovascular fitness. So, please just follow the plan. Each week, start by visiting the journal pages at the end of the weekly exercise lists and fill in Part 1. You'll fill in Part 2 at the end of the week. The journal is designed to create a sense of accountability to yourself and will build into a valuable record of your overall progress. It will help you pinpoint the challenges you're facing along the way and as well as increasing your self-awareness you'll be working out how to overcome those challenges – and celebrating every win too!

OK, let's start!

Here's a summary of your Week 1 programme:

Day 1	Home Workout 1
Day 2	Upper Body Weight Training Programme 1
Day 3	Home Workout 2
Day 4	Lower Body Weight Training Programme1
Day 5	Home Workout 3
Day 6	Home Workout 4
Day 7	OFF

Now follow your day-by-day exercises on the following pages.

DAY 1
HOME WORKOUT 1

Today's workout only lasts for 10 minutes to get you started, after which you will increase the duration and intensity of workouts day by day.

There are 4 exercises in this workout. You will perform each exercise for 20 seconds then rest for 20 seconds and move to the next exercise. You'll repeat this 4 times (4 sets).

The exercises are:

1. Squats — 20 secs on, 20 secs off
2. Horizontal Knees to Chest — 20 secs on, 20 secs off
3. Press-ups — 20 secs on, 20 secs off
4. High Knees — 20 secs on, 20 secs off

1. Squats

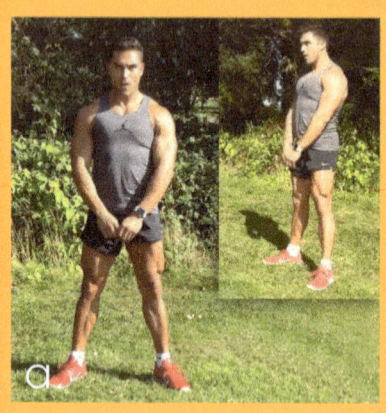

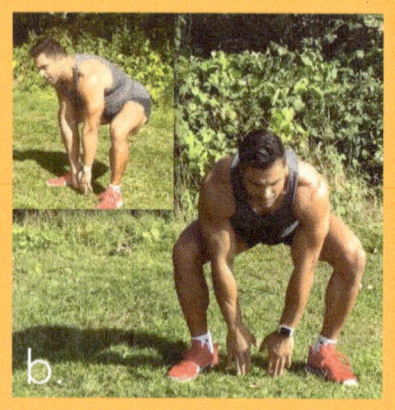

2. Horizontal Knees to Chest

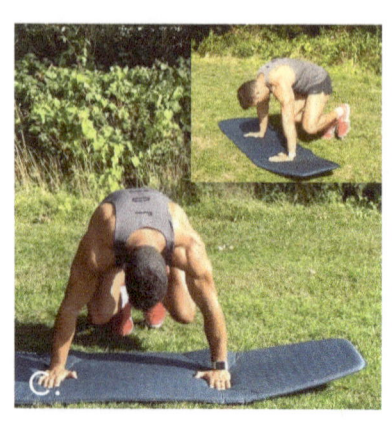

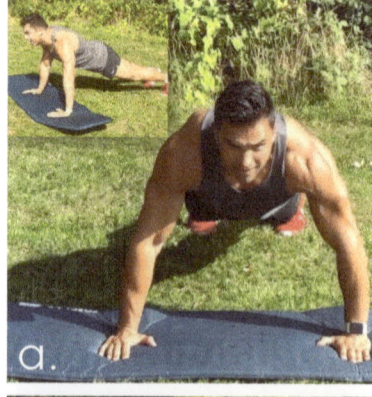

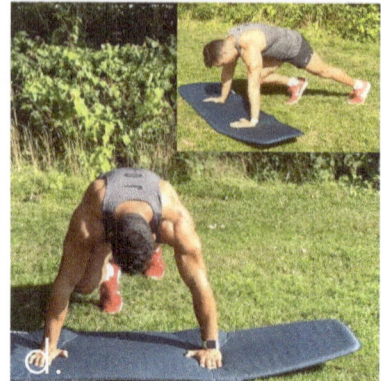

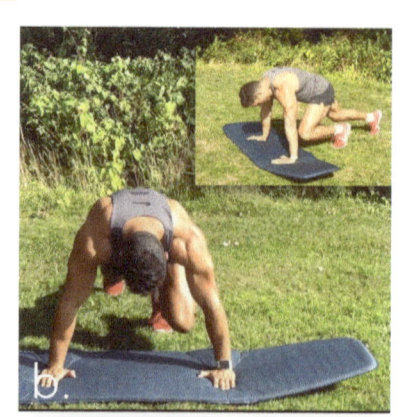

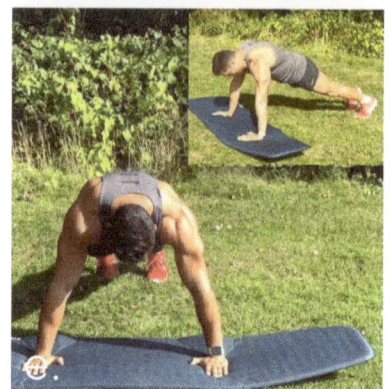

138 | GOKAY KURTULDUM

3. Press-ups (easier)

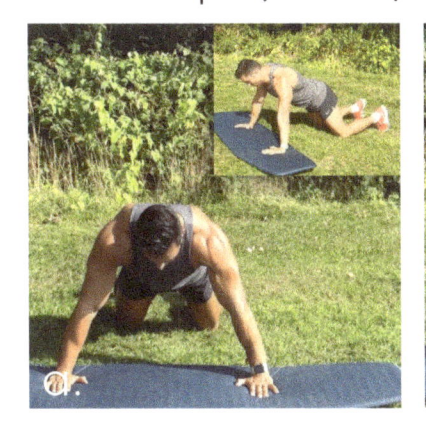

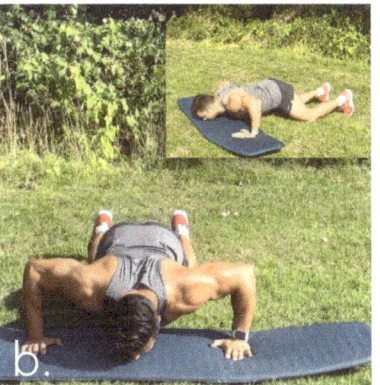

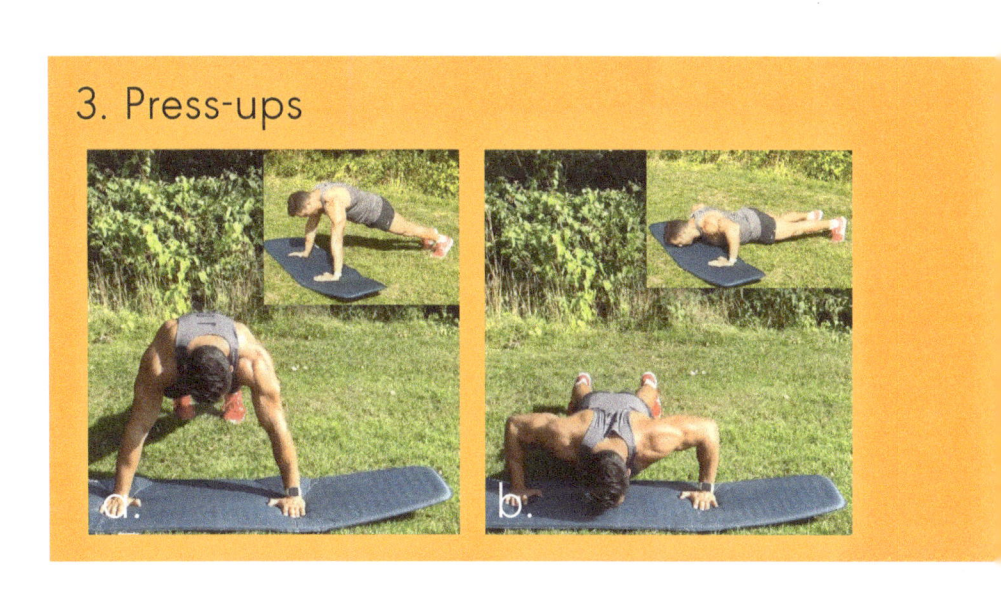

3. Press-ups

4. High Knees

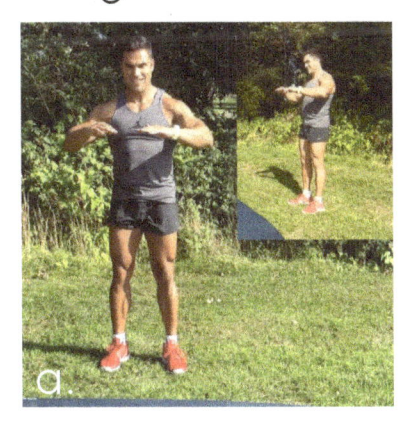

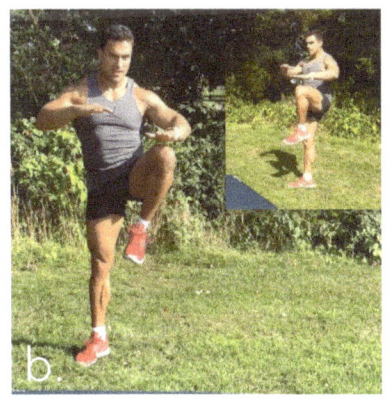

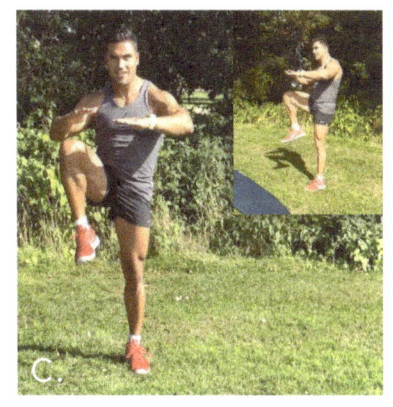

GET FIT, STAY FIT | 139

DAY 2
UPPER BODY WEIGHT TRAINING PROGRAMME 1

Day 2 involves a gym workout. There are 8 exercises, which you'll do in 3 sets with 45-60 seconds' rest between each set. The tempo for each repetition should be 1 second up, 1 second down (or vice versa).

1. Barbell Chest Press — 3 sets x 12 repetitions per set
2. Cable Fly — 3 sets x 12 reps
3. Lat Pull Down — 3 sets x 12 reps
4. Seated Rowing — 3 sets x 12 reps
5. Machine Shoulder Press — 3 sets x 12 reps
6. Barbell Biceps Curl — 3 sets x 12 reps
7. Cable V-Bar Triceps Extension — 3 sets x 12 reps
8. Plank — 3 sets x 30 seconds+

(feel free to stay in position for longer, as long as your posture is correct)

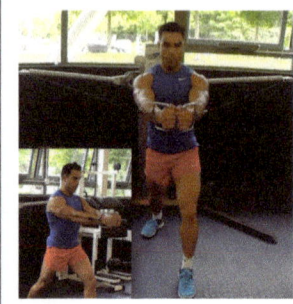

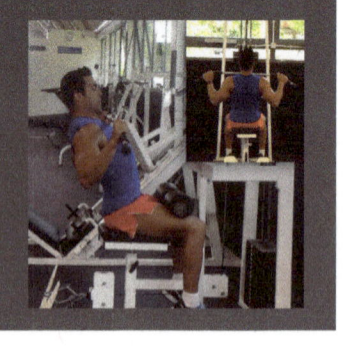

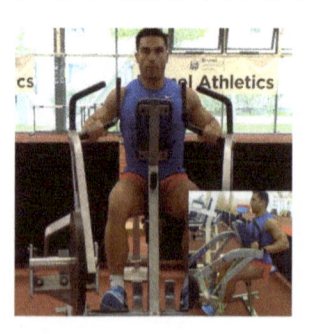

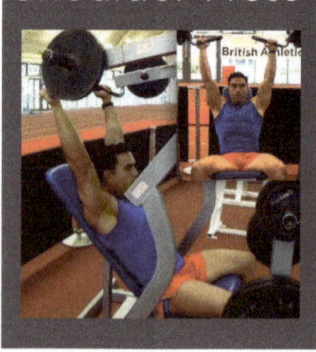

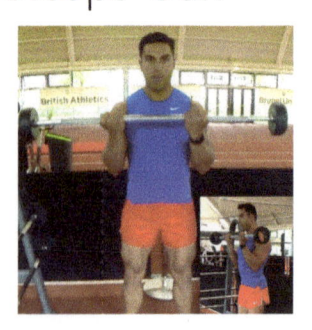

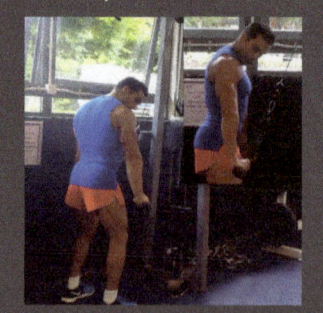

1. Barbell Chest Press
2. Cable Fly
3. Lat Pull Down
4. Seated Rowing
5. Machine Shoulder Press
6. Barbell Biceps Curl
7. Cable V-Bar Triceps Extension
8. Plank

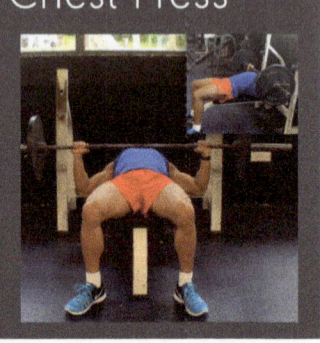

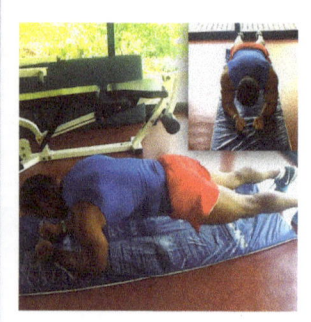

DAY 3
HOME WORKOUT 2

If you are feeling some stiffness in your muscles on Day 3, that's absolutely normal. Stretching always helps.

You will start with a cardio exercise, followed by a strength training exercise. There are 4 exercises, as on Day 1. You will perform each exercise for 20 seconds then rest for 20 seconds and move to the next exercise. Repeat this 4 times (4 sets).

1. Star Jumps — 20 secs on, 20 secs off
2. Alternating Backward Lunges — 20 secs on, 20 secs off
3. Hooks — 20 secs on, 20 secs off
4. Side Planks — 20 secs on, 20 secs off

1. Star Jumps

2. Alternating Backward Lunges

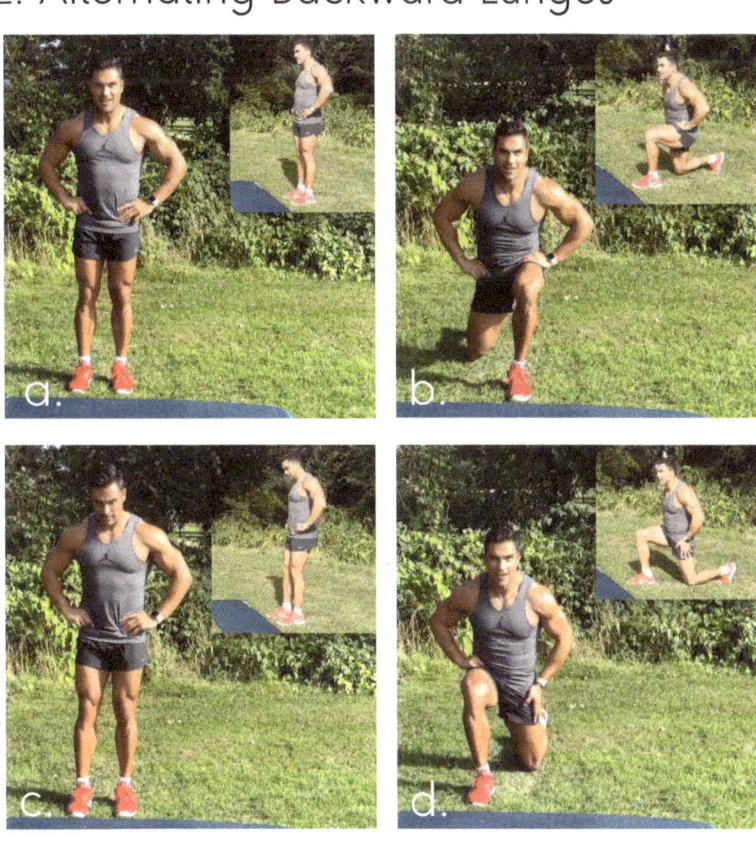

3. Hooks

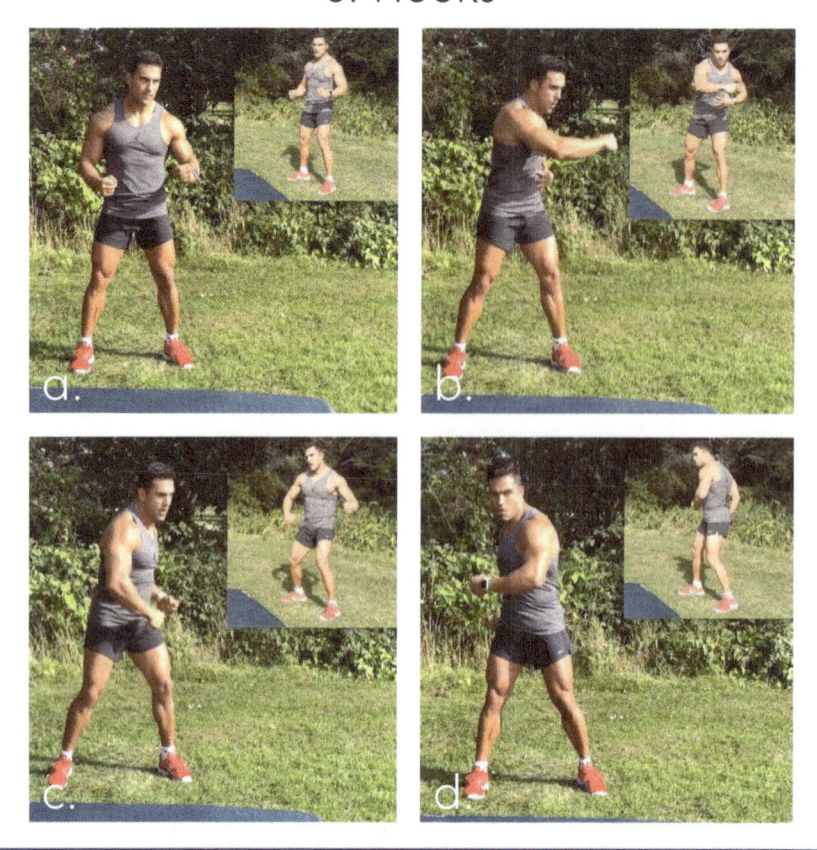

a.
b.
c.
d.

4. Side Planks

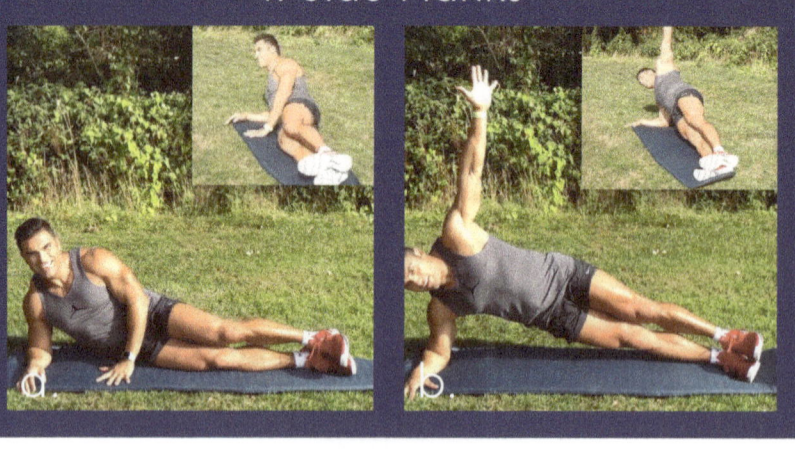

a.
b.

4b Easy Option

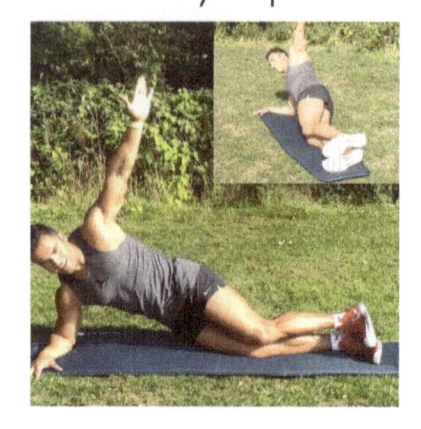

DAY 4
LOWER BODY WEIGHT TRAINING PROGRAMME 1

Today we are working our lower body at the gym. There are 7 exercises, which you'll do in 3 sets with 45-60 seconds' rest between each set. The tempo for each repetition should be 1 second up, 1 second down (or vice versa).

1.	Leg Extension	3 sets x 15 repetitions per set
2.	Leg Curl	3 sets x 15 reps
3.	Leg Press	3 sets x 12 reps
4.	Dumbbell Alternating Backward Lunges	3 sets x 10 reps
5.	Side Plank	3 sets x 30 secs each side
6.	Abs Vertical Scissors	3 sets x 30 secs
7.	Abs Crunches with Hands on Thighs	3 sets x 20 reps

1. Leg Extension

2. Leg Curl

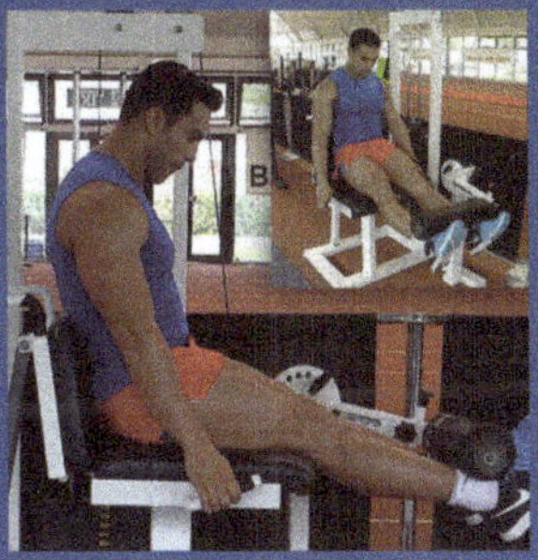

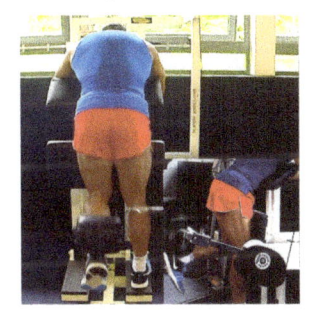

3. Leg Press

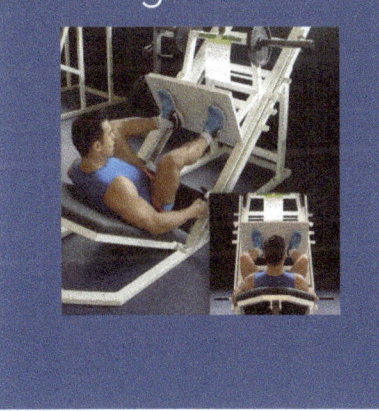

4. Dumbbell Alternating Backward Lunges

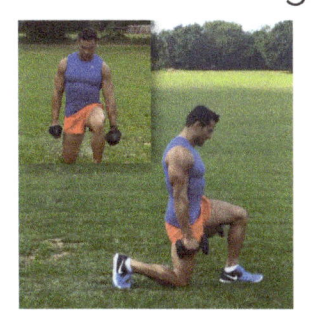

5. Side Plank

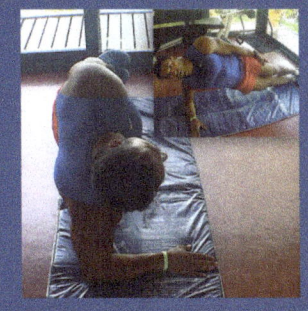

6. Abs Vertical Scissors

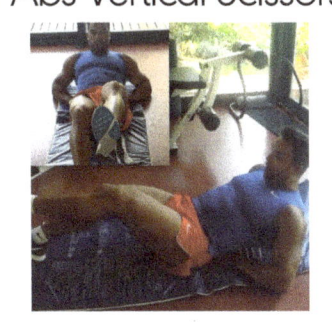

7. Abs Crunches

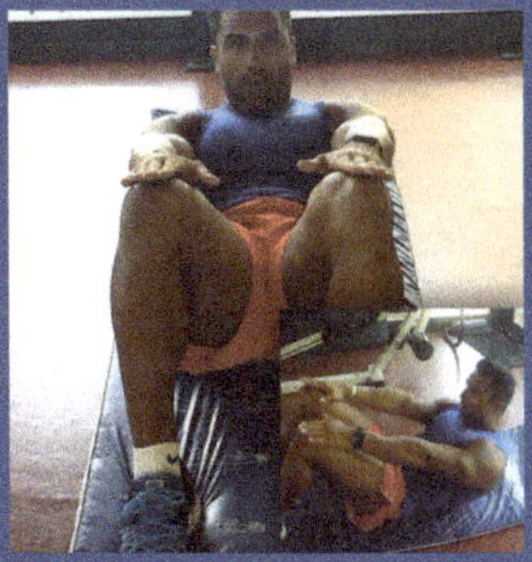

GET FIT, STAY FIT

DAY 5
HOME WORKOUT 3

Day 5's workout focuses on abdominals and core muscles. There are 5 exercises, each one lasting 20 seconds, but there will be only 10 seconds' rest in between. The first 4 exercises are for your core and the last one is a cardio exercise, just to keep you on your toes! You will do these for 4 sets.

1. Oblique Curl Right — 20 secs on, 10 secs off
2. Oblique Curl Left — 20 secs on, 10 secs off
3. Cycling in the Air — 20 secs on, 10 secs off
4. Plank — 20 secs on, 10 secs off
5. Side Touch Shuttles — 20 secs on, 10 secs off

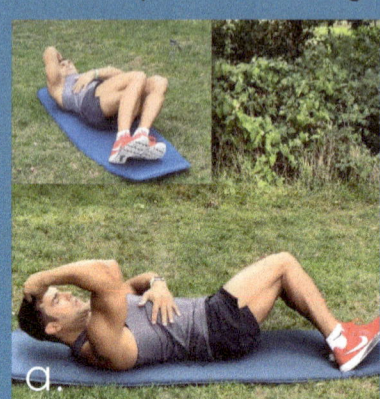

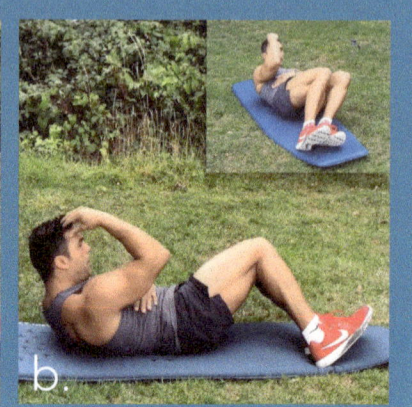

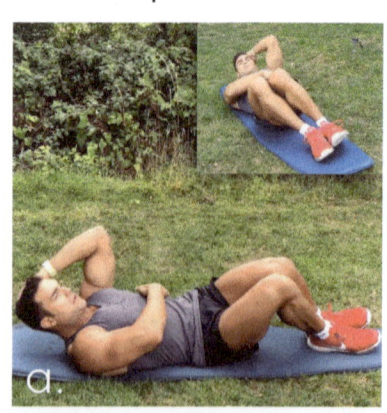

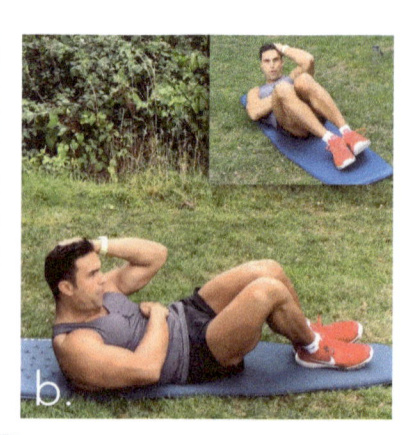

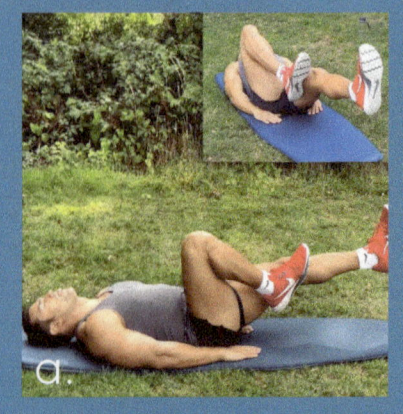

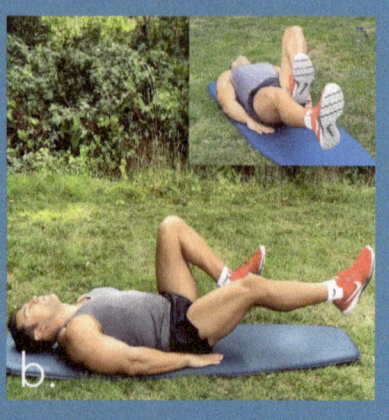

1. Oblique Curl Right

2. Oblique Curl Left

3. Cycling in the Air

4. Plank

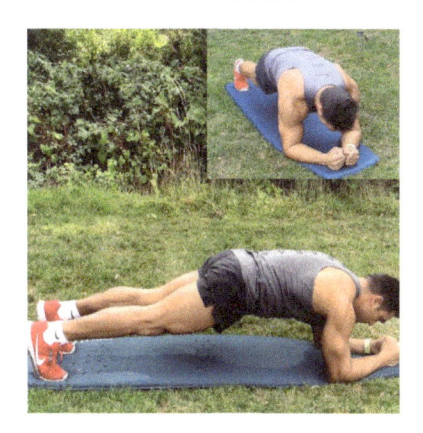

5. Side Touch Shuttles

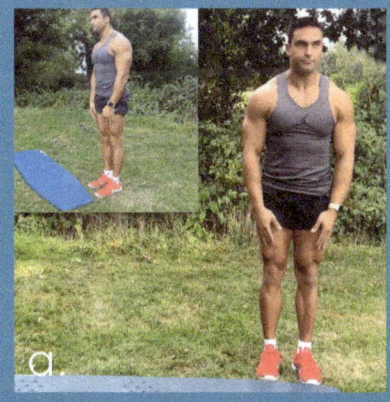

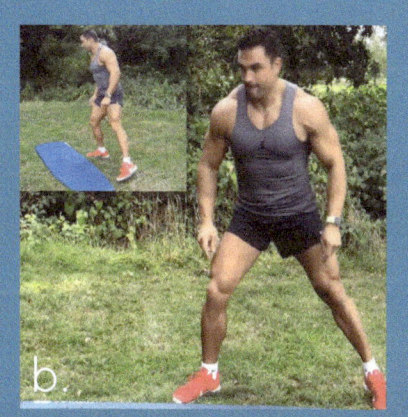

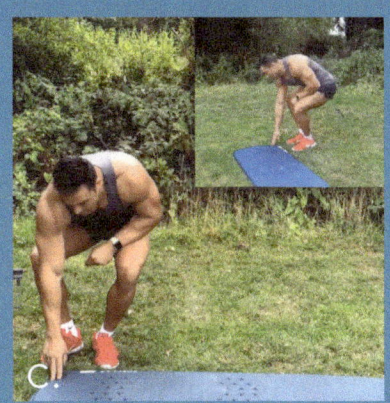

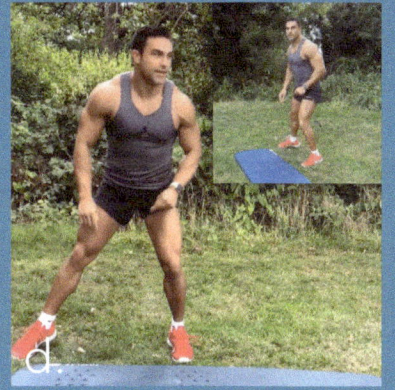

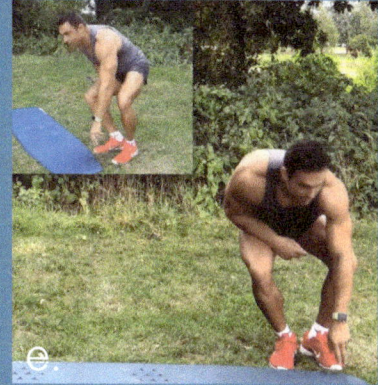

a.
b.
c.
d.
e.

GET FIT, STAY FIT | 145

DAY 6
HOME WORKOUT 4

Day 6 involves doing a leg exercise with some cardio and abs. Once again, each exercise lasts for 20 seconds, with 20 seconds' rest. You will do these for 4 sets.

1. Side Lunges — 20 secs on, 20 secs off
2. Horizontal Side Jumps — 20 secs on, 20 secs off
3. Heel Touches — 20 secs on, 20 secs off
4. Leg Kicks — 20 secs on, 20 secs off, switch legs after each set

1. Side Lunges

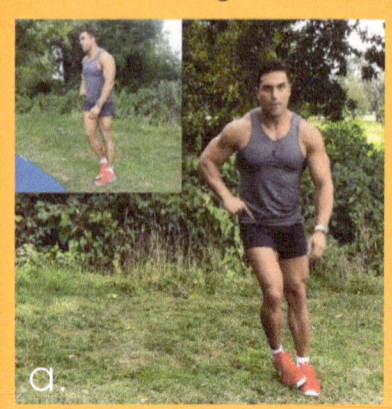

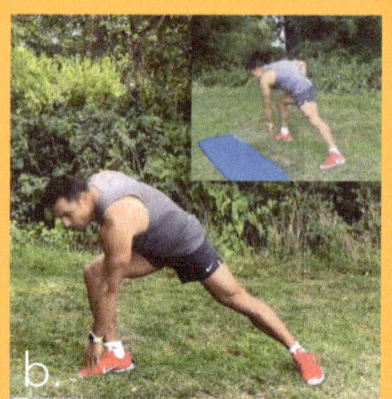

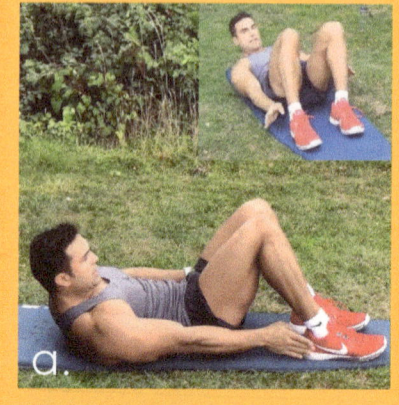

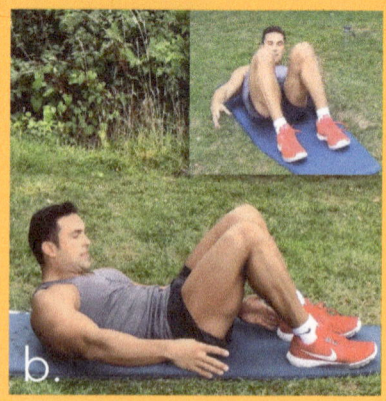

2. Horizontal Side Jumps

3. Heel Touches

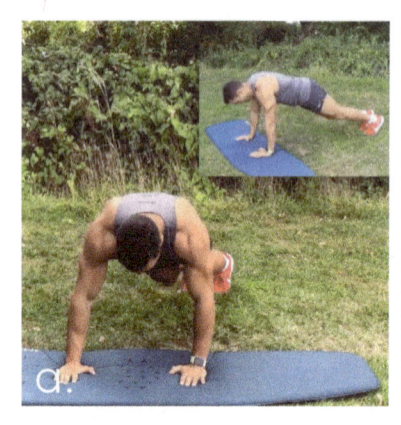

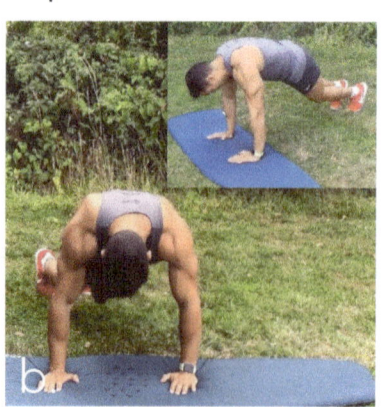

4. Leg Kicks

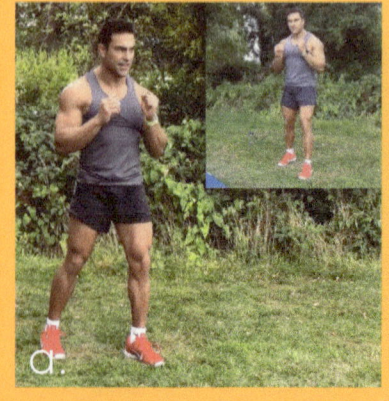

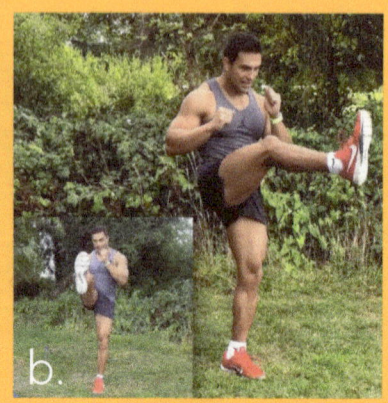

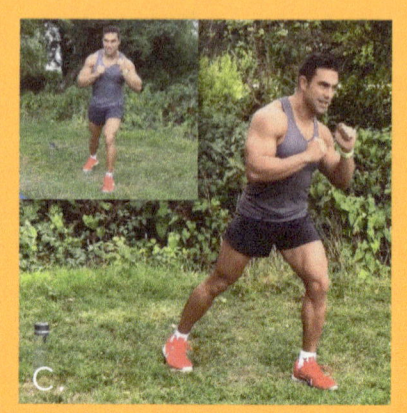

146 | GOKAY KURTULDUM

DAY 7 OFF

WEEK 1 PROGRESS JOURNAL

Use these pages to set your intentions at the start of the week and record and reflect on your progress at the end of the week. Alternatively, use a special notebook for this purpose.

PART 1: INTENTIONS/PLANNING

My starting weight this week: _____

My starting waist measurement: _____

My goal weight at the end of this week: _____

My goal waist measurement at the end of this week: _____

Any other goals for the week (e.g. no alcohol during the week and no more than 14 units during the weekend or going to bed early weekdays and sleep minimum 7 hours etc.)

_____

_____

Which days are going to be tricky this week and why? (E.g. client dinner on Thursday which involves drinking alcohol)

_____

How will I deal with this? _____

_____

GET FIT, STAY FIT | 147

Any other notes/thoughts:

PART 2: RECORD/REFLECTIONS

At the end of this week how many goals did I achieve? _____

How many did I come close to? _____

How am I feeling about my progress? _____

Which goals did I not reach? _____

Why was that? Family commitments, too much work and no time, not motivated enough? Can I define exactly what hindered my progress? Can I take action on that next week?

What actions can I take next week to improve on this?

What were my wins this week? (e.g. weight loss, mileage run etc?)

I've achieved

Give marks out of 10 for progress this week

8.5 WEEK 2 PROGRAMME AND JOURNAL PAGES

In this week's programme you have the same gym workouts as last week. The duration of your home workouts is starting to increase, so by Day 10 you'll be doing 15 minutes of exercise. These workouts are perfect for people like you who are busy and want to fit a workout into a tight schedule. The beauty of my workout plan is that you exercise most days; the sessions are brief enough for you to complete them without fail while still finding them highly effective.

Once again, start by filling in the Intentions/Planning section of your journal pages, after the week's exercise listings.

Here's a summary of your Week 2 programme:

Day 8	Home Workout 5
Day 9	Upper Body Weight Training P1
Day 10	Home Workout 6
Day 11	Lower Body Weight Training P1
Day 12	Home Workout 7
Day 13	Home Workout 8
Day 14	OFF

Now follow the day-by-day exercises on the following pages.

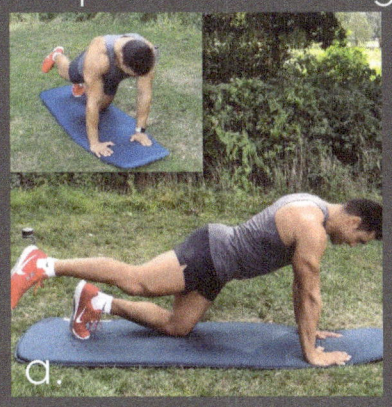

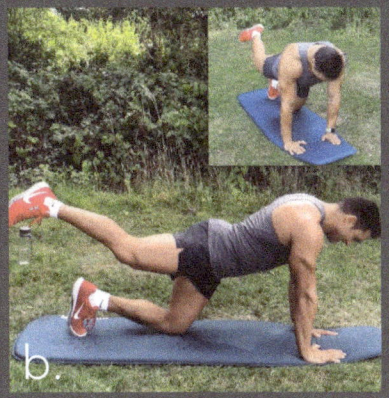

DAY 8
HOME WORKOUT 5

This workout is designed to work your gluteus muscles and abs, along with a bit of cardio to keep your heart rate up. You will do these for 4 sets.

1. Hip Extensions Right — 20 secs on, 20 secs off
2. Hip Extensions Left — 20 secs on, 20 secs off
3. Burpees — 20 secs on, 20 secs off
4. Leg Raises — 20 secs on, 20 secs off

1. Hip Extensions Right

2. Hip Extensions Left

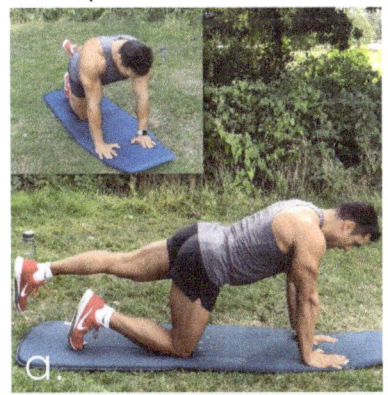

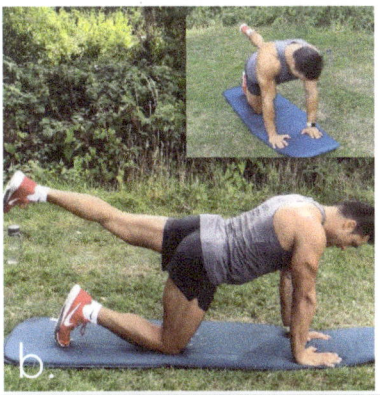

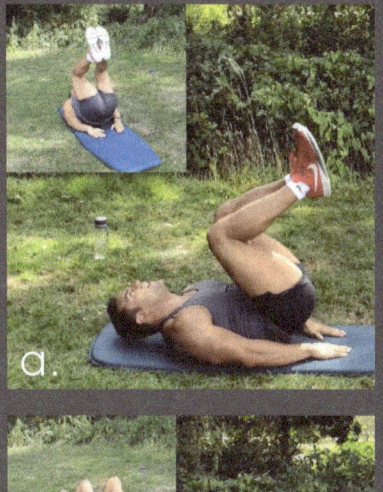

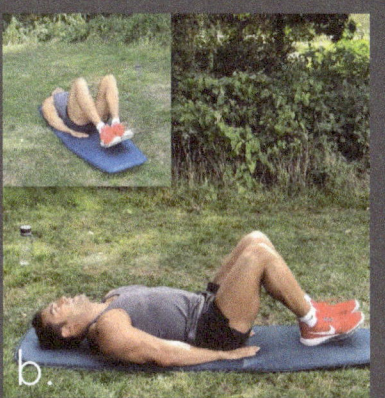

3. Burpees

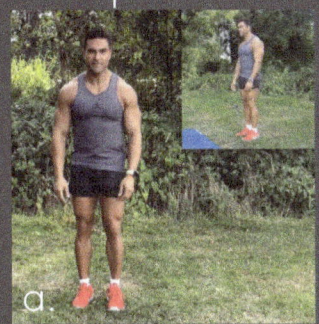

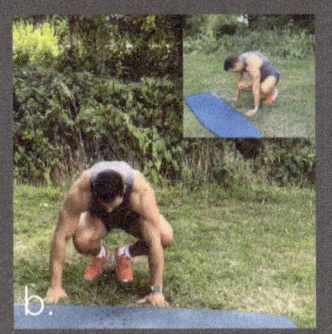

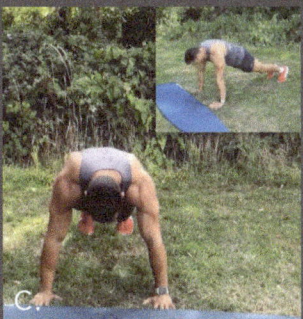

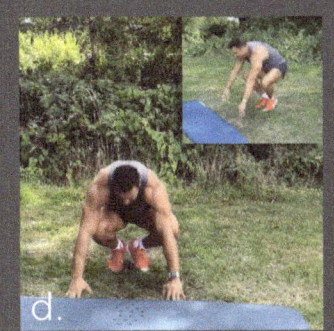

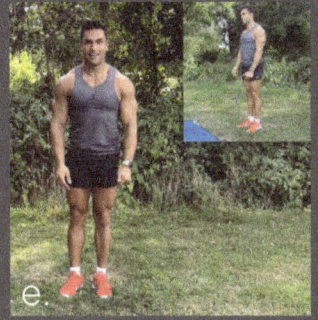

4. Leg Raises

DAY 9
UPPER BODY WEIGHT TRAINING PROGRAMME 1

Day 9 involves a gym workout. This is the same workout you did on Day 2. There are 8 exercises, which you'll do in 3 sets with 45-60 seconds' rest between each set. The tempo for each repetition should be 1 second up, 1 second down (or vice versa).

1. Barbell Chest Press — 3 sets x 12 repetitions per set
2. Cable Fly — 3 sets x 12 reps
3. Lat Pull Down — 3 sets x 12 reps
4. Seated Rowing — 3 sets x 12 reps
5. Machine Shoulder Press — 3 sets x 12 reps
6. Barbell Biceps Curl — 3 sets x 12 reps
7. Cable V-Bar Triceps Extension — 3 sets x 12 reps
8. Plank — 3 sets x 30 secs+ (feel free to stay longer, as long as your posture is correct)

1. Barbell Chest Press

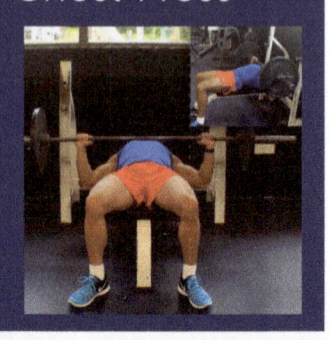

2. Cable Fly

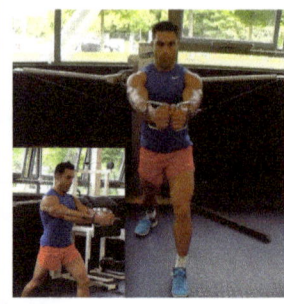

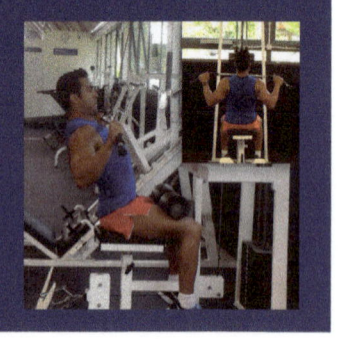

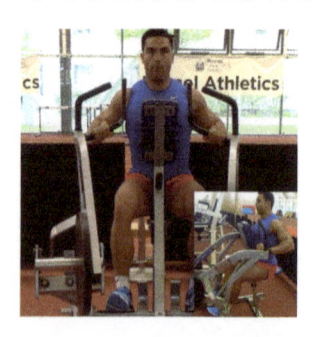

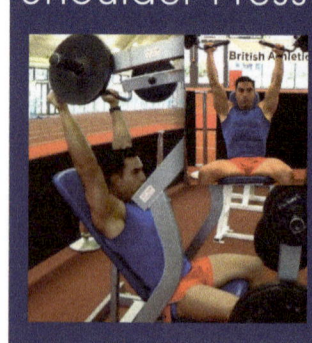

3. Lat Pull Down

4. Seated Rowing

5. Machine Shoulder Press

6. Barbell Biceps Curl

7. Cable V-Bar Triceps Extension

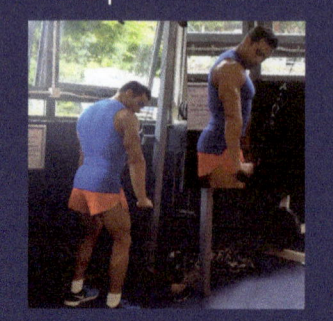

8. Plank

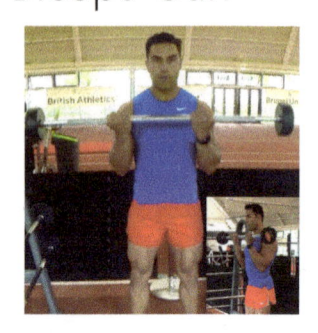

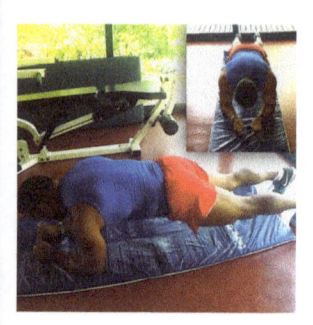

152 | GOKAY KURTULDUM

DAY 10
HOME WORKOUT 6

This workout involves 6 exercises, not 4, and each exercise is going to be for 30 seconds with a 20 second break in between. You will do these for 3 sets.

1. Squats — 30 secs on, 20 secs off
2. Alternating Backward Lunges — 30 secs on, 20 secs off
3. Upper Cuts — 30 secs on, 20 secs off
4. Lateral Plank Walks — 30 secs on, 20 secs off
5. Rhomboid Squeezes — 30 secs on, 20 secs off
6. Arm Circles — 30 secs on, 20 secs off

1. Squats

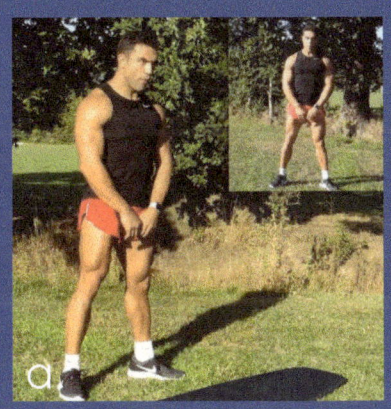

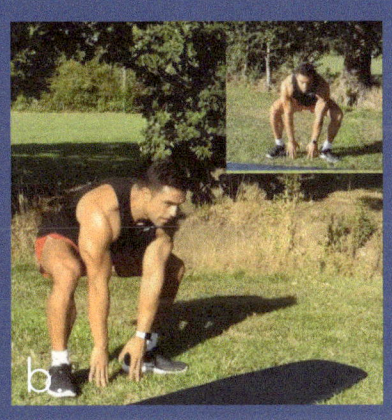

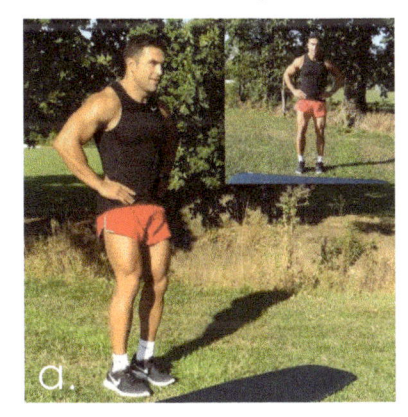

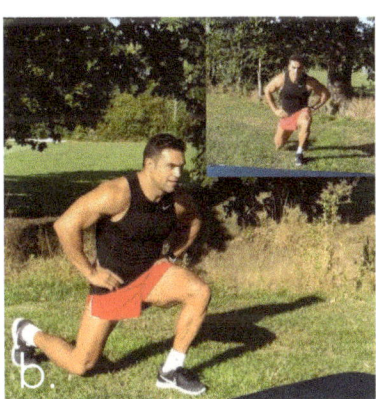

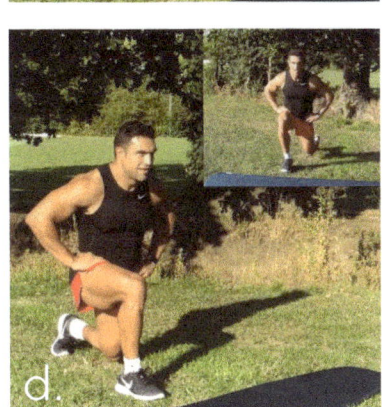

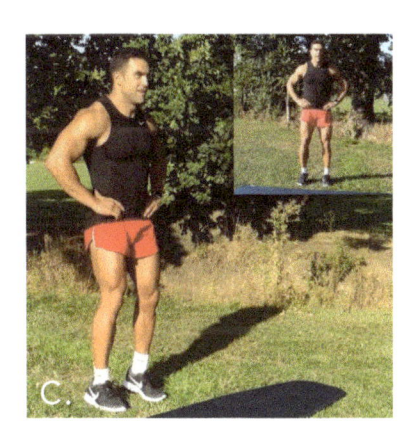

2. Alternating Backward Lunges

GET FIT, STAY FIT | 153

3. Upper Cuts

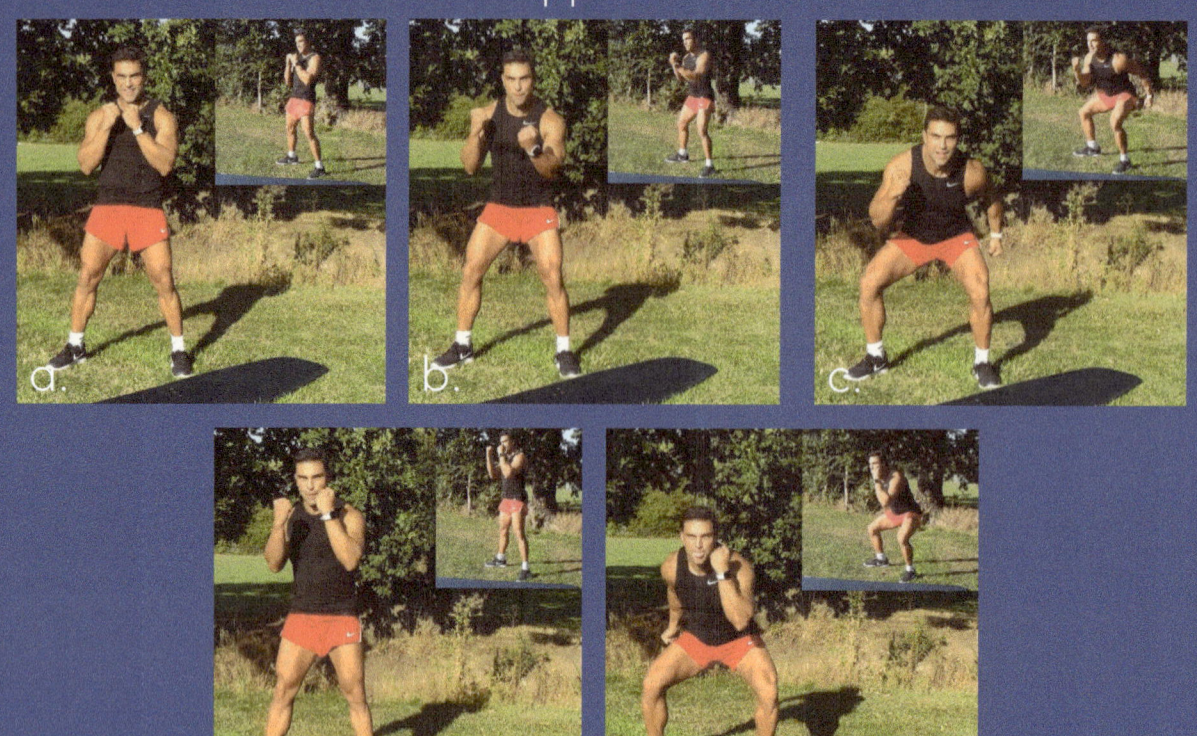

a.

b.

c.

d.

e.

4. Lateral Plank Walks

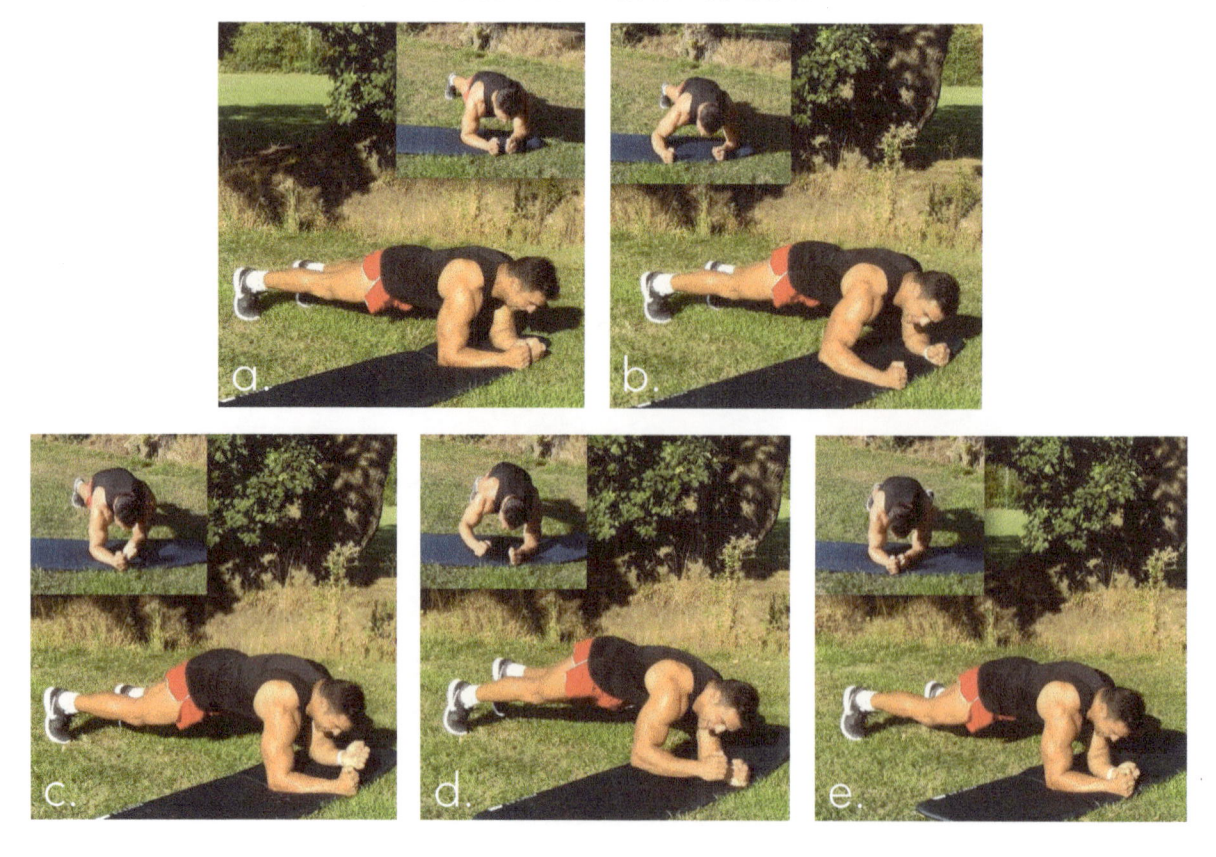

a.

b.

c.

d.

e.

5. Rhomboid Squeezes

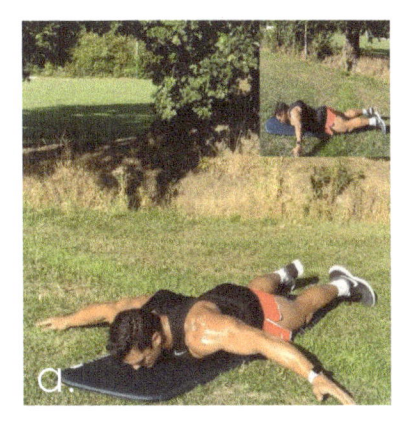

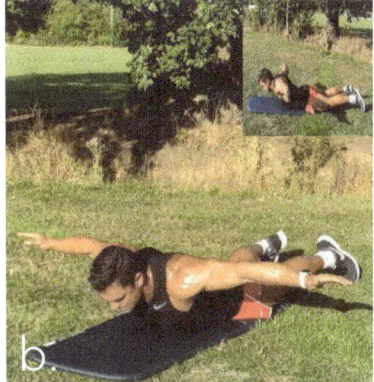

6. Arm Circles

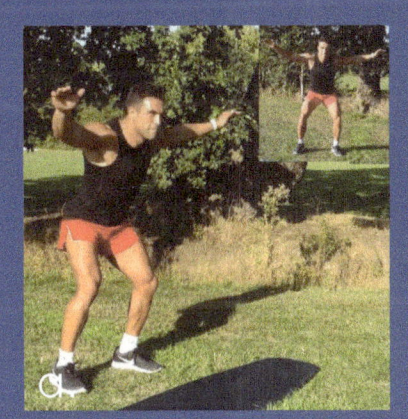

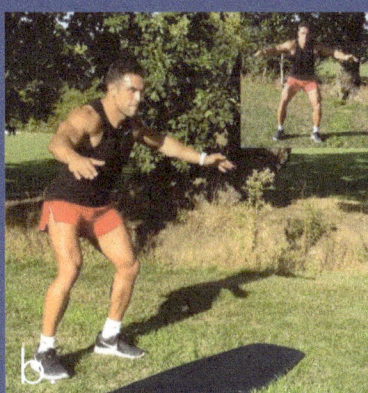

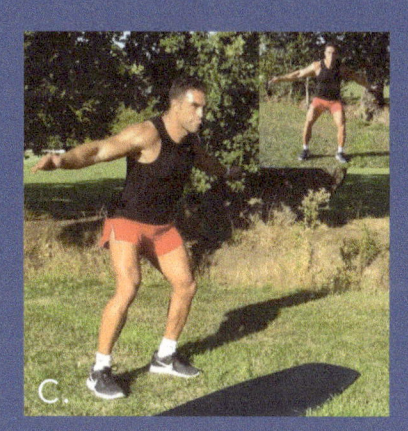

GET FIT, STAY FIT | 155

DAY 11
LOWER BODY WEIGHT TRAINING PROGRAMME 1

Today you are working your lower body at the gym. The same workout you did on Day 4. There are 7 exercises, which you'll do in 3 sets with 45-60 seconds' rest between each set. The tempo for each repetition should be 1 second up, 1 second down (or vice versa).

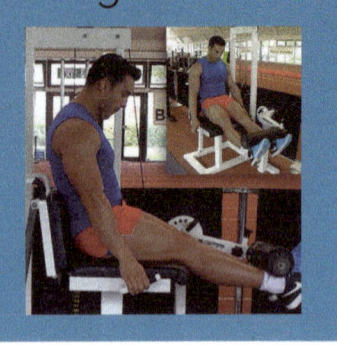

1. Leg Extension — 3 sets x 15 repetitions per set
2. Leg Curl — 3 sets x 15 reps
3. Leg Press — 3 sets x 12 reps
4. Dumbbell Alternating Backward Lunges — 3 sets x 10 reps
5. Side Plank — 3 sets x 30 secs each side
6. Abs Vertical Scissors — 3 sets x 30 secs
7. Abs Crunches with Hands on Thighs — 3 sets x 20 reps

1. Leg Extension

2. Leg Curl

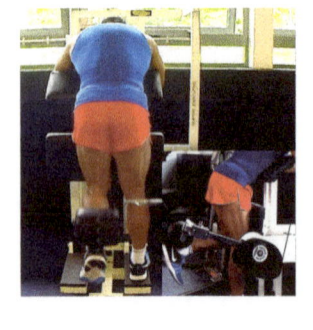

3. Leg Press

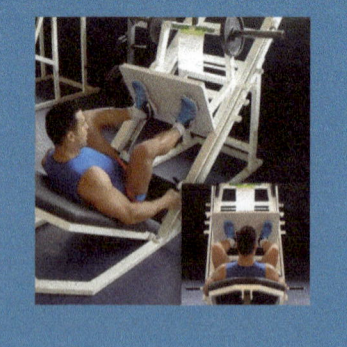

4. Dumbbell Alternating Backward Lunges

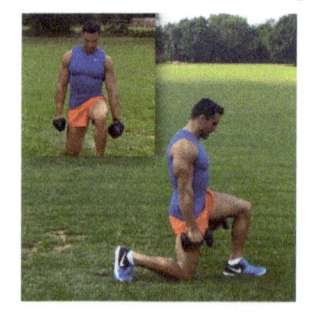

5. Side Plank

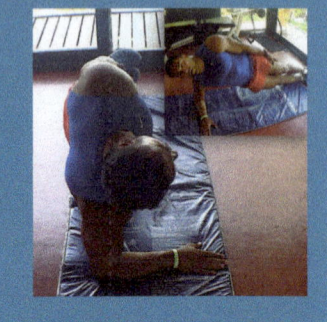

6. Abs Vertical Scissors

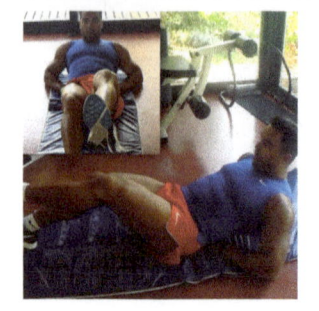

7. Abs Crunches

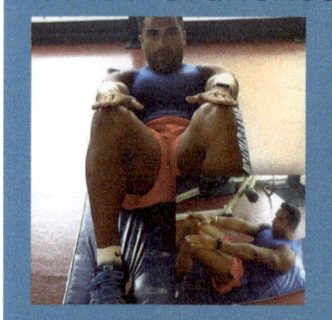

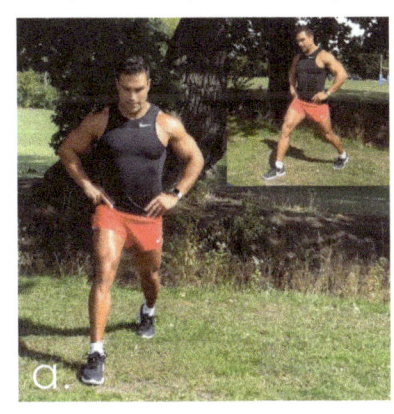

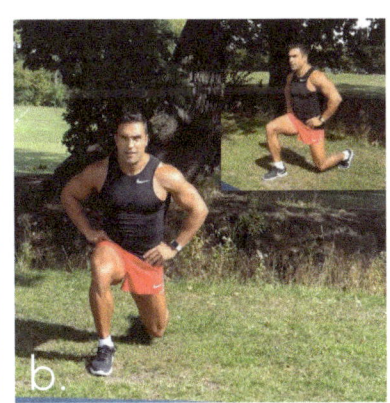

DAY 12
HOME WORKOUT 7

As with Day 10, Day 12 gives you 6 exercises to do. Each one is for 30 seconds with 20 second rests in between. You will do this for 3 sets.

1. Split Squats Right — 30 secs on, 20 secs off
2. Split Squats Left — 30 secs on, 20 secs off
3. Dead Bug — 30 secs on, 20 secs off
4. Press-ups and Rotate — 30 secs on, 20 secs off
5. Slalom Side-hops — 30 secs on, 20 secs off
6. Plank Step In and Out — 30 secs on, 20 secs off

1. Split Squats Right

2. Split Squats Left

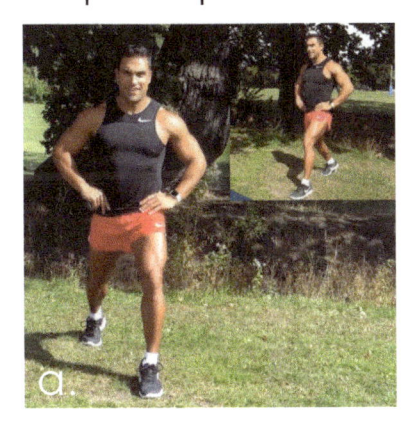

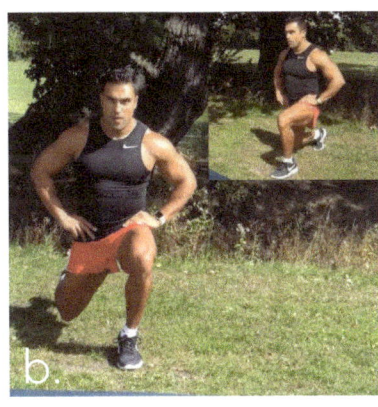

3. Dead Bug

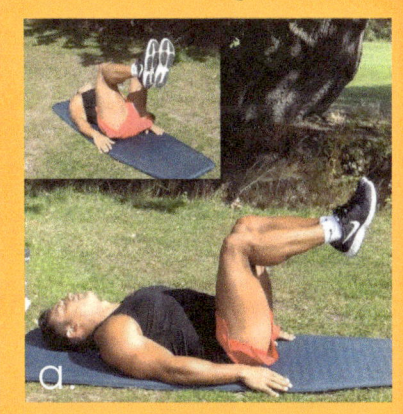

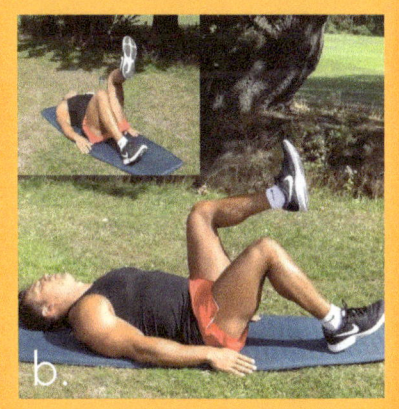

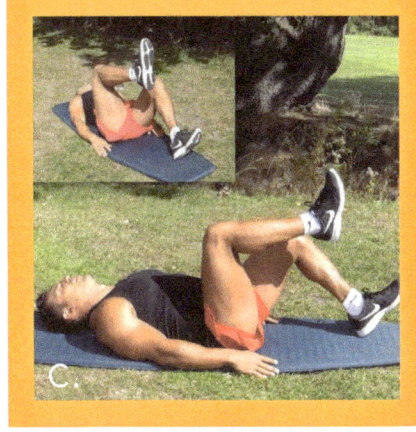

GET FIT, STAY FIT | 157

4. Press-ups and Rotate

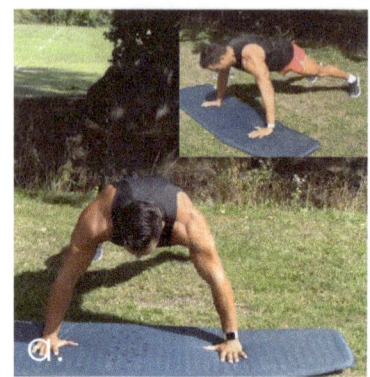

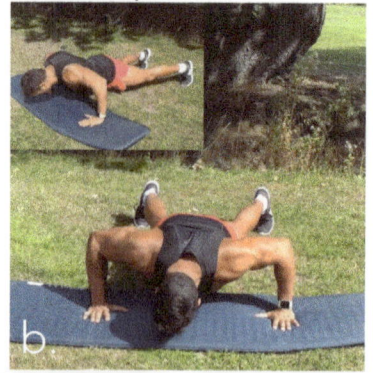

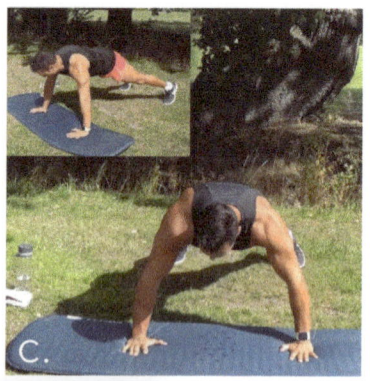

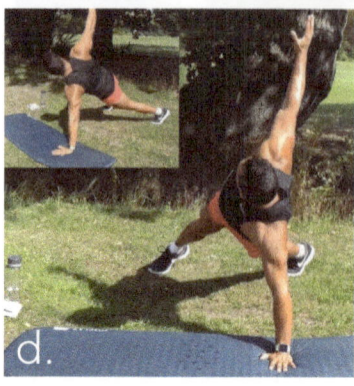

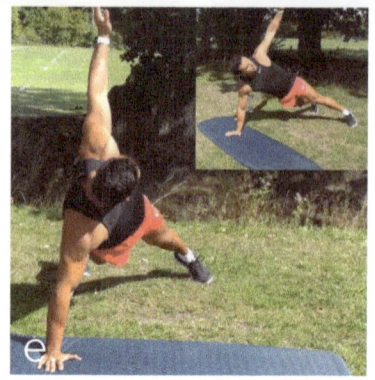

5. Slalom Side-hops

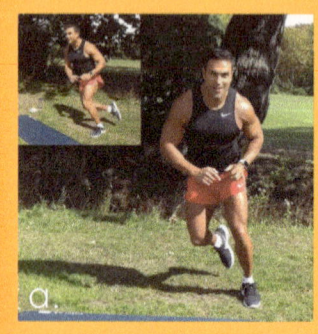

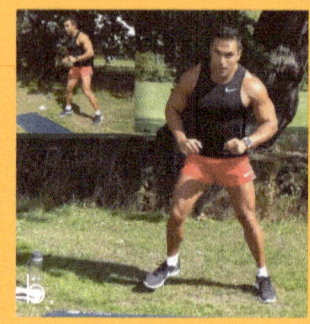

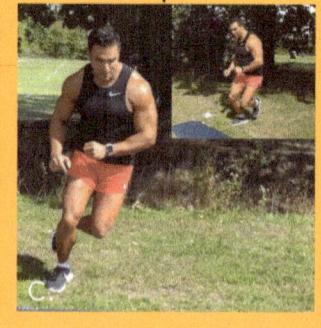

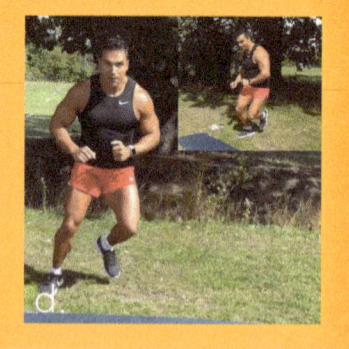

6. Plank Step In and Out

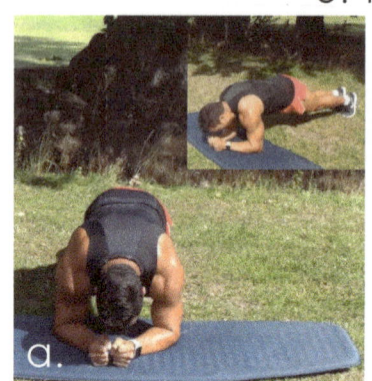

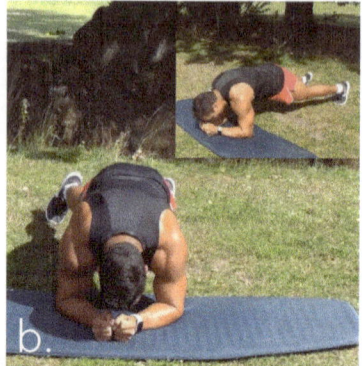

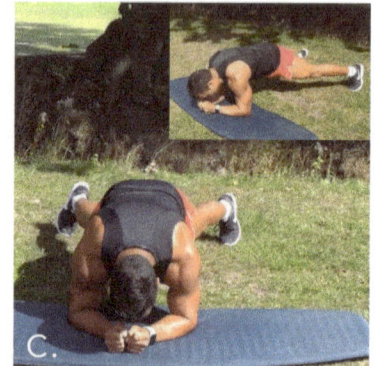

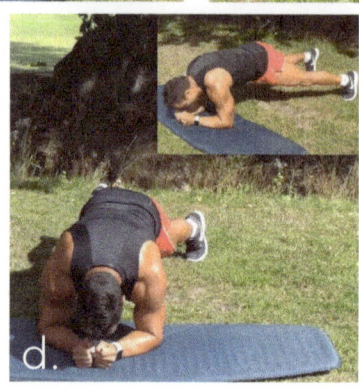

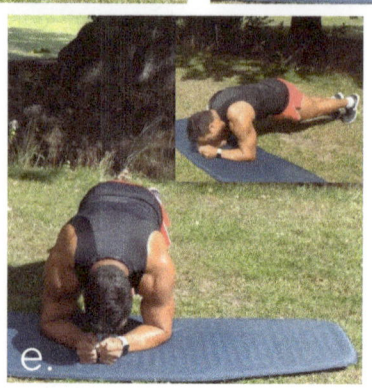

DAY 13
HOME WORKOUT 8

Today, 3 of the 6 exercises are cardio exercises. Again, each exercise lasts for 30 seconds with 20 seconds' rest in between. Do 3 sets.

1. Good Morning — 30 secs on, 20 secs off
2. Side Touch Shuttles — 30 secs on, 20 secs off
3. Plank with Knee Flexion — 30 secs on, 20 secs off
4. Squat and Jump — 30 secs on, 20 secs off
5. Floor Triceps Dips — 30 secs on, 20 secs off
6. Spotty Dog — 30 secs on, 20 secs off

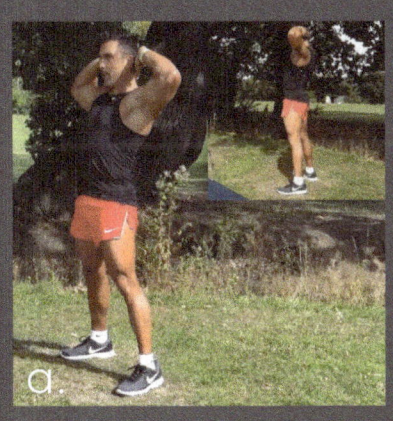

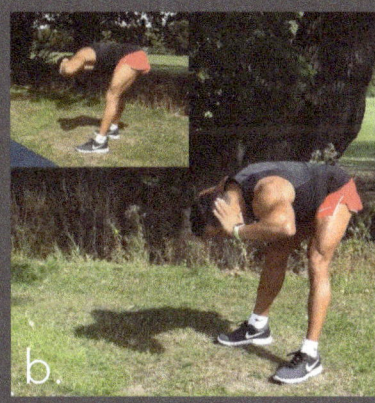

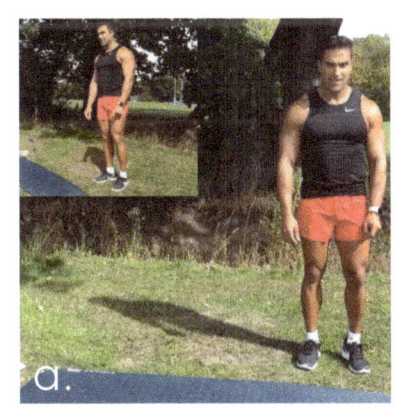

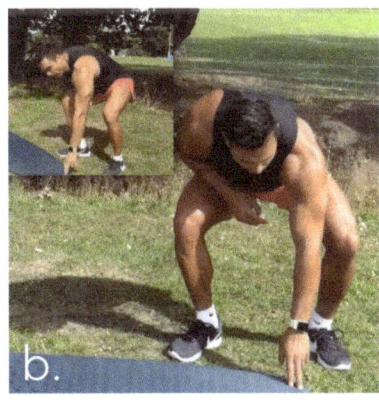

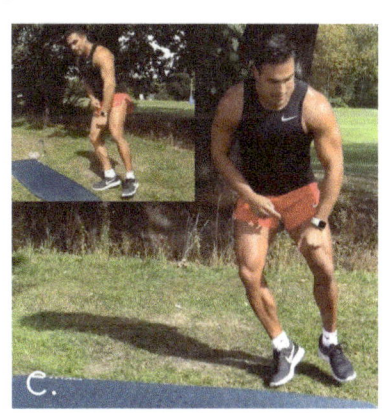

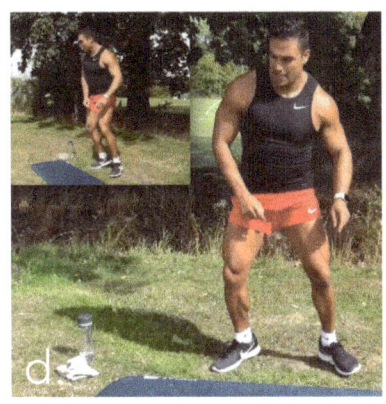

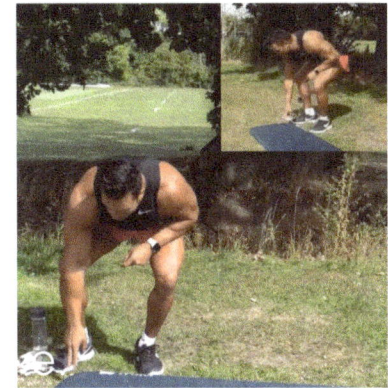

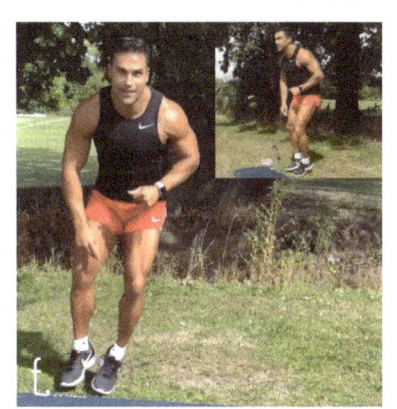

1. Good Morning

2. Side Touch Shuttles

GET FIT, STAY FIT | 159

3. Plank with Knee Flexion

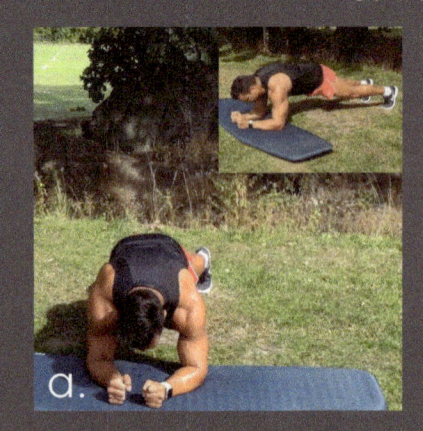

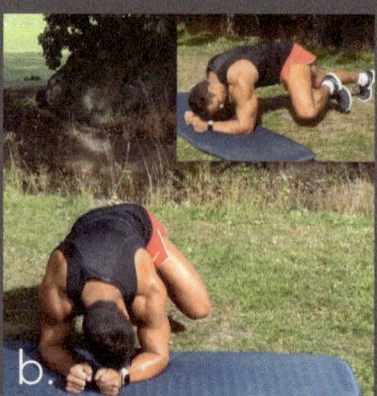

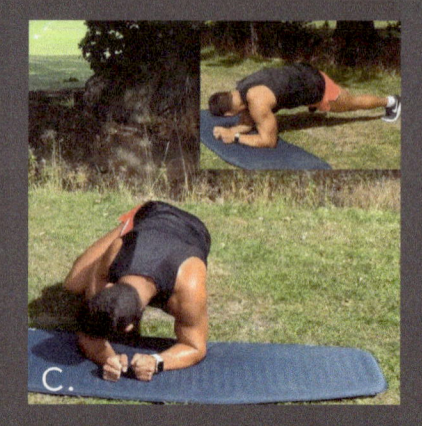

4. Squat and Jump

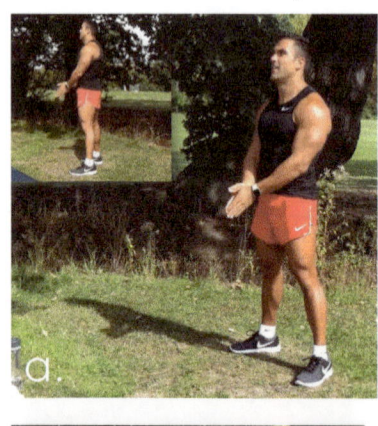

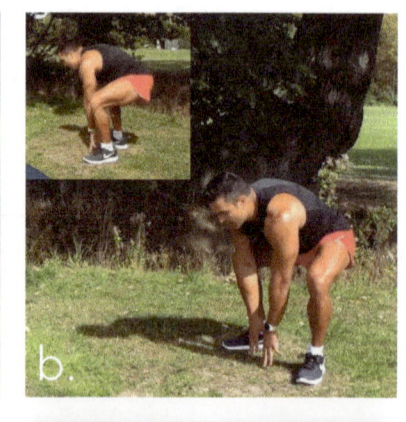

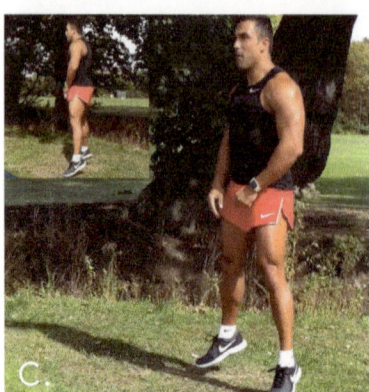

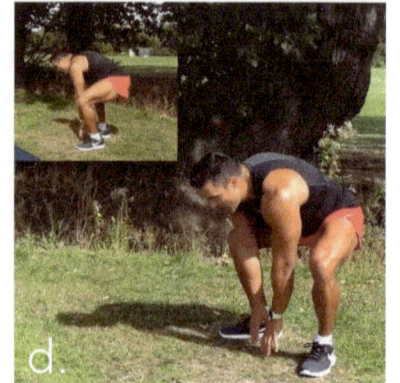

5. Floor Triceps Dips

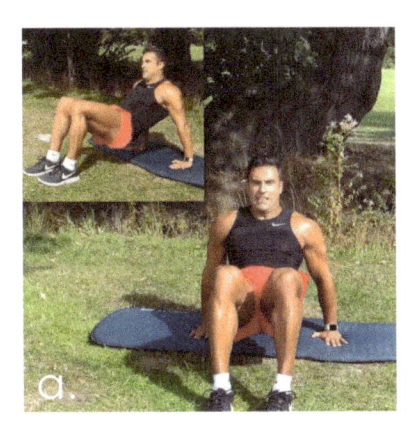

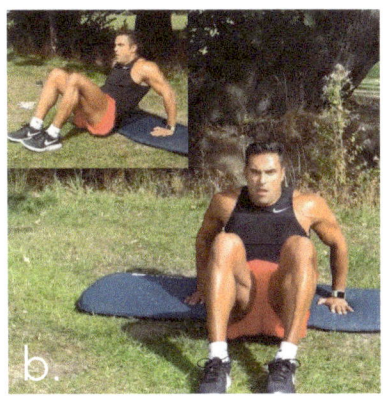

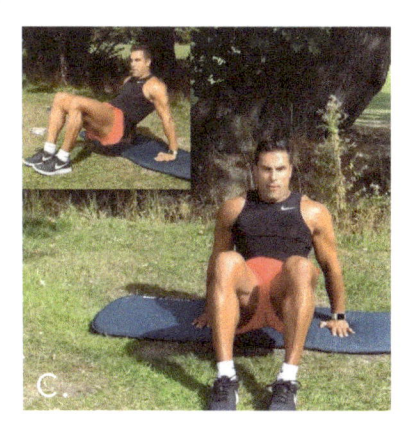

6. Spotty Dog

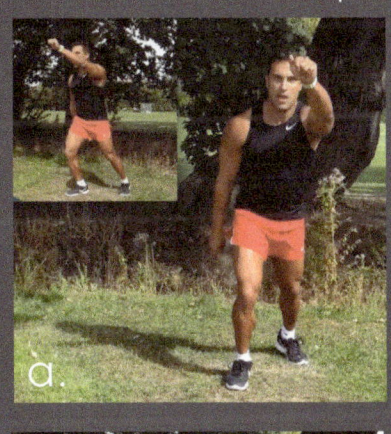

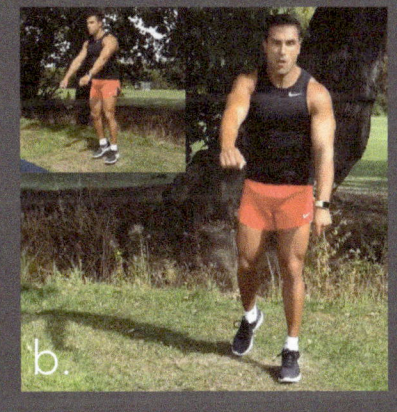

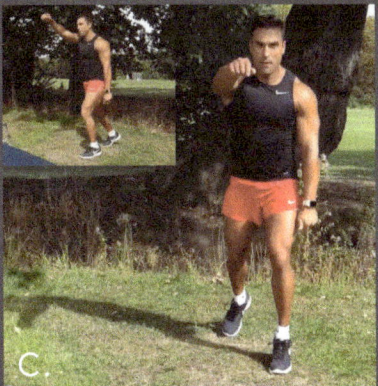

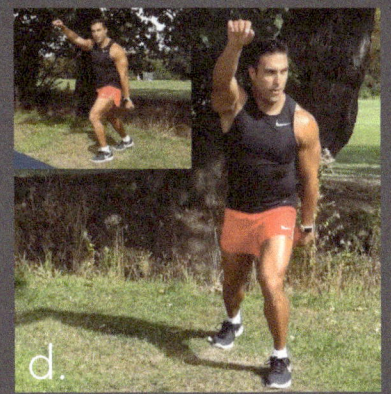

GET FIT, STAY FIT | 161

DAY 14 OFF

WEEK 2 PROGRESS JOURNAL

Use these pages to set your intentions at the start of the week and record and reflect on your progress at the end of the week. Alternatively, use a special notebook for this purpose.

PART 1: INTENTIONS/PLANNING

My starting weight this week: _____

My starting waist measurement: _____

My goal weight at the end of this week: _____

My goal waist measurement at the end of this week: _____

Any other goals for the week (e.g. no alcohol during the week and no more than 14 units during the weekend or going to bed early weekdays and sleep minimum 7 hours etc.)

_____

_____

Which days are going to be tricky this week and why? (E.g. client dinner on Thursday which involves drinking alcohol)

_____

How will I deal with this? _____

_____

Any other notes/thoughts:

PART 2: RECORD/REFLECTIONS

At the end of this week how many goals did I achieve? _____

How many did I come close to? _____

How am I feeling about my progress? _____

Which goals did I not reach? _____

Why was that? Family commitments, too much work and no time, not motivated enough? Can I define exactly what hindered my progress? Can I take action on that next week?

What actions can I take next week to improve on this?

What were my wins this week? (e.g. weight loss, mileage run etc?)

I've achieved

Give marks out of 10 for progress this week

8.6 WEEK 3 PROGRAMME AND JOURNAL PAGES

This week you have the same gym routine as last time and the home workouts continue to last for 15 minutes. Once again, start with Part 1 of your journal before embarking on the first day's exercises.

Here's a summary of your Week 3 programme:

Day 15	Home Workout 9
Day 16	Upper Body Weight Training P1
Day 17	Home Workout 10 (Pyramid)
Day 18	Lower Body Weight Training P1
Day 19	Home Workout 6
Day 20	Home Workout 7
Day 21	OFF

Now follow your day-by-day exercises on the next pages.

DAY 15
HOME WORKOUT 9

I have good news for you. Day 15 is about doing loads of floor exercises so you won't be moving much. These exercises will work your gluteus (bum) and also your back. There are 8 exercises and each one is for 30 seconds but with only an 8 second rest in between. Do 3 sets.

1. Clams Right — 30 secs on, 8 secs off
2. Clams Left — 30 secs on, 8 secs off
3. Bridge — 30 secs on, 8 secs off
4. Leg Kicks Right — 30 secs on, 8 secs off
5. Leg Kicks Left — 30 secs on, 8 secs off
6. Skydiver — 30 secs on, 8 secs off
7. Side Leg Kicks Right — 30 secs on, 8 secs off
8. Side Leg Kicks Left — 30 secs on, 8 secs off

1. Clams Right

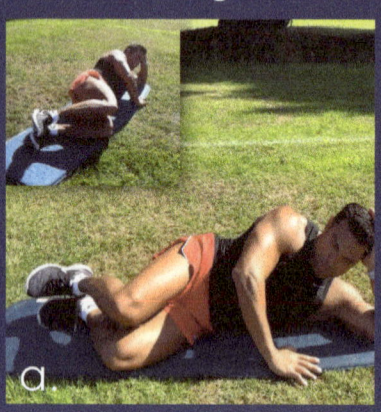

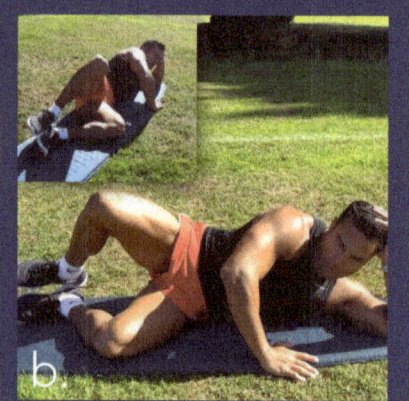

2. Clams Left

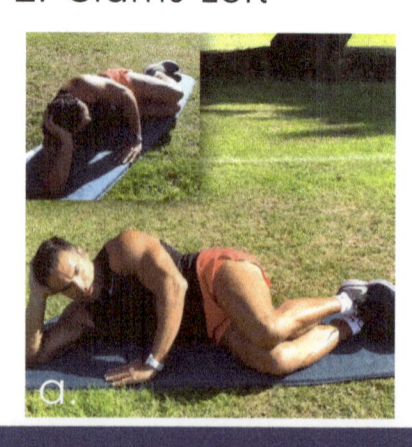

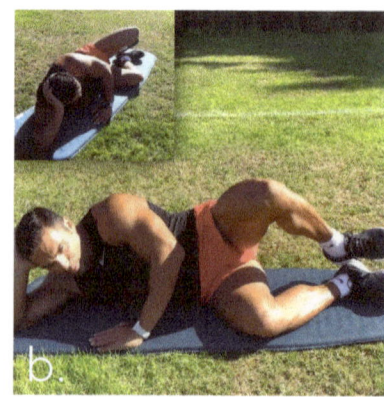

3. Bridge

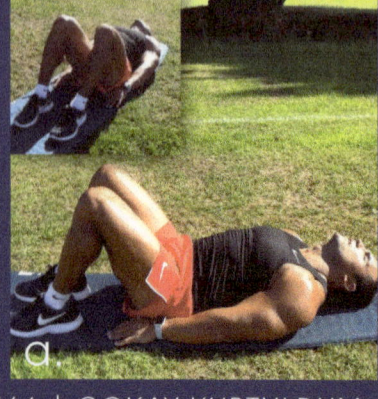

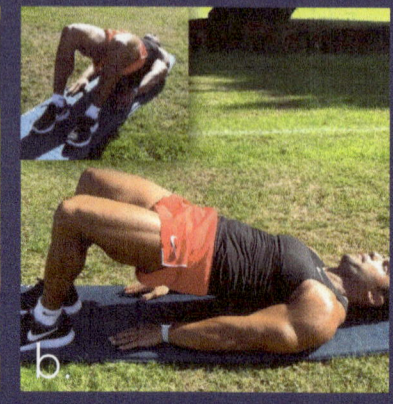

166 | GOKAY KURTULDUM

4. Leg Kicks Right

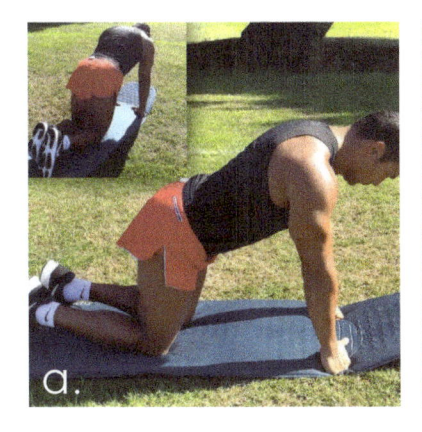

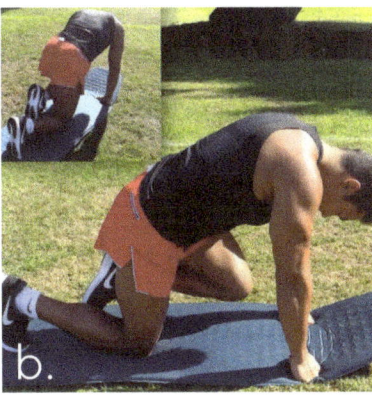

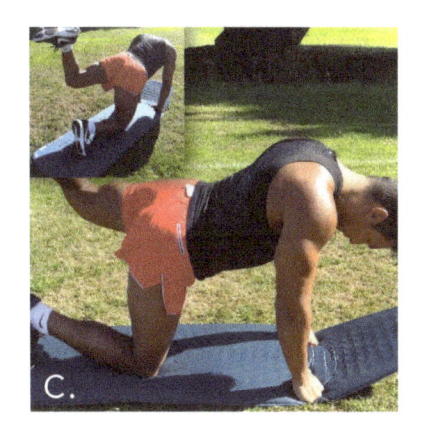

a.   b.   c.

5. Leg Kicks Left

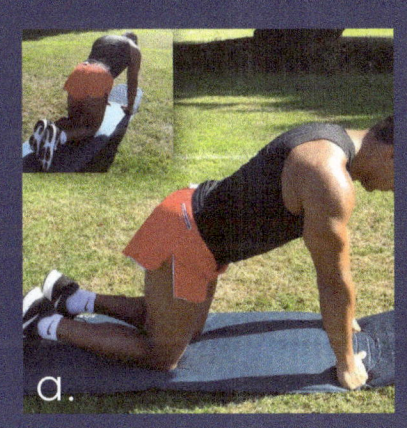

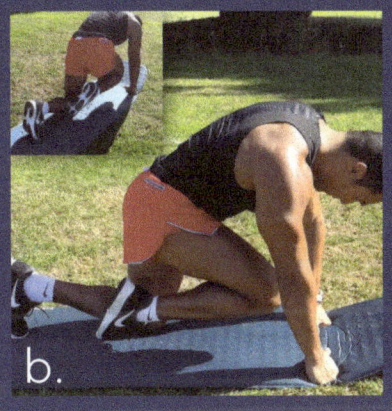

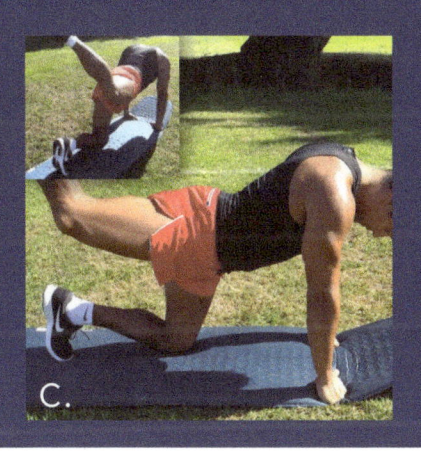

a.   b.   c.

6. Skydiver

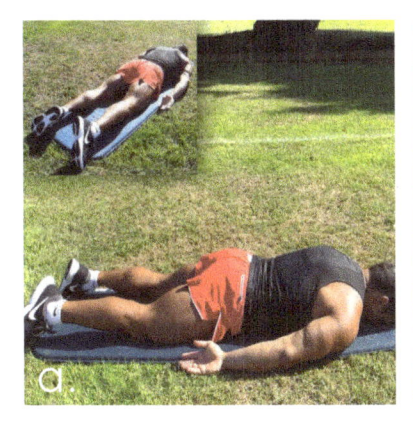

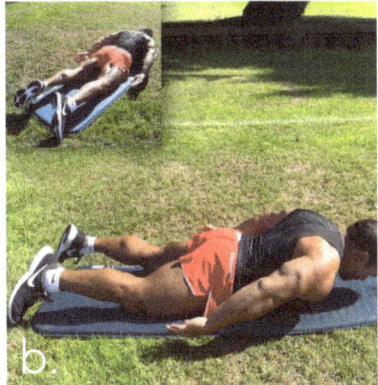

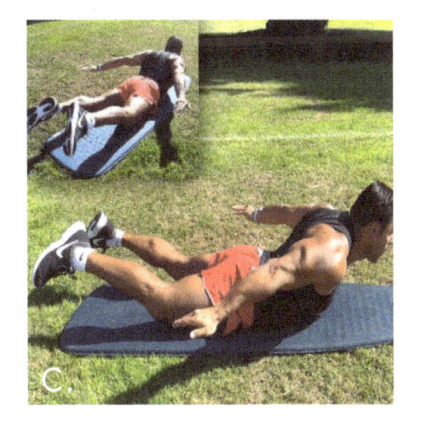

a.   b.   c.

GET FIT, STAY FIT | 167

7. Side Leg Kicks Right

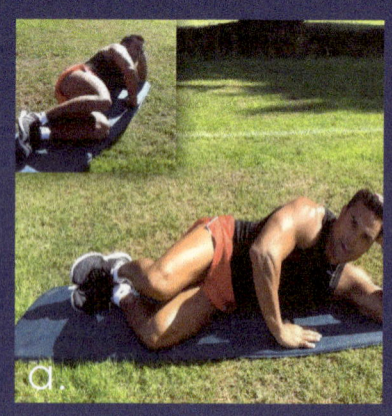

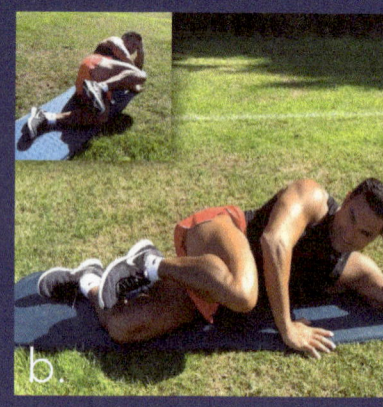

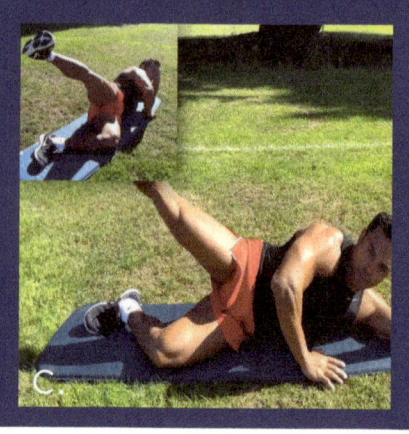

8. Side Leg Kicks Left

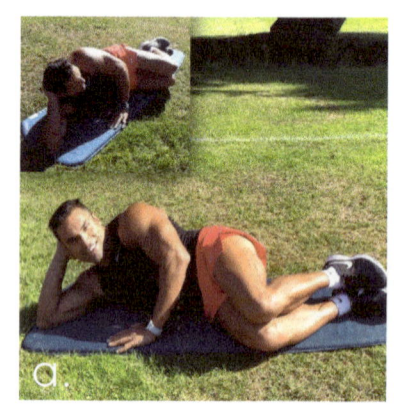

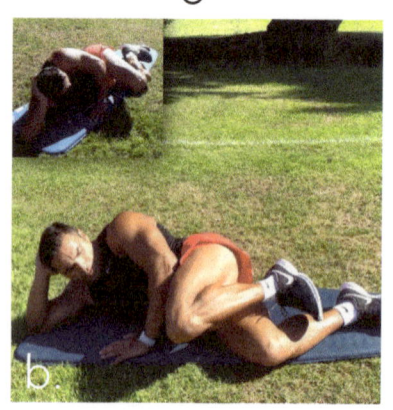

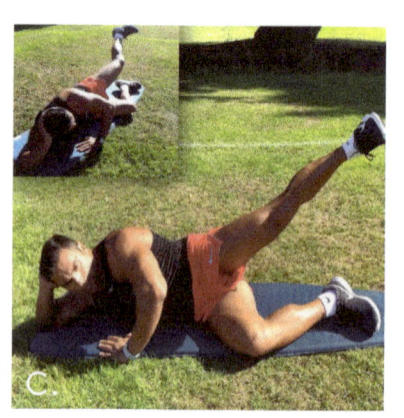

DAY 16
UPPER BODY WEIGHT TRAINING PROGRAMME 1

Day 16 involves a gym workout. This is the same as the workout you did on Day 2 and Day 9. However, you will do these for 4 sets and the duration of the Plank is a bit longer. You will again rest 45-60 seconds between each set. The tempo for each repetition should be 1 second up, 1 second down (or vice versa).

1.	Barbell Chest Press	4 sets x 12 repetitions per set
2.	Cable Fly	4 sets x 12 reps
3.	Lat Pull Down	4 sets x 12 reps
4.	Seated Rowing	4 sets x 12 reps
5.	Machine Shoulder Press	4 sets x 12 reps
6.	Barbell Biceps Curl	4 sets x 12 reps
7.	Cable V-Bar Triceps Extension	4 sets x 12 reps
8.	Plank	4 sets x 45 secs+ (feel free to stay longer, as long as your posture is correct)

1. Barbell Chest Press

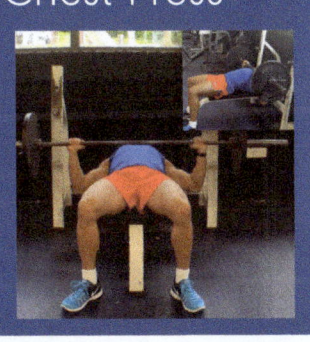

2. Cable Fly

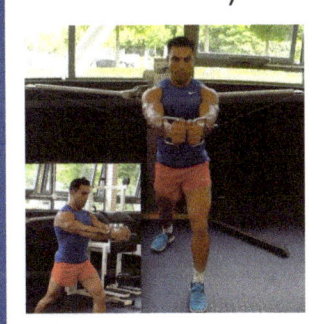

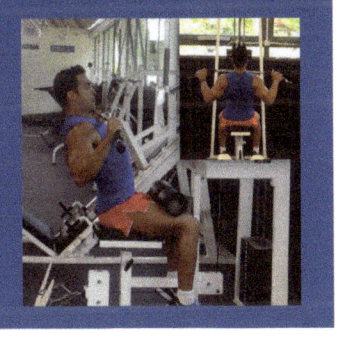

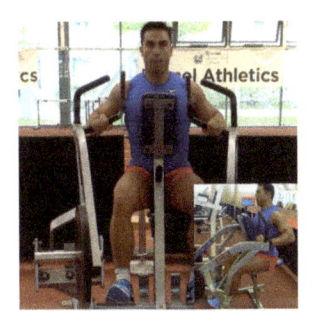

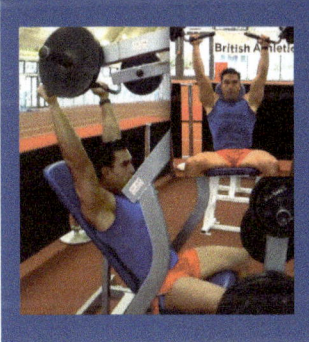

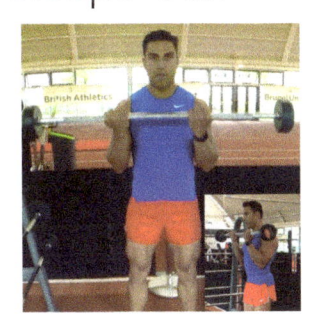

3. Lat Pull Down

4. Seated Rowing

5. Machine Shoulder Press

6. Barbell Biceps Curl

7. Cable V-Bar Triceps Extension

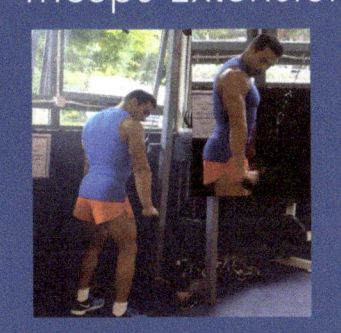

8. Plank

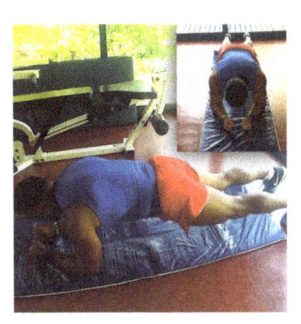

GET FIT, STAY FIT | 169

DAY 17
HOME WORKOUT 10 (PYRAMID)

Day 17's workout is a challenging one, descending pyramid-style, with 3 exercises.

You will start with press-ups for 30 seconds (press-ups on knees are allowed!) then take a 15 second rest. Set 2 is press-ups for 20 seconds with a 15 second rest again, then press-ups for 10 seconds. This is followed by 30 seconds of Abs Scissors, lasting 20 and 10 seconds with a 15 second break between each set. The final exercise is Horizontal Side Jumps, the cardio aspect for the day, again for 30, 20 and 10 seconds with 15 seconds' break between every set. Do 3 sets.

1. Press-ups — 30 secs on, 15 secs off
2. Press-ups — 20 secs on, 15 secs off
3. Press-ups — 10 secs on, 15 secs off
4. Abs Scissors — 30 secs on, 15 secs off
5. Abs Scissors — 20 secs on, 15 secs off
6. Abs Scissors — 10 secs on, 15 secs off
7. Horizontal Side Jumps — 30 secs on, 15 secs off
8. Horizontal Side Jumps — 20 secs on, 15 secs off
9. Horizontal Side Jumps — 10 secs on, 15 secs off

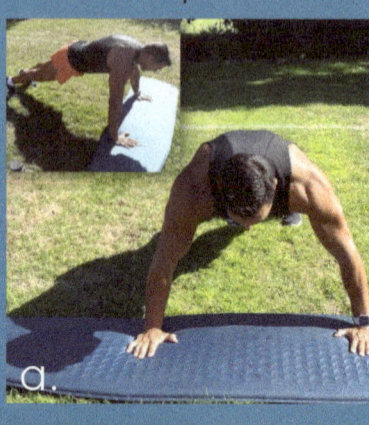

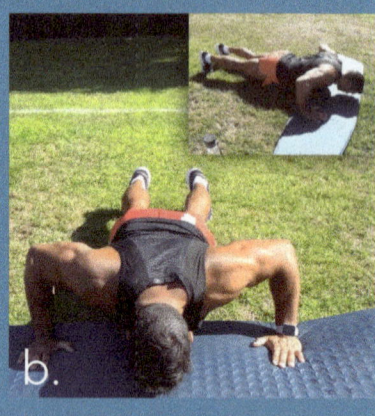

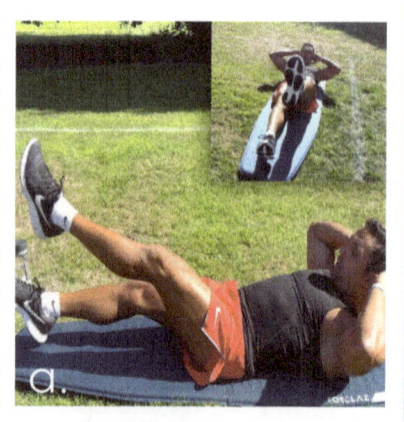

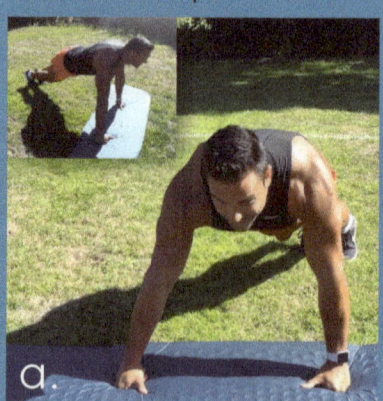

1. Press-ups

2. Abs Scissors

3. Horizontal Side Jumps

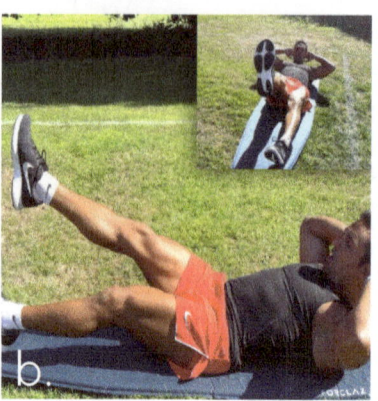

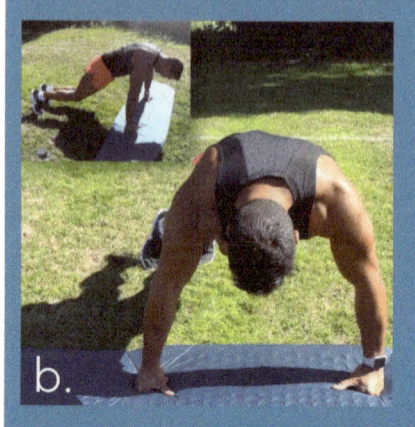

170 | GOKAY KURTULDUM

DAY 18
LOWER BODY WEIGHT TRAINING PROGRAMME 1

Today you'll be working your lower body at the gym. The same workout you did on Day 4 and Day 11. However, you will do 4 sets today. The rest is the same as last time: 45-60 seconds between each set. The tempo for each repetition should be 1 second up, 1 second down (or vice versa).

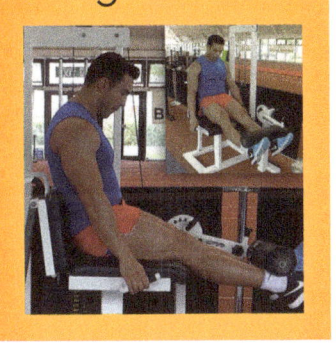

1. Leg Extension — 4 sets x 15 repetitions per set
2. Leg Curl — 4 sets x 15 reps
3. Leg Press — 4 sets x 12 reps
4. Dumbbell Alternating Backward Lunges — 4 sets x 10 reps
5. Side Plank — 4 sets x 40 secs each side
6. Abs Vertical Scissors — 4 sets x 40 secs
7. Abs Crunches with Hands on Thighs — 4 sets x 30 reps

1. Leg Extension

2. Leg Curl

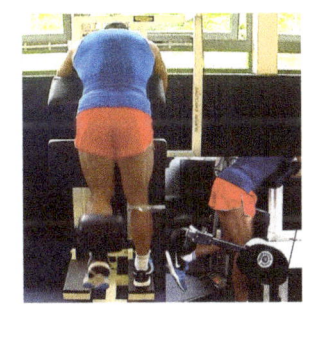

3. Leg Press

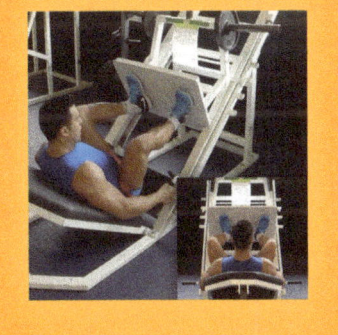

4. Dumbbell Alternating Backward Lunges

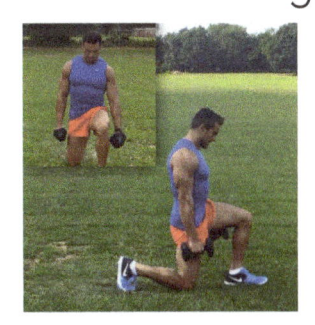

5. Side Plank

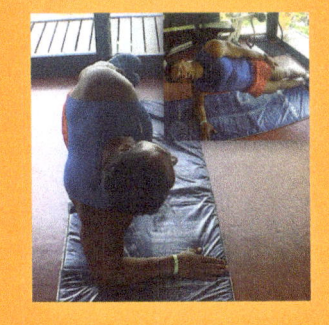

6. Abs Vertical Scissors

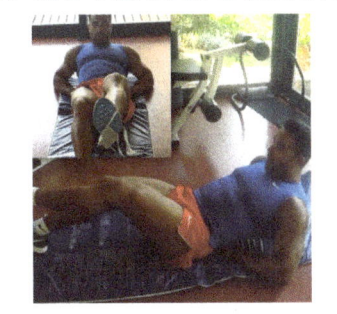

7. Abs Crunches

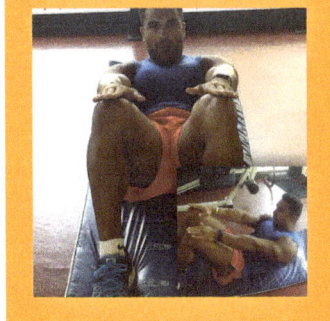

GET FIT, STAY FIT | 171

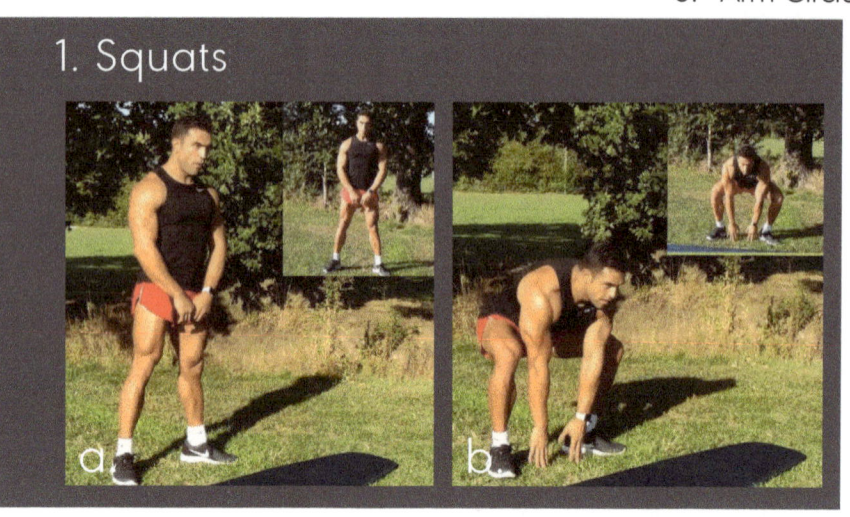

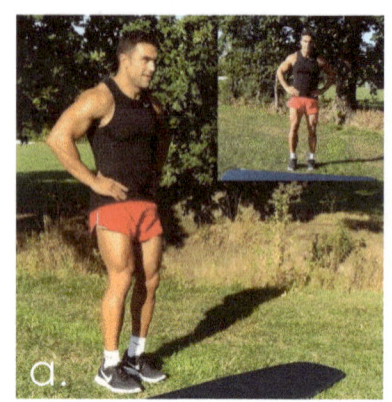

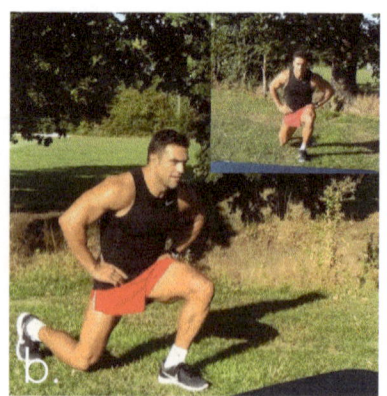

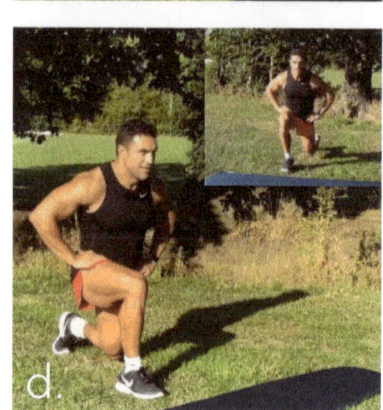

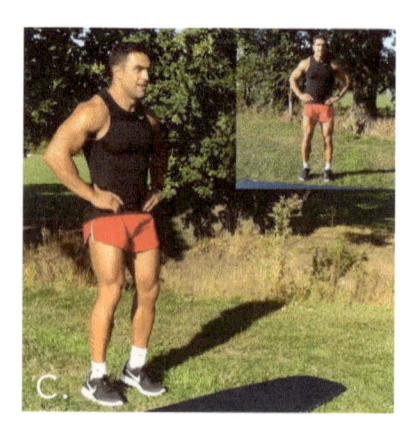

DAY 19
HOME WORKOUT 6

This workout involves 6 exercises, not 4, and each exercise is going to be for 30 seconds with a 20 second break in between. You will do these for 3 sets.

1. Squats — 30 secs on, 20 secs off
2. Alternating Backward Lunges — 30 secs on, 20 secs off
3. Upper Cuts — 30 secs on, 20 secs off
4. Lateral Plank Walks — 30 secs on, 20 secs off
5. Rhomboid Squeezes — 30 secs on, 20 secs off
6. Arm Circles — 30 secs on, 20 secs off

1. Squats

2. Alternating Backward Lunges

172 | GOKAY KURTULDUM

3. Upper Cuts

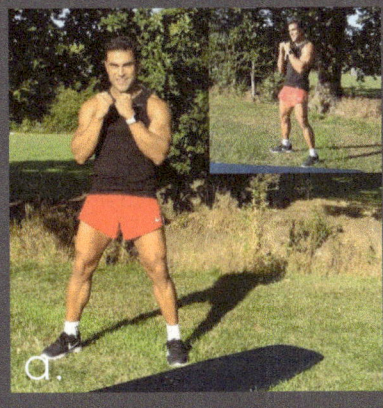

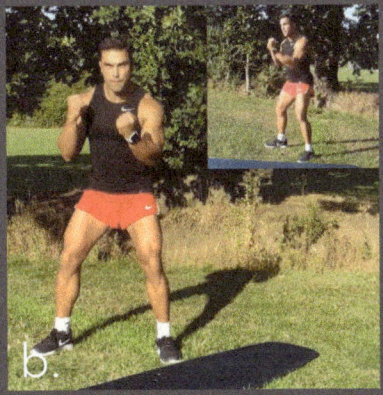

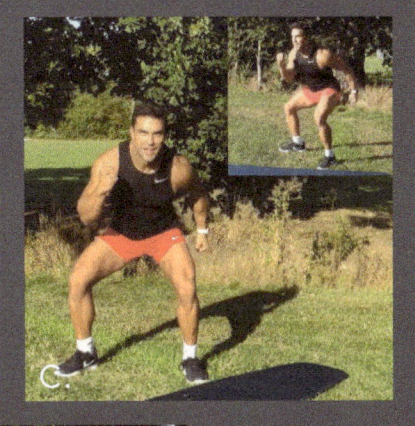

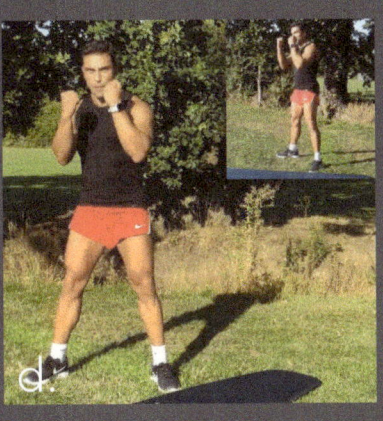

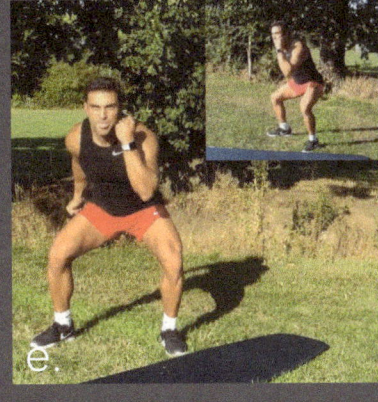

4. Lateral Plank Walks

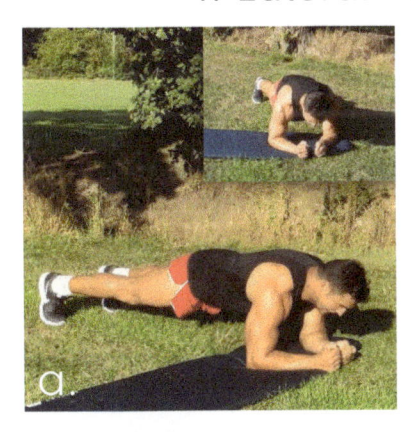

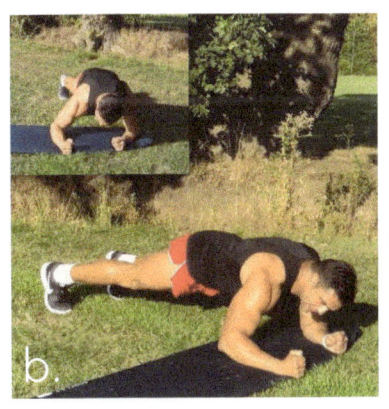

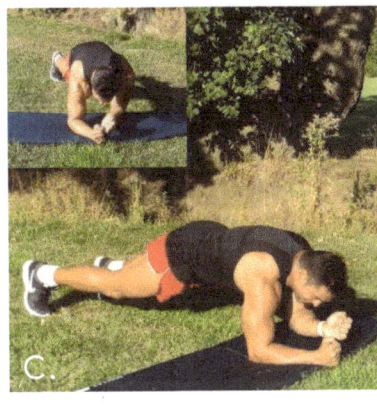

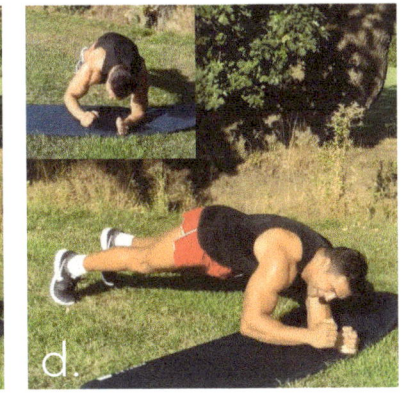

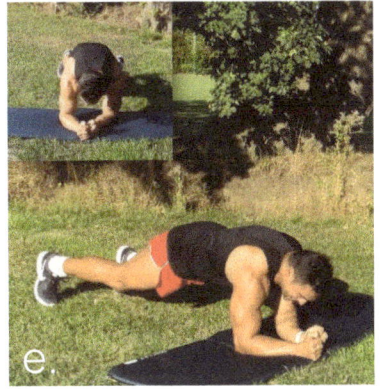

GET FIT, STAY FIT | 173

5. Rhomboid Squeezes

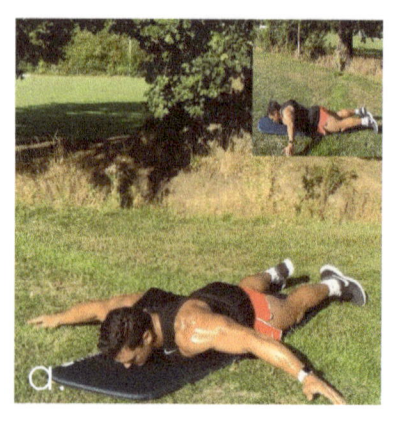

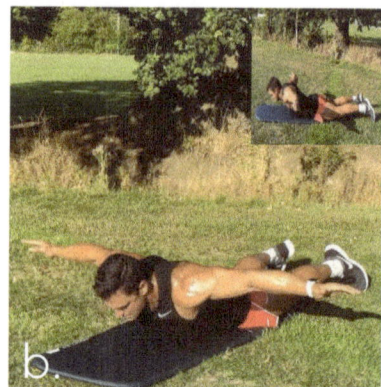

6. Arm Circles

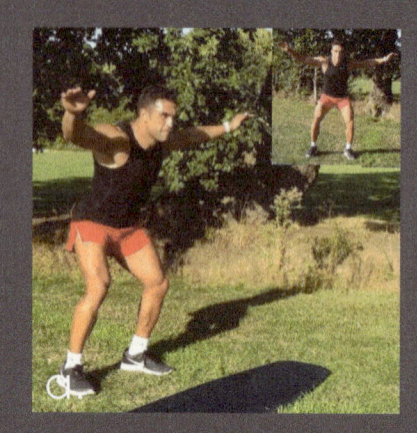

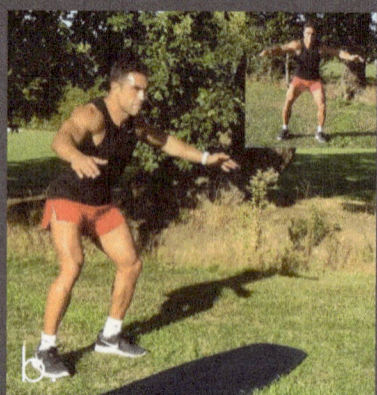

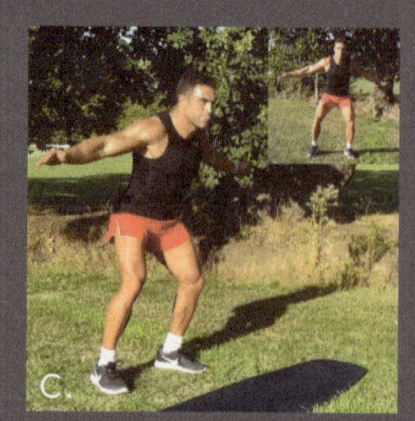

DAY 20
HOME WORKOUT 7

As with Day 19, you have 6 exercises today. Each one is for 30 seconds with 20 seconds' rest in between. You will do 3 sets.

1. Split Squats Right — 30 secs on, 20 secs off
2. Split Squats Left — 30 secs on, 20 secs off
3. Dead Bug — 30 secs on, 20 secs off
4. Press-ups and Rotate — 30 secs on, 20 secs off
5. Slalom Side-hops — 30 secs on, 20 secs off
6. Plank Step In and Out — 30 secs on, 20 secs off

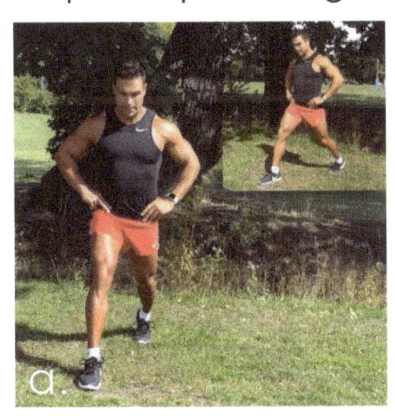

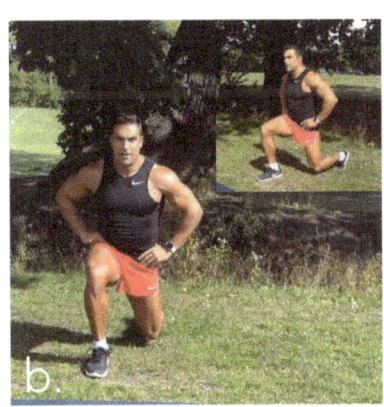

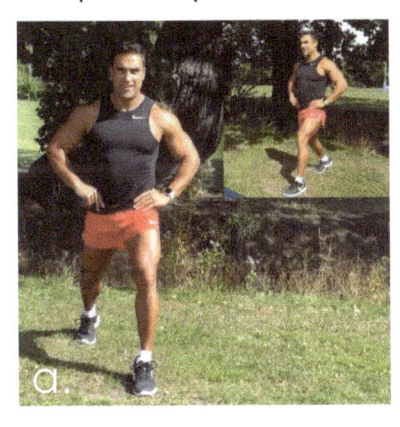

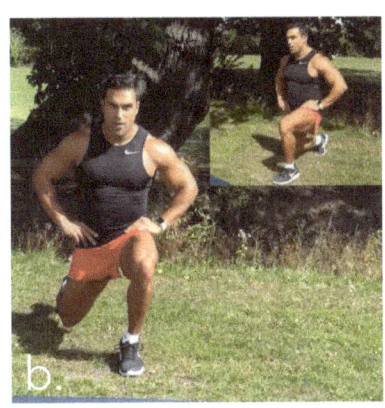

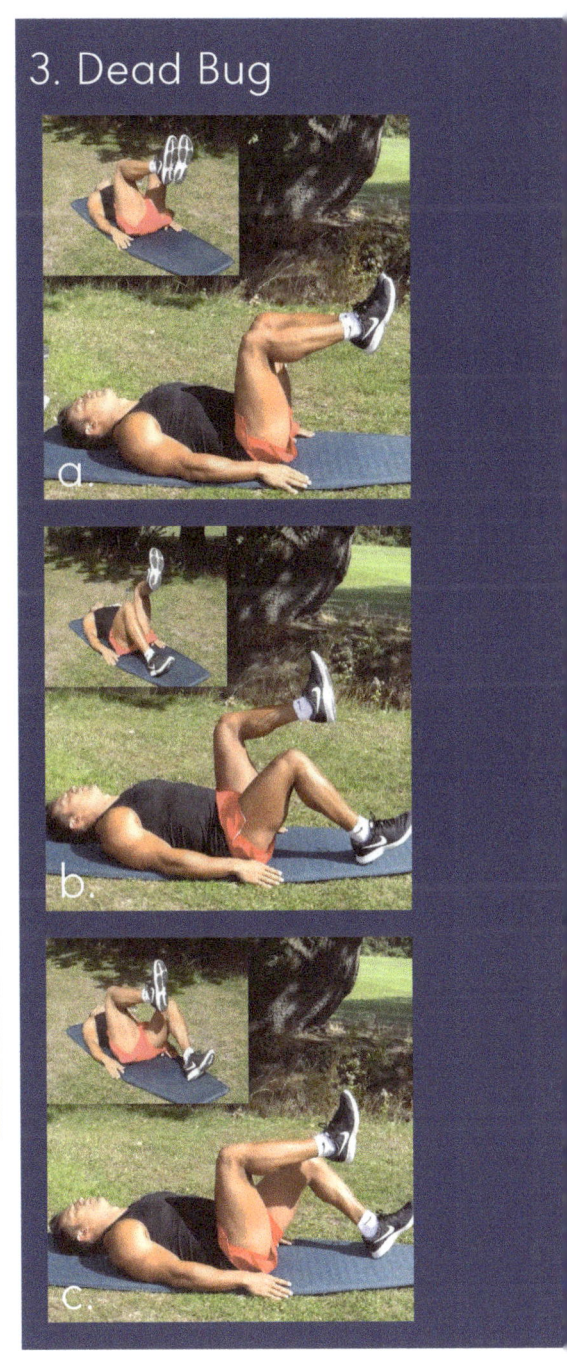

1. Split Squats Right

2. Split Squats Left

3. Dead Bug

GET FIT, STAY FIT | 175

4. Press-ups and Rotate

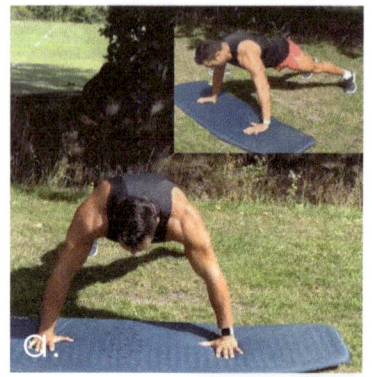

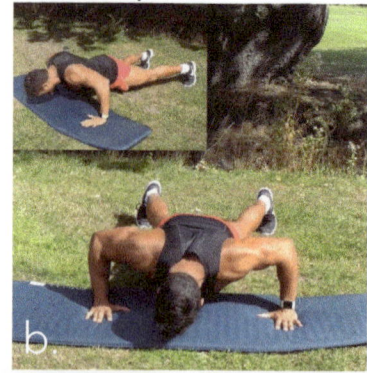

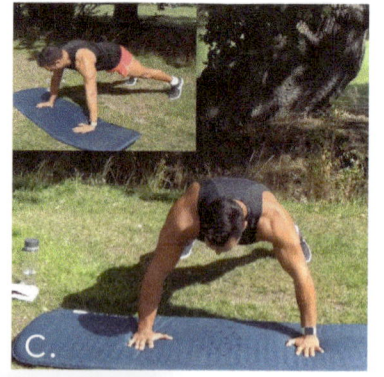

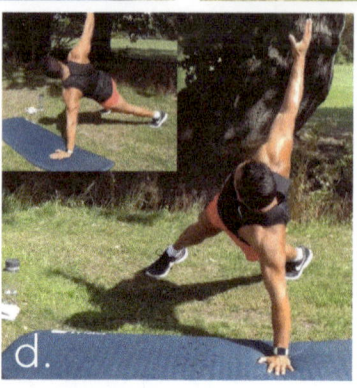

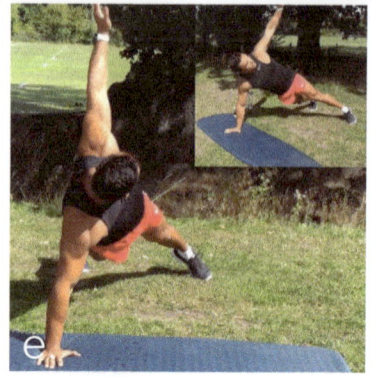

a.
b.
c.
d.
e.

5. Slalom Side-hops

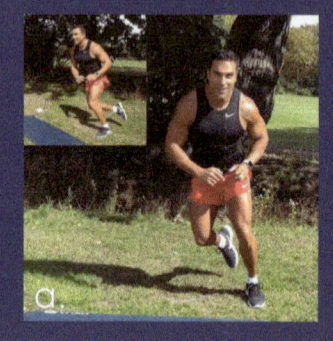

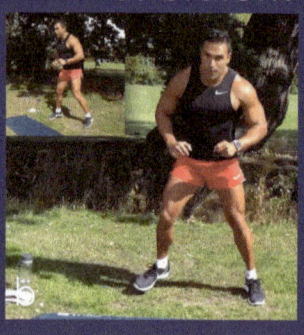

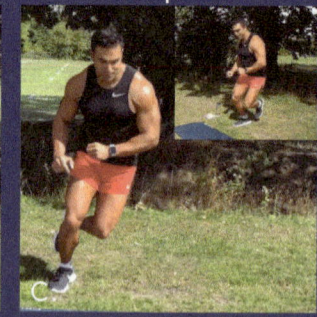

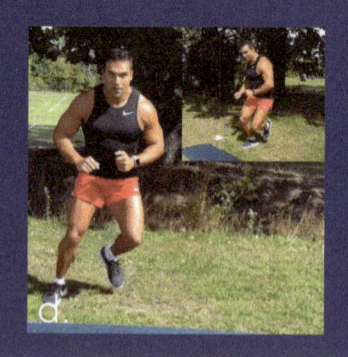

a.
b.
c.
d.

6. Plank Step In and Out

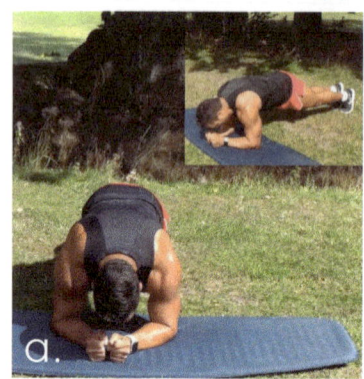

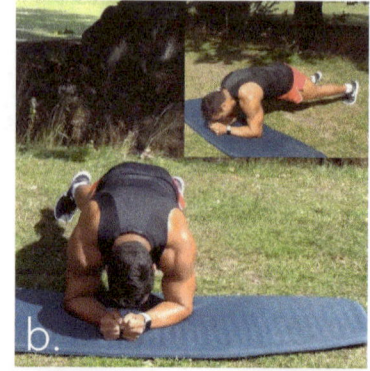

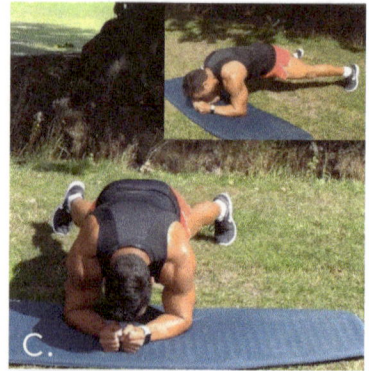

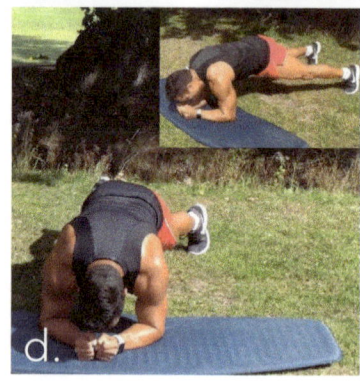

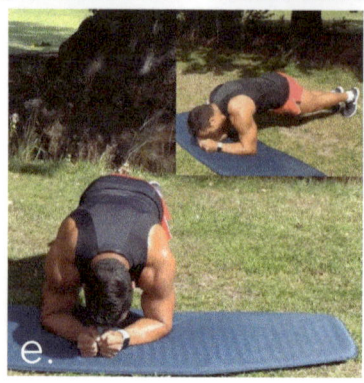

a.
b.
c.
d.
e.

DAY 21 OFF

WEEK 3 PROGRESS JOURNAL

Use these pages to set your intentions at the start of the week and record and reflect on your progress at the end of the week. Alternatively, use a special notebook for this purpose.

PART 1: INTENTIONS/PLANNING

My starting weight this week: _____

My starting waist measurement: _____

My goal weight at the end of this week: _____

My goal waist measurement at the end of this week: _____

Any other goals for the week (e.g. no alcohol during the week and no more than 14 units during the weekend or going to bed early weekdays and sleep minimum 7 hours etc.)

_____

_____

Which days are going to be tricky this week and why? (E.g. client dinner on Thursday which involves drinking alcohol)

_____

How will I deal with this? _____

_____

GET FIT, STAY FIT | 177

Any other notes/thoughts:

PART 2: RECORD/REFLECTIONS

At the end of this week how many goals did I achieve? _____

How many did I come close to? _____

How am I feeling about my progress? _____

Which goals did I not reach? _____

Why was that? Family commitments, too much work and no time, not motivated enough? Can I define exactly what hindered my progress? Can I take action on that next week?

What actions can I take next week to improve on this?

What were my wins this week? (e.g. weight loss, mileage run etc?)

I've achieved

Give marks out of 10 for progress this week

8.7 WEEK 4 PROGRAMME AND JOURNAL PAGES

This week, your gym workouts change and it may take you a little while to get to know the exercises you are doing for your upper and lower body. But once you've done them a few times, you'll become familiar with the names. Please pay close attention to the exercise instructions in Chapter 11: they point out the correct techniques which are so important when it comes to maximising benefits as well as minimising the risk of injury. In addition, you have only one home workout this week, again for 15 minutes. You will have 2 days off this week. Start with Part 1 of this week's journal, as usual.

Here's a summary of your Week 4 programme:

Day 22	Upper Body Weight Training P2(a)
Day 23	Lower Body Weight Training P2(a)
Day 24	Home Workout 8
Day 25	Upper Body Weight Training P2(b)
Day 26	Lower Body Weight Training P2(b)
Day 27	OFF
Day 28	OFF

Now do the day-by-day exercises on the following pages.

DAY 22
UPPER BODY WEIGHT TRAINING PROGRAMME 2(A)

Today is a gym session. You are going to change the upper body programme. This is more advanced than Upper Body Programme 1. The tempo for each repetition should be 1 second up, 1 second down (or vice versa). You will do these for 3 sets.

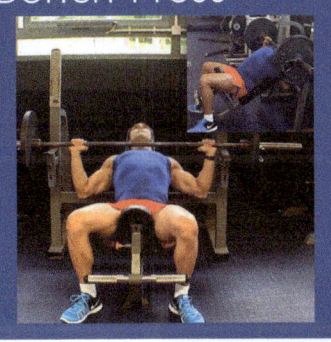

1. Inclined Barbell Bench Press — 3 sets x 12 repetitions
2. Dumbbells Chest Fly — 3 sets x 12 reps
3. Dumbbells Inclined Bench Press — 3 sets x 12 reps
4. Dumbbell One Arm Rowing — 3 sets x 12 reps
5. Cable Reverse Fly (Back Extension) — 3 sets x 12 reps
6. Lat Pull Down Wide Overhand Grip — 3 sets x 12 reps
7. Cable Crunches — 3 sets x 20 reps
8. Leg Raises — 3 sets x 20 reps

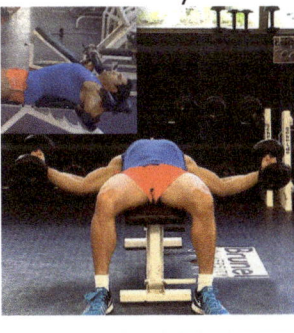

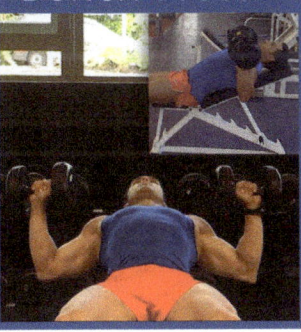

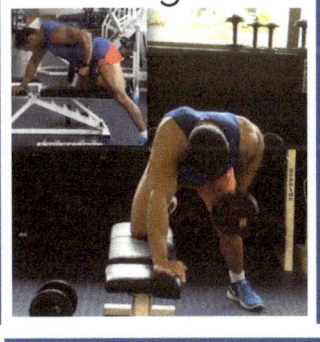

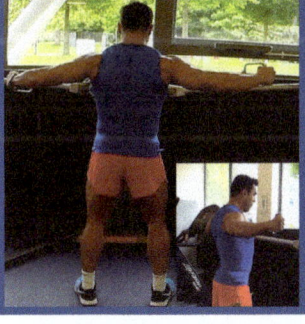

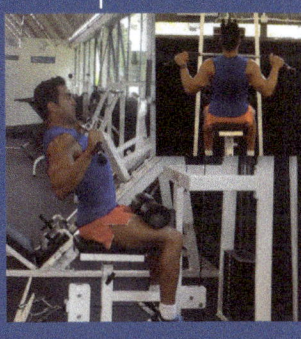

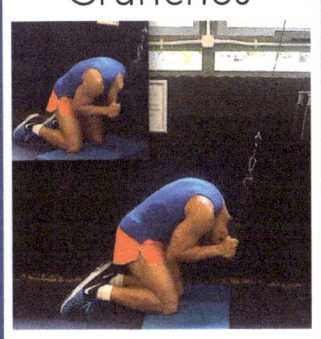

1. Inclined Barbell Bench Press
2. Dumbbells Chest Fly
3. Dumbbells Inclined Bench Press
4. Dumbbell One Arm Rowing
5. Cable Reverse Fly
6. Lat Pull Down Wide Overhand Grip
7. Cable Crunches
8. Leg Raises

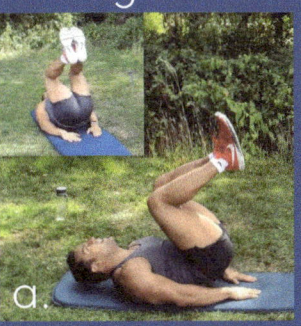

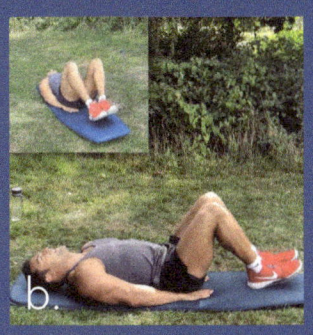

GET FIT, STAY FIT | 181

DAY 23
LOWER BODY WEIGHT TRAINING PROGRAMME 2(A)

Today is another gym day. As with yesterday's session, I've changed your lower body programme to a more advanced session. The tempo for each repetition should be 1 second up, 1 second down (or vice versa). There are 7 exercises only so you'll do 4 sets of leg exercises and 3 sets of core.

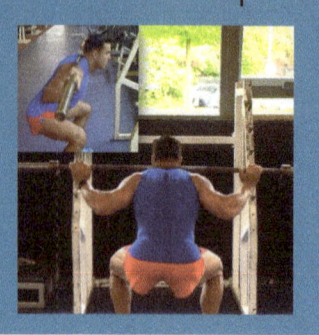

1. Barbell Squats — 4 sets x 12 repetitions
2. Side Lunges — 4 sets x 15 reps each side
3. Barbell Deadlift — 4 sets x 12 reps
4. Oblique (Russian) Twist — 3 sets x 20 reps each side
5. Plank — 3 sets x 45 secs
6. Oblique Crunches — 3 sets x 25 reps each side
7. Slow Release Sit-ups — 3 sets x 20 reps

1. Barbell Squats

2. Side Lunges

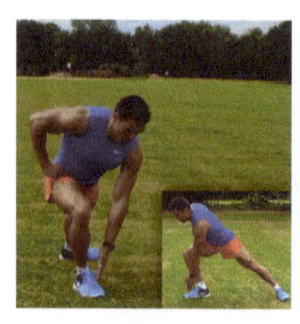

3. Barbell Deadlift

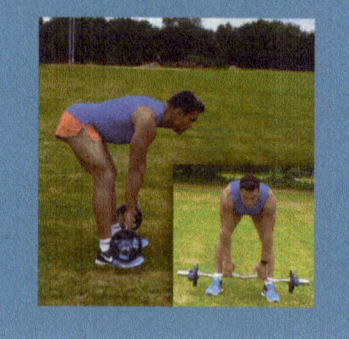

4. Oblique (Russian) Twist

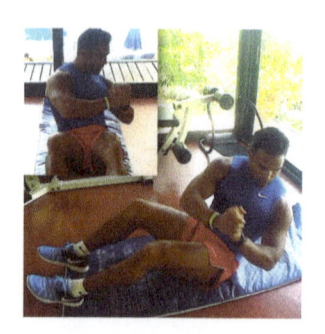

5. Plank

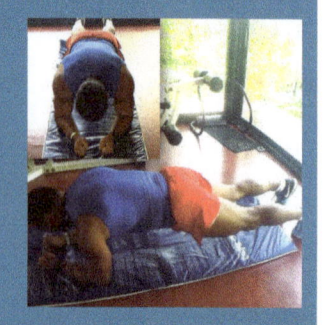

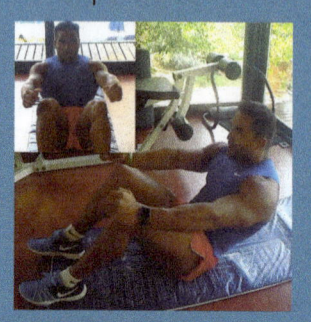

6. Oblique Crunches

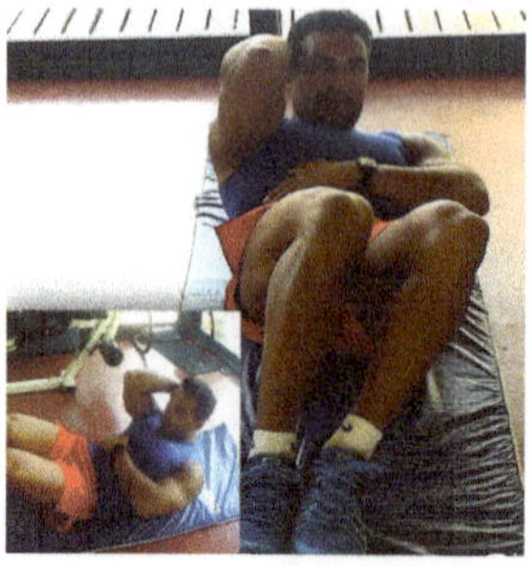

7. Slow Release Sit-ups

DAY 24
HOME WORKOUT 8

Today you'll repeat the workout you did on Day 13.

3 of the 6 exercises are cardio exercises. Each exercise lasts for 30 seconds with 20 seconds' rest.

1. Good Morning — 30 secs on, 20 secs off
2. Side Touch Shuttles — 30 secs on, 20 secs off
3. Plank with Knee Flexion — 30 secs on, 20 secs off
4. Squat and Jump — 30 secs on, 20 secs off
5. Floor Triceps Dips — 30 secs on, 20 secs off
6. Spotty Dog — 30 secs on, 20 secs off

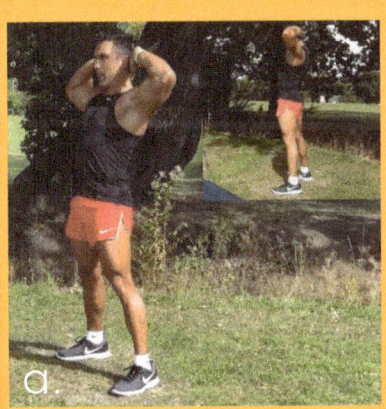

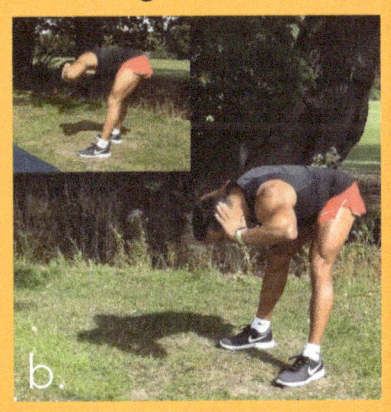

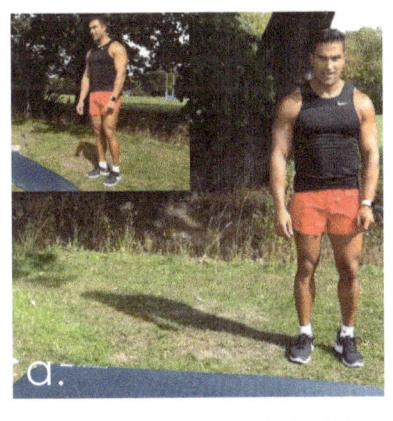

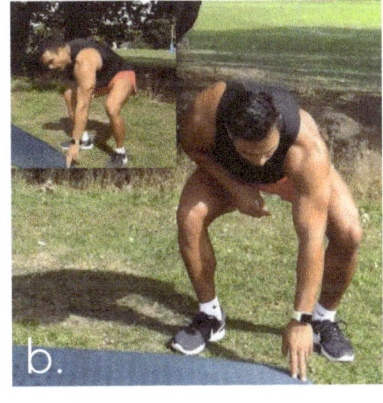

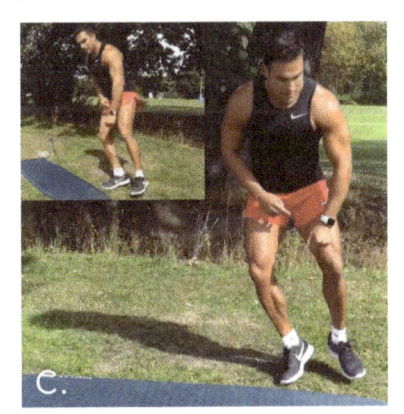

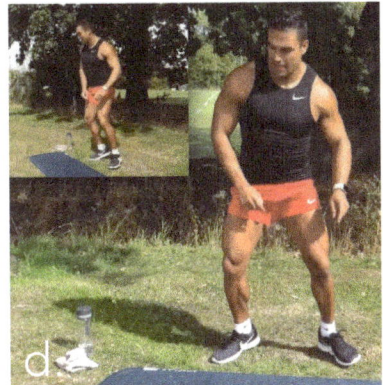

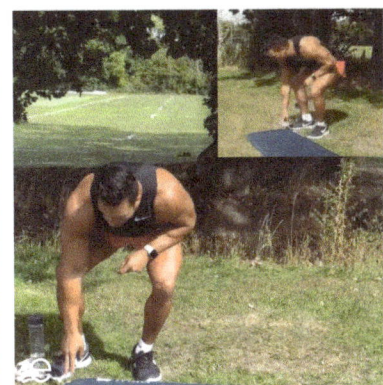

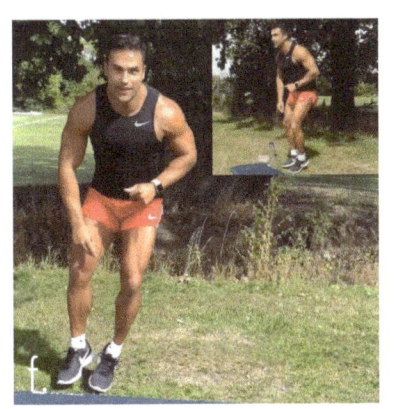

1. Good Morning

2. Side Touch Shuttles

GET FIT, STAY FIT | 183

3. Plank with Knee Flexion

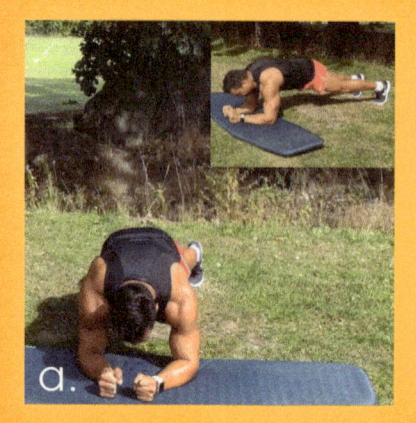

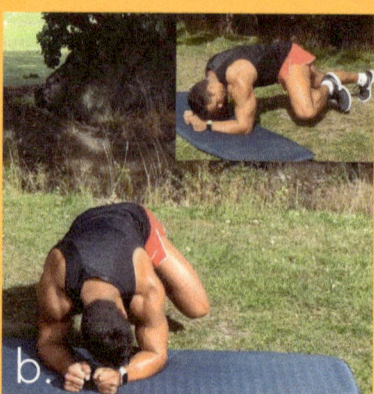

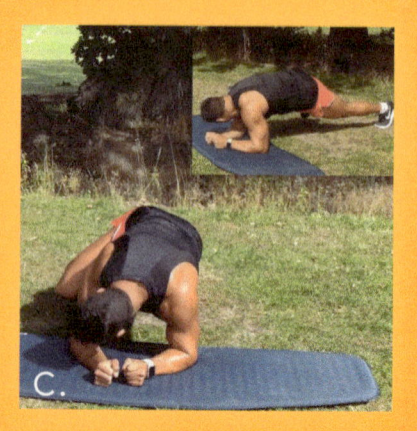

4. Squat and Jump

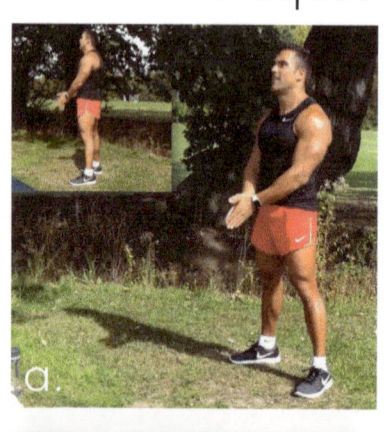

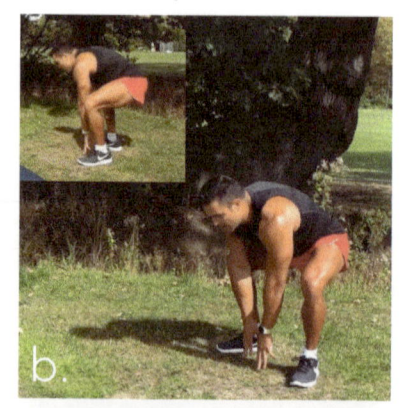

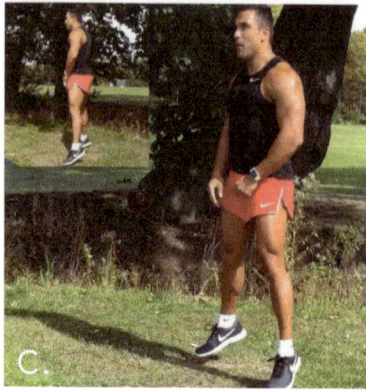

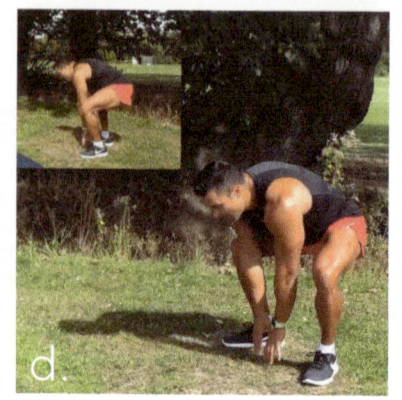

184 | GOKAY KURTULDUM

5. Floor Triceps Dips

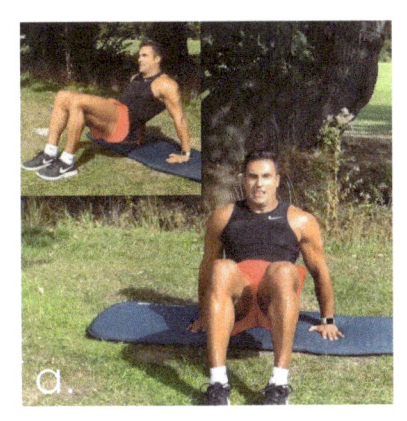

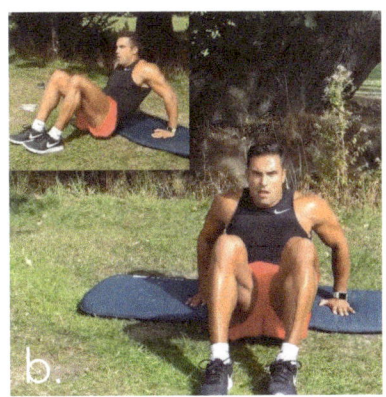

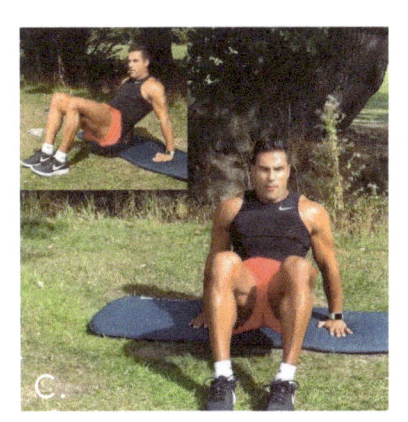

6. Spotty Dog

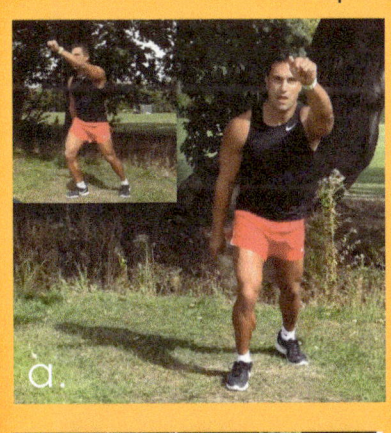

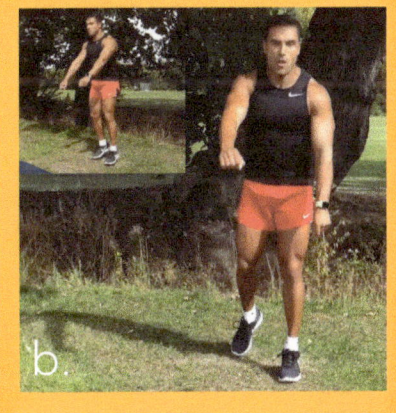

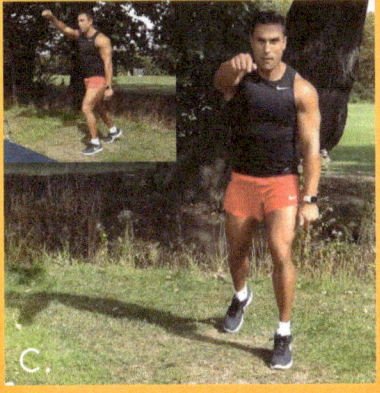

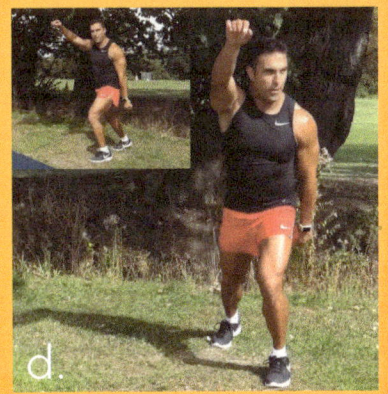

GET FIT, STAY FIT | 185

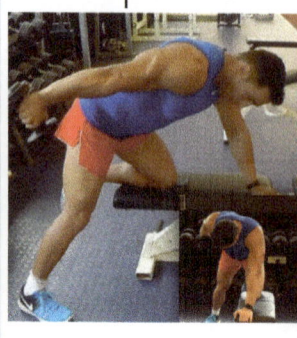

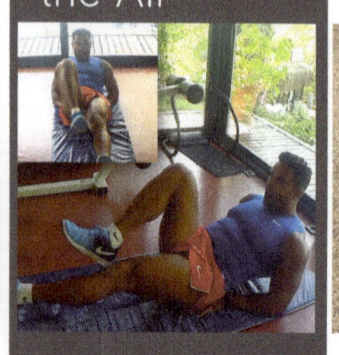

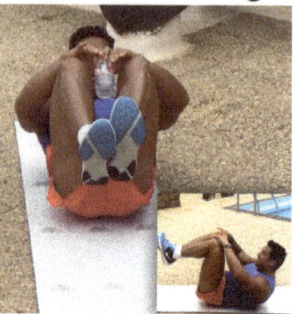

DAY 25
UPPER BODY WEIGHT TRAINING PROGRAMME 2(B)

I've split your advanced upper body programme into two sections, (a) and (b). So today we will do Upper Body Programme 2(b). The tempo for each repetition should be 1 second up, 1 second down (or vice versa).

1. Barbell Shoulder Press — 4 sets x 12 repetitions
2. Dumbbell Side Laterals — 4 sets x 12 reps
3. Cable Front Raise — 3 sets x 12 reps
4. EZ Barbell Biceps Curl — 3 sets x 12 reps
5. Dumbbell Inclined Biceps Curl — 3 sets x 12 reps
6. Standing EZ Bar Triceps Extension — 3 sets x 12 reps
7. Dumbbell One Arm Triceps Kick — 3 sets x 12 reps each side
8. Cycling in the Air — 3 sets x 30 secs
9. Dead Bug — 3 sets x 15 reps each side

1. Barbell Shoulder Press
2. Dumbbells Side Laterals
3. Cable Front Raise
4. EZ Barbell Biceps Curl
5. Dumbbell Inclined Biceps Curl
6. Standing EZ Bar Triceps Extension
7. Dumbbell One Arm Triceps Kick
8. Cycling in the Air
9. Dead Bug

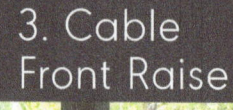

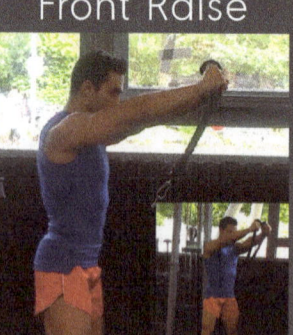

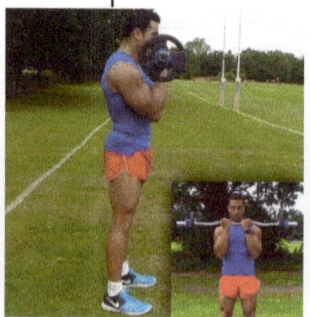

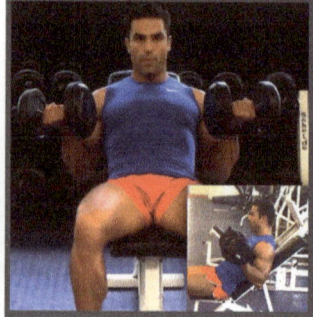

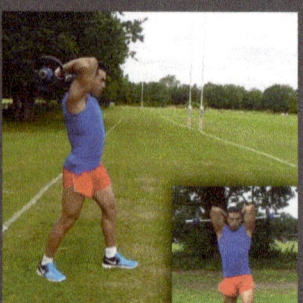

DAY 26
LOWER BODY WEIGHT TRAINING PROGRAMME 2(B)

I've split your advanced lower body programme into two sections, (a) and (b). So today we will do Lower Body Programme 2(b). The tempo for each repetition should be 1 second up, 1 second down (or vice versa).

1. Leg Extension — 3 sets x 15 repetitions
2. TRX Squat Jumps — 3 sets x 15 reps
3. Leg Curl — 3 sets x 15 reps
4. Split Squats — 3 sets x 15 reps each side
5. Abdominal Crunches with Raised Arms — 3 sets x 30 reps
6. Abs Scissors Heel Taps — 3 sets x 20 reps each side
7. Oblique Crunches — 3 sets x 30 reps each side
8. Plank Weight Rotation — 3 sets x 10 each direction

1. Leg Extension

2. TRX Squat Jumps

3. Leg Curl

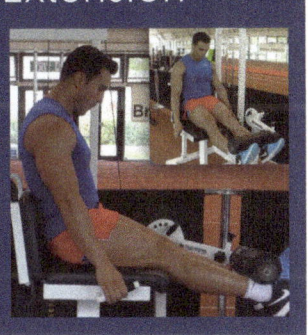

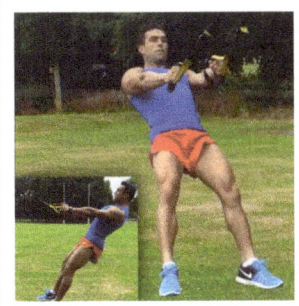

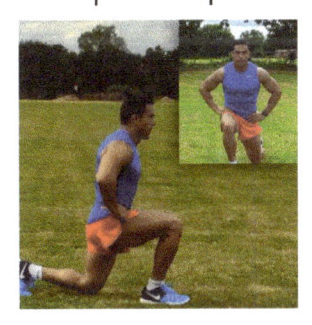

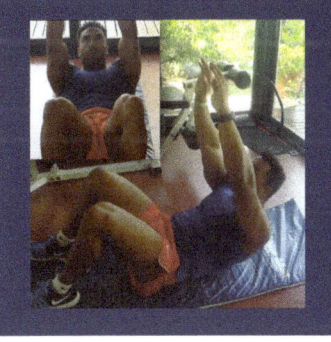

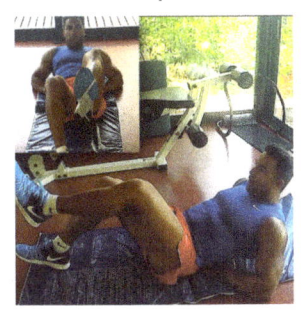

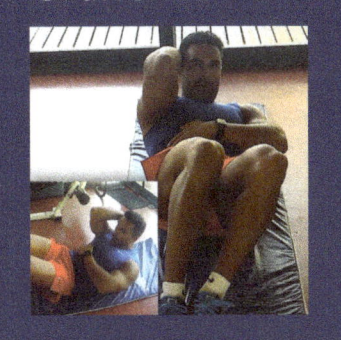

4. Split Squats

5. Abdominal Crunches with Raised Arms

6. Abs Scissors Heel Taps

7. Oblique Crunches

8. Plank Weight Rotation

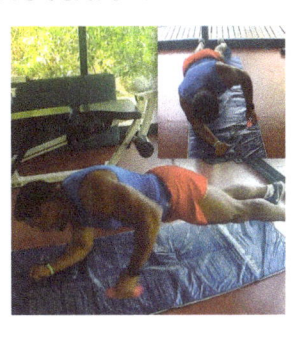

GET FIT, STAY FIT | 187

DAY 27 AND 28 OFF

WEEK 4 PROGRESS JOURNAL

Use these pages to set your intentions at the start of the week and record and reflect on your progress at the end of the week. Alternatively, use a special notebook for this purpose.

PART 1: INTENTIONS/PLANNING

My starting weight this week: _____

My starting waist measurement: _____

My goal weight at the end of this week: _____

My goal waist measurement at the end of this week: _____

Any other goals for the week (e.g. no alcohol during the week and no more than 14 units during the weekend or going to bed early weekdays and sleep minimum 7 hours etc.)

_____

_____

Which days are going to be tricky this week and why? (E.g. client dinner on Thursday which involves drinking alcohol)

_____

How will I deal with this? _____

_____

Any other notes/thoughts:

PART 2: RECORD/REFLECTIONS

At the end of this week how many goals did I achieve? _____

How many did I come close to? _____

How am I feeling about my progress? _____

Which goals did I not reach? _____

Why was that? Family commitments, too much work and no time, not motivated enough? Can I define exactly what hindered my progress? Can I take action on that next week?

What actions can I take next week to improve on this?

What were my wins this week? (e.g. weight loss, mileage run etc?)

I've achieved

Give marks out of 10 for progress this week

8.8 WEEK 5 PROGRAMME AND JOURNAL PAGES

During this week, home workouts are prioritised. This will save you time if you happen to have a busy week. You'll work your muscles at the gym twice this week, to build muscle and strength. You will notice that two of the home workouts are now 20 minutes long – you are building stamina! Turn to Part 1 of your journal first.

Here's a summary of your Week 5 programme:

Day 29   Home Workout 9
Day 30   Upper Body Weight Training P2(a)
Day 31   Home Workout 10 (Pyramid)
Day 32   Lower Body Weight Training P2(a)
Day 33   Home Workout 11
Day 34   Home Workout 12
Day 35   OFF

Now complete your day-by-day exercises on the following pages.

DAY 29
HOME WORKOUT 9

Here you repeat the workout you did on Day 15.

This involves loads of floor exercises so you won't be moving about much. You'll work your gluteus (bum) a lot and also your back. There are 8 exercises and each one is for 30 seconds but with only 8 seconds' rest. Do 3 sets.

1. Clams Right — 30 secs on, 8 secs off
2. Clams Left — 30 secs on, 8 secs off
3. Bridge — 30 secs on, 8 secs off
4. Leg Kicks Right — 30 secs on, 8 secs off
5. Leg Kicks Left — 30 secs on, 8 secs off
6. Skydiver — 30 secs on, 8 secs off
7. Side Leg Kicks Right — 30 secs on, 8 secs off
8. Side Leg Kicks Left — 30 secs on, 8 secs off

1. Clams Right

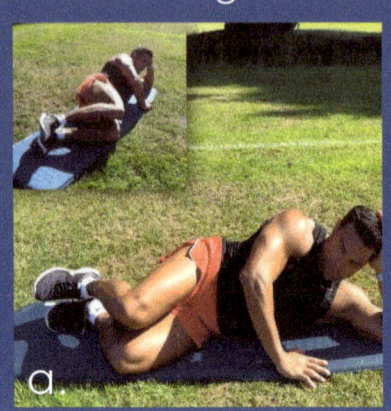

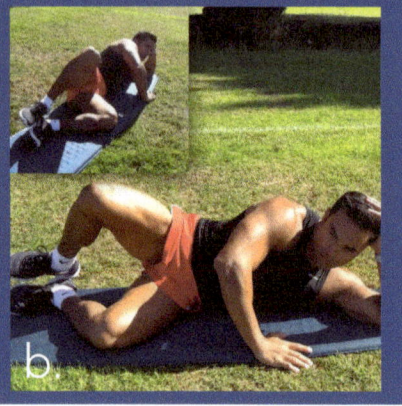

2. Clams Left

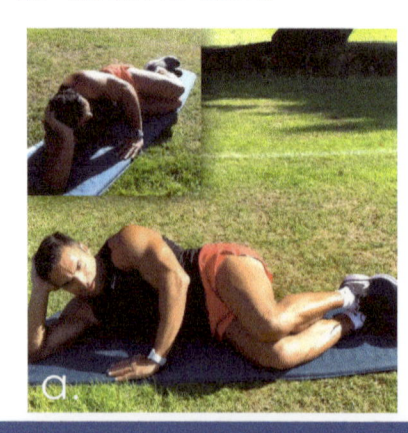

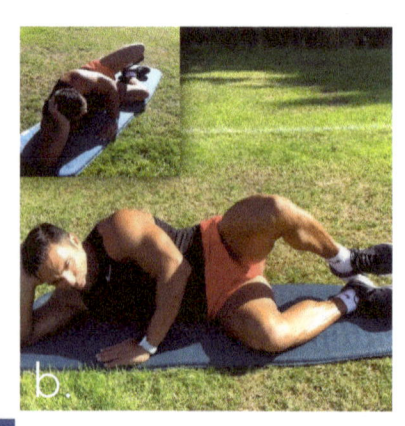

3. Bridge

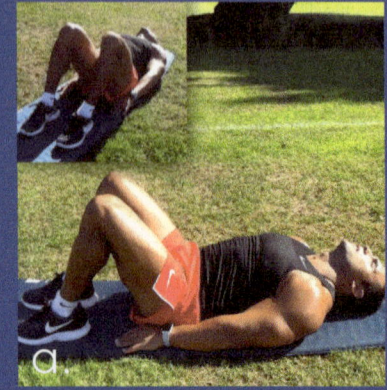

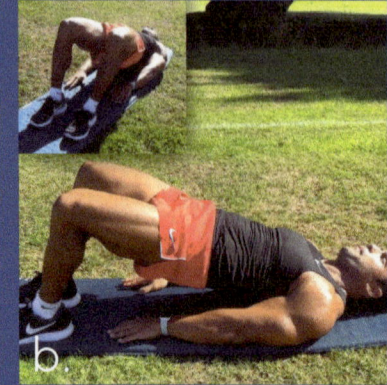

192 | GOKAY KURTULDUM

4. Leg Kicks Right

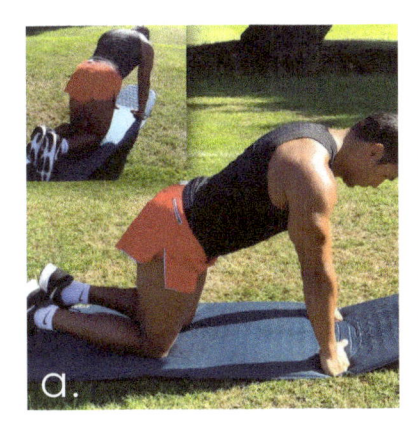

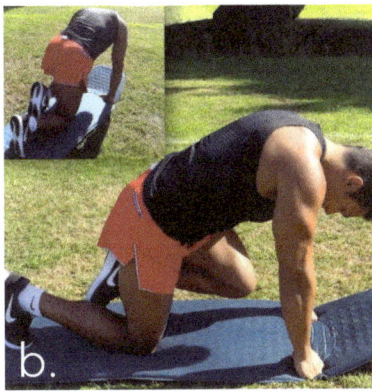

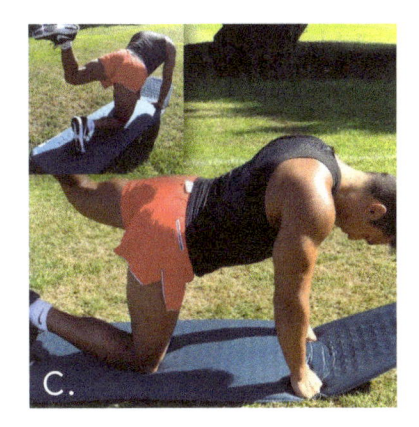

a.   b.   c.

5. Leg Kicks Left

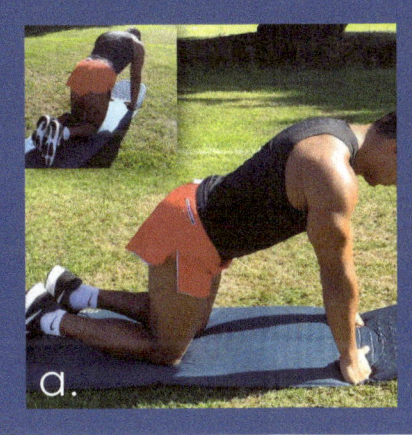

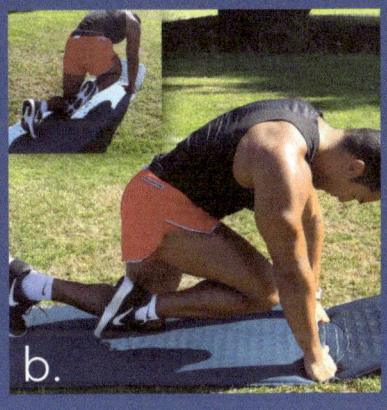

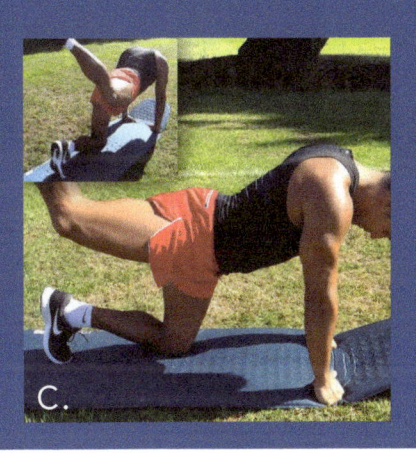

a.   b.   c.

6. Skydiver

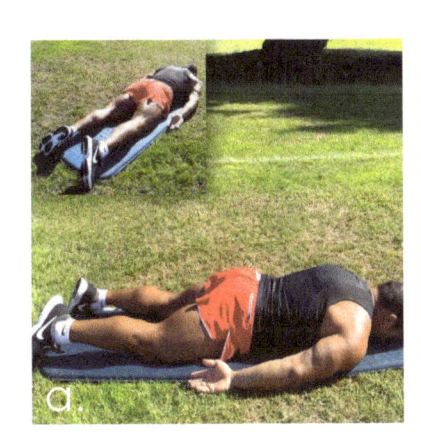

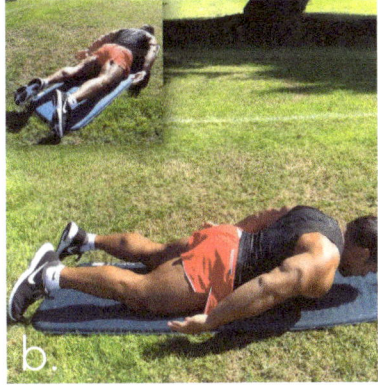

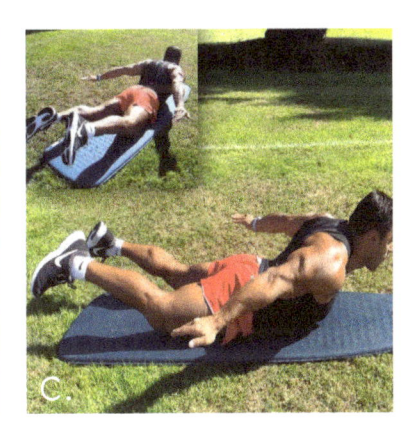

a.   b.   c.

GET FIT, STAY FIT | 193

7. Side Leg Kicks Right

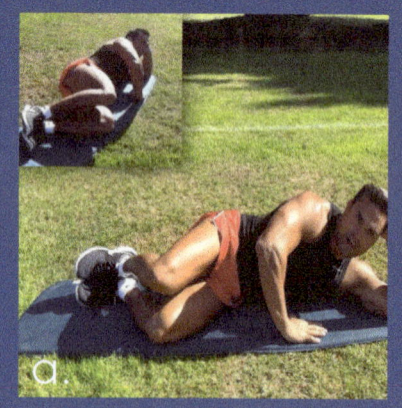

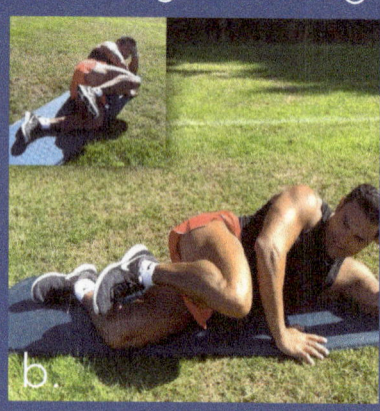

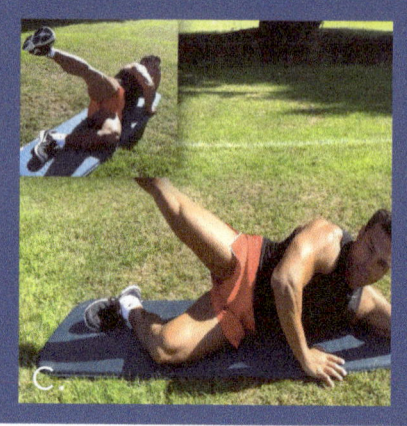

8. Side Leg Kicks Left

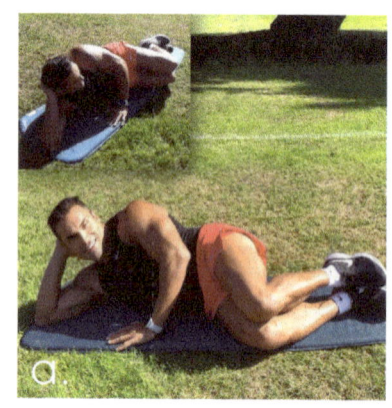

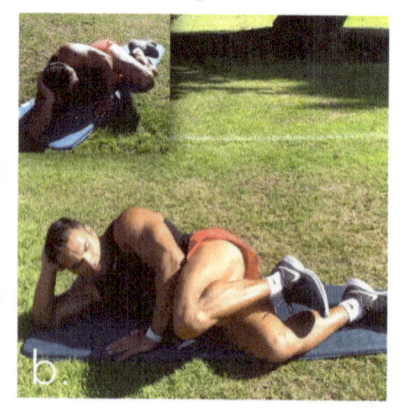

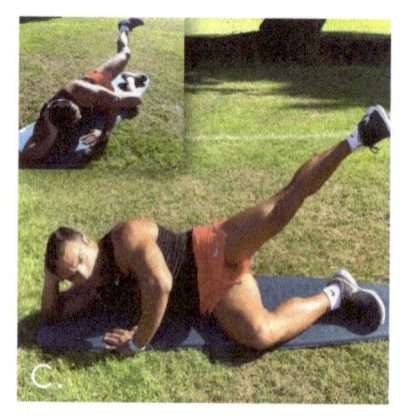

DAY 30
UPPER BODY WEIGHT TRAINING PROGRAMME 2(A)

This is the same as the workout you did on Day 22. However, you will do these for 4 sets. The tempo for each repetition should be 1 second up, 1 second down (or vice versa).

1. Inclined Barbell Bench Press — 4 sets x 12 repetitions
2. Dumbbells Chest Fly — 4 sets x 12 reps
3. Dumbbells Inclined Bench Press — 4 sets x 12 reps
4. Dumbbell One Arm Rowing — 4 sets x 12 reps
5. Cable Reverse Fly (Back Extension) — 4 sets x 12 reps
6. Lat Pull Down Wide Overhand Grip — 4 sets x 12 reps
7. Cable Crunches — 4 sets x 25 reps
8. Leg Raises — 4 sets x 25 reps

1. Inclined Barbell Bench Press

2. Dumbbells Chest Fly

3. Dumbbells Inclined Bench Press

4. Dumbbell One Arm Rowing

5. Cable Reverse Fly

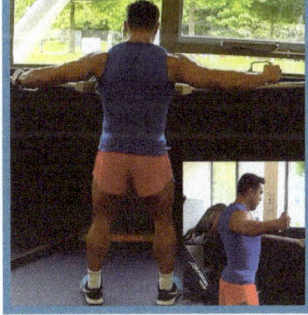

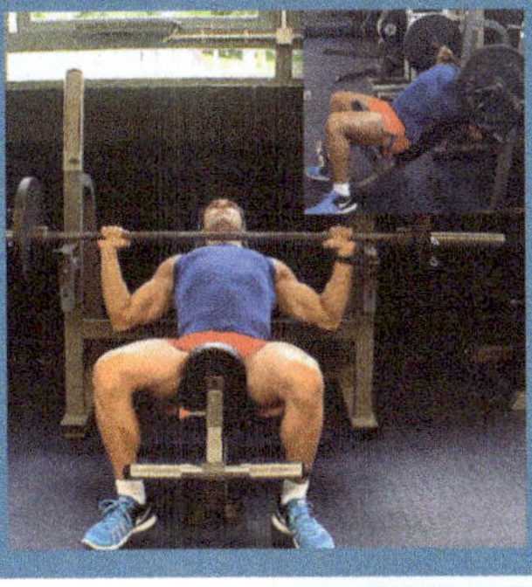

6. Lat Pull Down Wide Overhand Grip

7. Cable Crunches

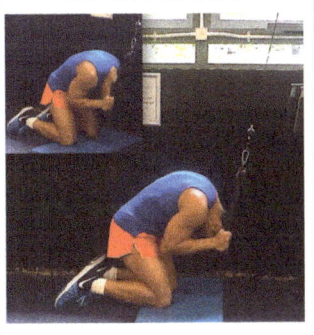

8. Leg Raises

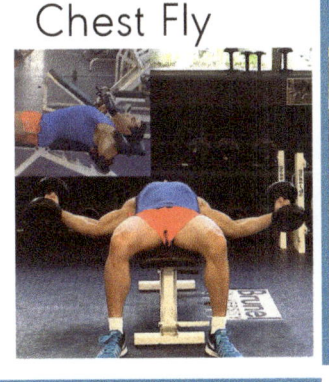

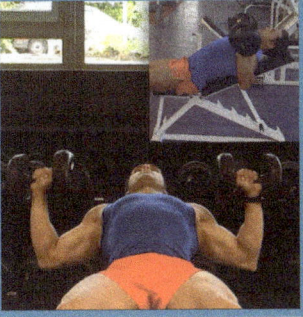

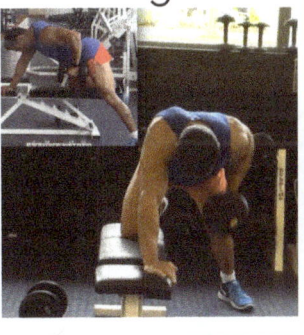

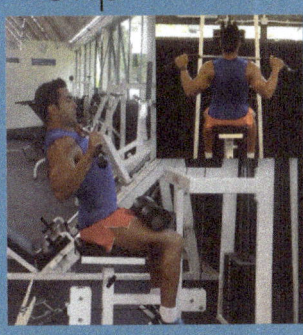

a.

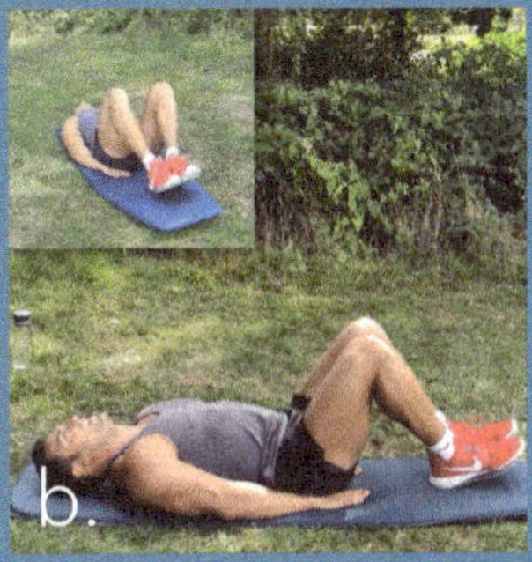

b.

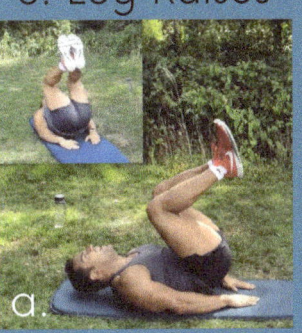

GET FIT, STAY FIT

DAY 31
HOME WORKOUT 10 (PYRAMID)

This is a repeat of the workout on Day 17. It's a hard workout! I do like this workout. It descends pyramid-style, through 3 exercises, in 3 sets.

1.	Press-ups	30 secs on, 15 secs off
2.	Press-ups	20 secs on, 15 secs off
3.	Press-ups	10 secs on, 15 secs off
4.	Abs Scissors	30 secs on, 15 secs off
5.	Abs Scissors	20 secs on, 15 secs off
6.	Abs Scissors	10 secs on, 15 secs off
7.	Horizontal Side Jumps	30 secs on, 15 secs off
8.	Horizontal Side Jumps	20 secs on, 15 secs off
9.	Horizontal Side Jumps	10 secs on, 15 secs off

1. Press-ups

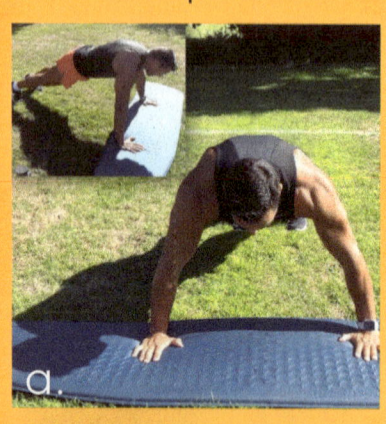

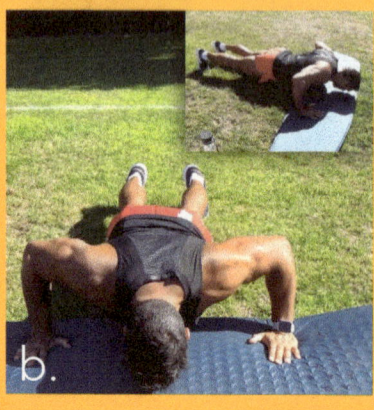

2. Abs Scissors

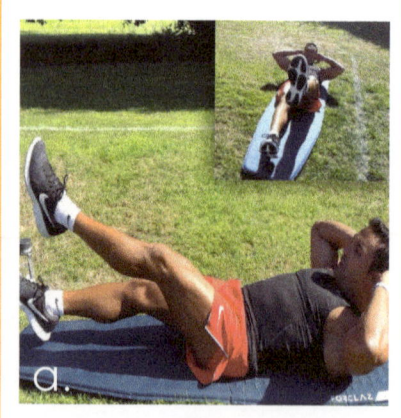

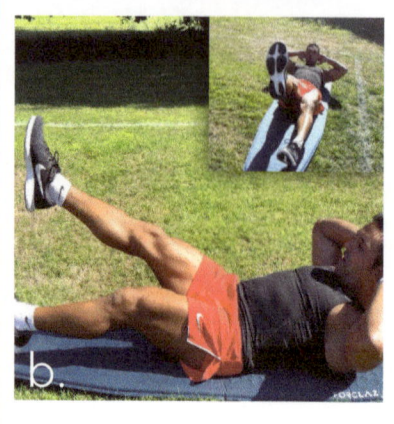

3. Horizontal Side Jumps

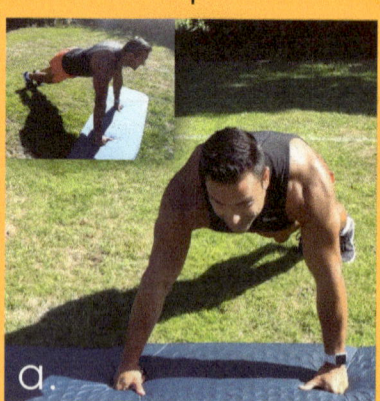

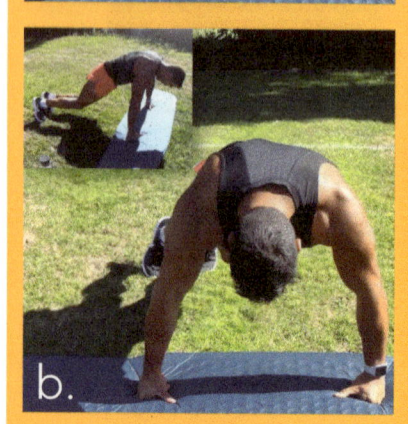

196 | GOKAY KURTULDUM

DAY 32
LOWER BODY WEIGHT TRAINING PROGRAMME 2(A)

This is the same workout you did on Day 23. The tempo for each repetition should be 1 second up, 1 second down (or vice versa). There are 7 exercises only so you will do 4 sets of leg exercises and 3 sets of core.

1. Barbell Squats — 4 sets x 12 repetitions
2. Side Lunges — 4 sets x 15 reps each side
3. Barbell Deadlift — 4 sets x 12 reps
4. Oblique (Russian) Twist — 3 sets x 20 reps each side
5. Plank — 3 sets x 45 secs
6. Oblique Crunches — 3 sets x 25 reps each side
7. Slow Release Sit-ups — 3 sets x 20 reps

1. Barbell Squats

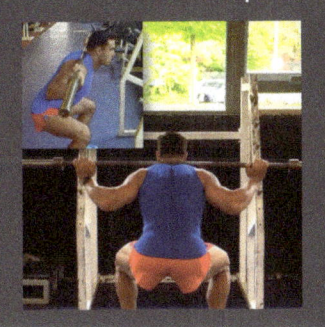

2. Side Lunges

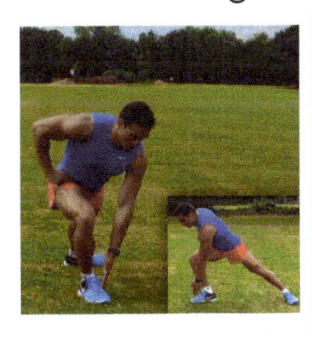

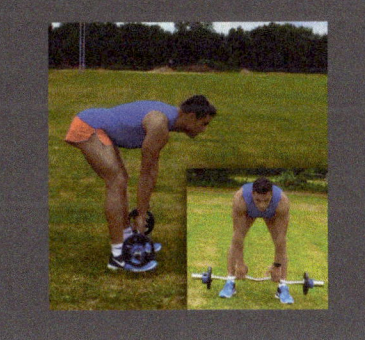

3. Barbell Deadlift

4. Oblique (Russian) Twist

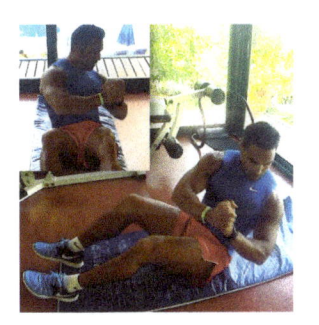

5. Plank

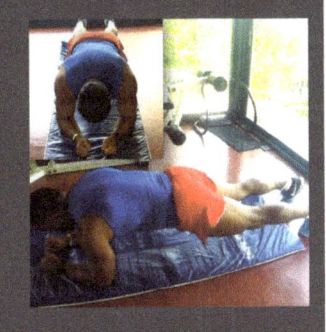

6. Oblique Crunches

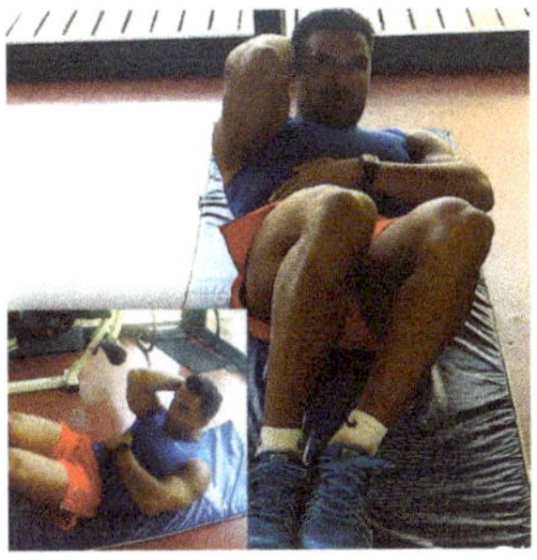

7. Slow Release Sit-ups

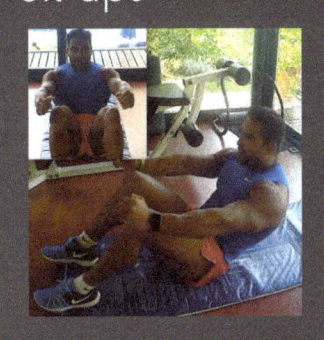

GET FIT, STAY FIT | 197

DAY 33
HOME WORKOUT 11

Today's workout contains 6 exercises, performed in a descending pyramid. For Set 1, each exercise will last for 50 seconds, Set 2 is 40 seconds, Set 3 is 30 seconds, all the way down to 10 seconds each in 5 sets. The rest time between each exercise is 10 seconds.

Set 1: each exercise for 50 secs
Set 2: each exercise for 40 secs
Set 3: each exercise for 30 secs
Set 4: each exercise for 20 secs
Set 5: each exercise for 10 secs

1. Lunge Back and Side

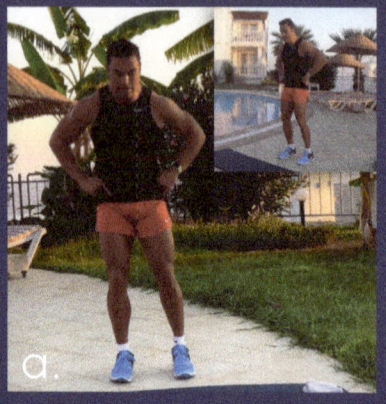

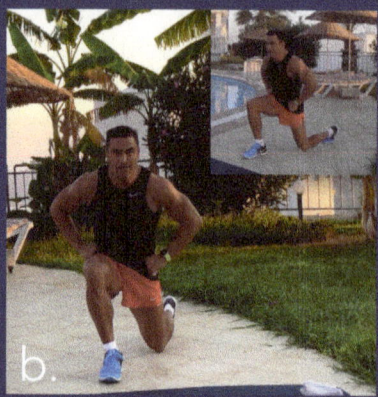

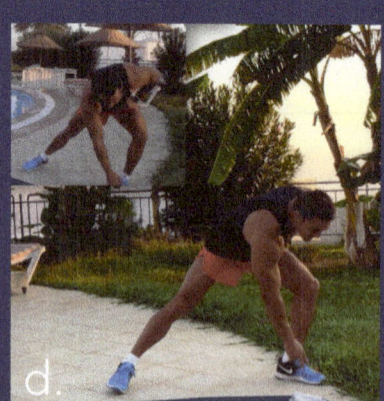

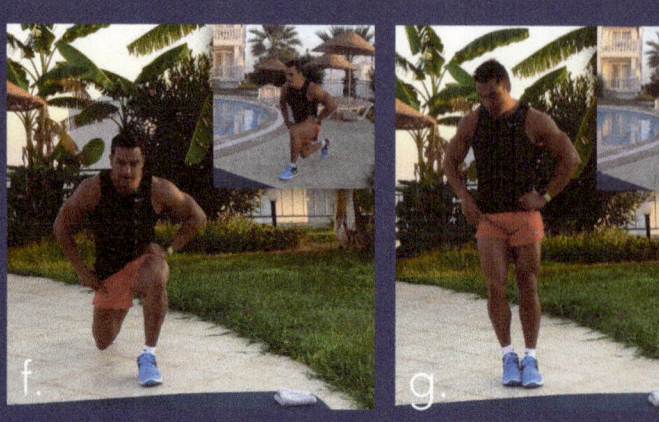

These are the exercises:

1. Lunge Back and Side
2. Squat Thrust to Sides
3. Scissors
4. Duck Squats
5. Dynamic Plank to Press-ups with a Jump
6. Knee Hits

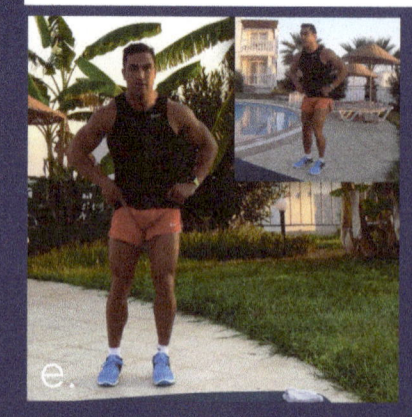

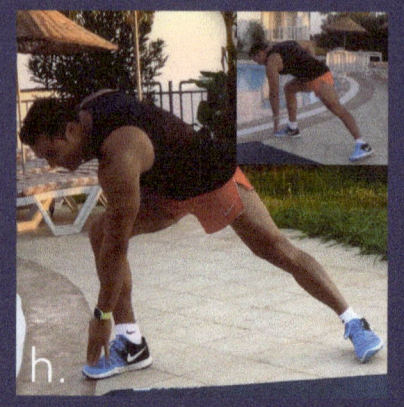

198 | GOKAY KURTULDUM

2. Squat Thrust to Sides

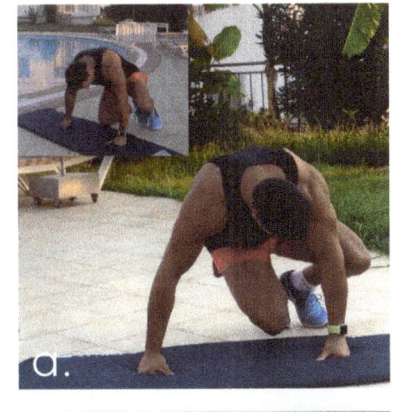

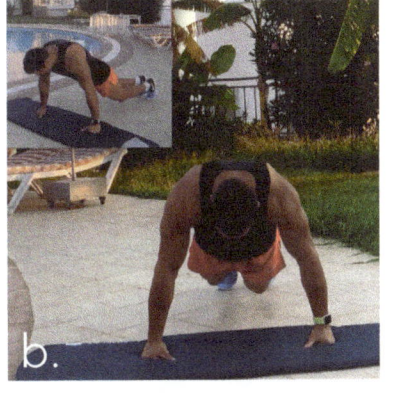

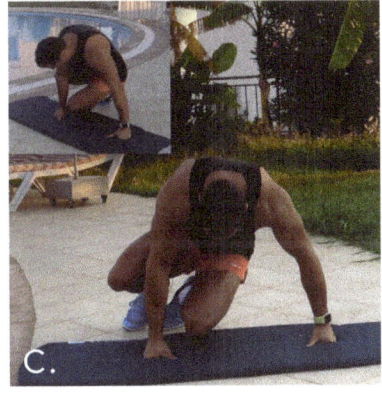

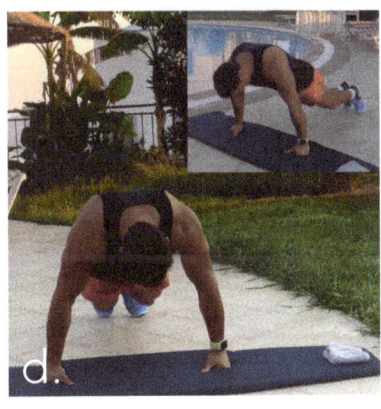

a.
b.
c.
d.

3. Scissors

a.
b.
c.

4. Duck Squats

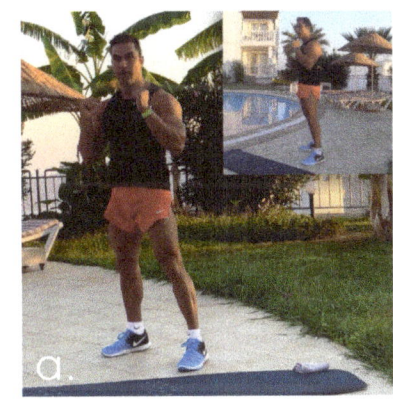

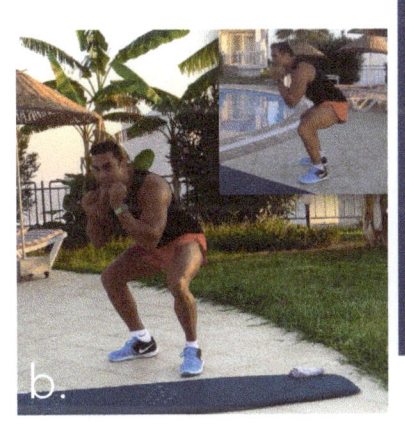

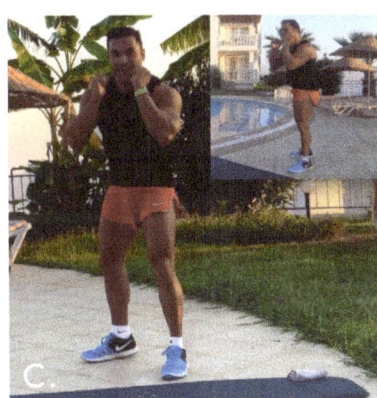

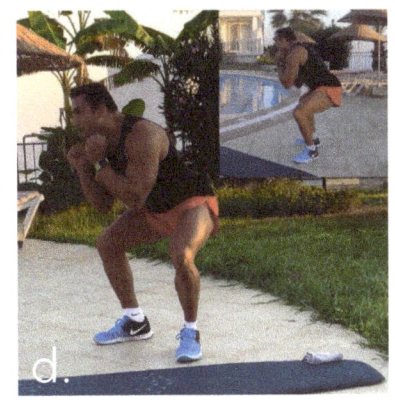

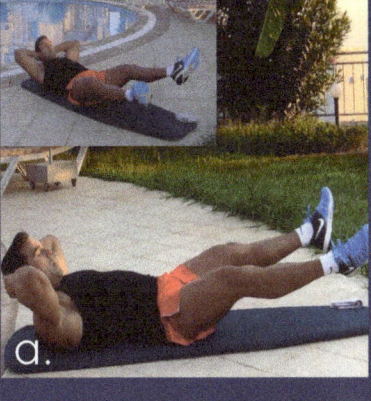

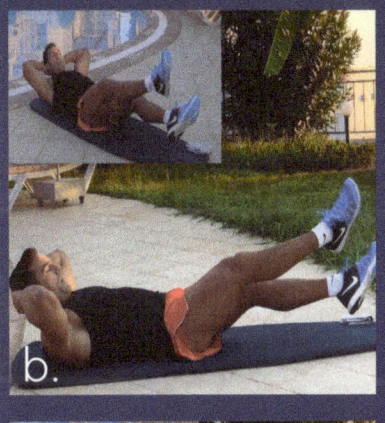

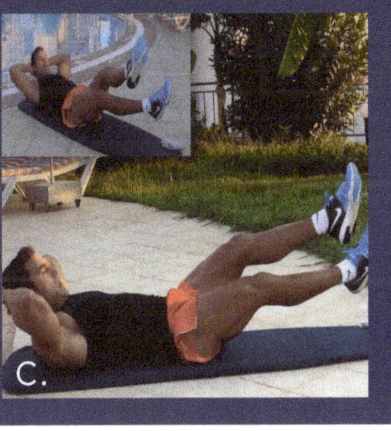

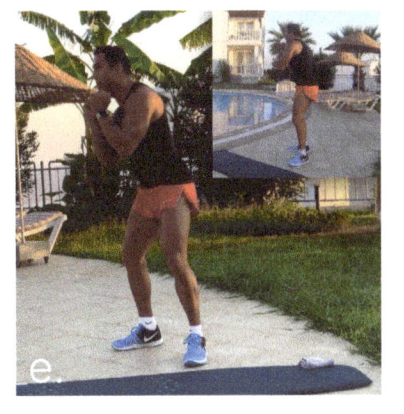

a.
b.
c.
d.
e.

GET FIT, STAY FIT | 199

5. Dynamic Plank to Press-ups with a Jump

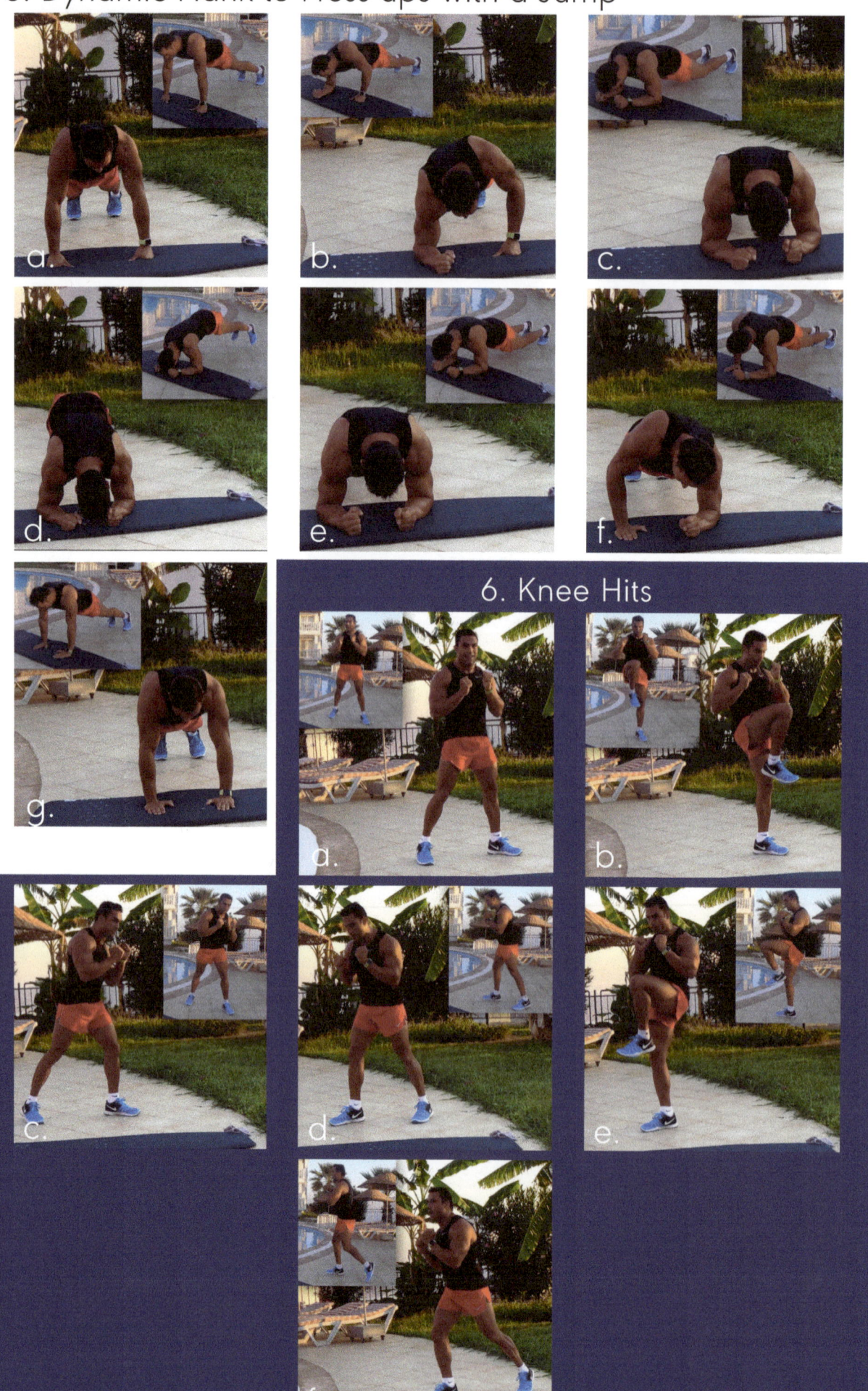

6. Knee Hits

200 | GOKAY KURTULDUM

DAY 34
HOME WORKOUT 12

There are 6 exercises today, as yesterday. Each exercise lasts for 40 seconds and the rest time between sets is 10 seconds only! Do 4 sets.

1. Skiing Torso Rotation — 40 secs on, 10 secs off
2. Squats Increasing Claps — 40 secs on, 10 secs off
3. Leg Kick, Tap with Opposite Hand — 40 secs on, 10 secs off
4. Reverse Crunches with Knee Flexion — 40 secs on, 10 secs off
5. Side Tap, Side Laterals — 40 secs on, 10 secs off
6. Burpees and Forward Lunges — 40 secs on, 10 secs off

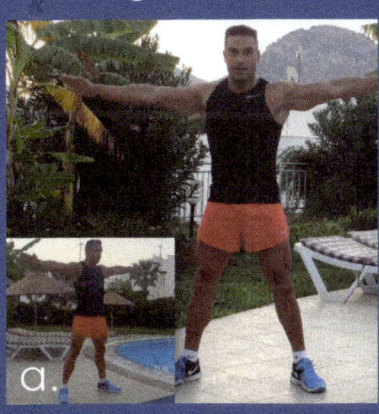

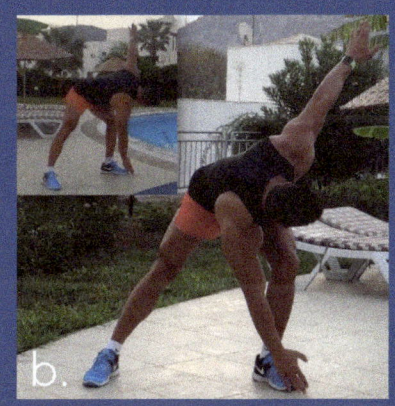

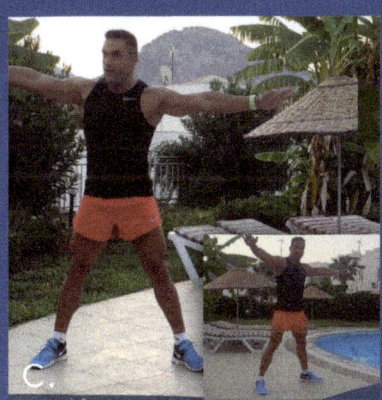

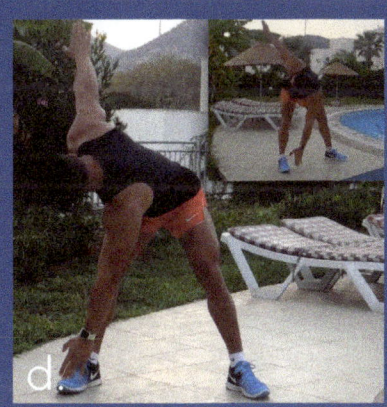

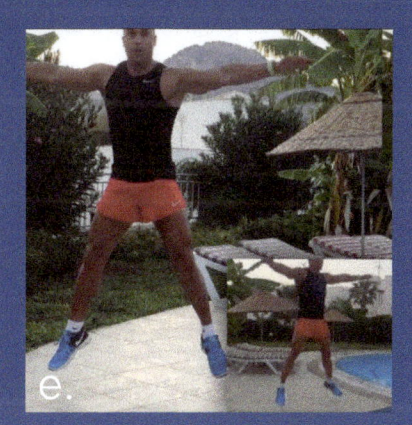

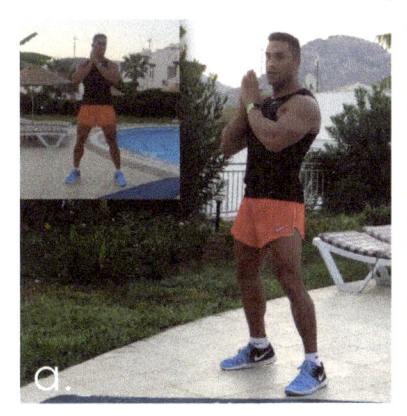

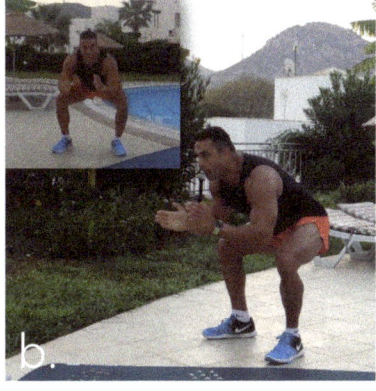

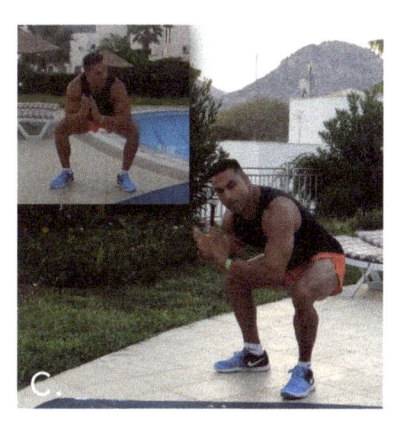

1. Skiing Torso Rotation

2. Squats Increasing Claps

GET FIT, STAY FIT | 201

3. Leg Kick, Tap with Opposite Hand

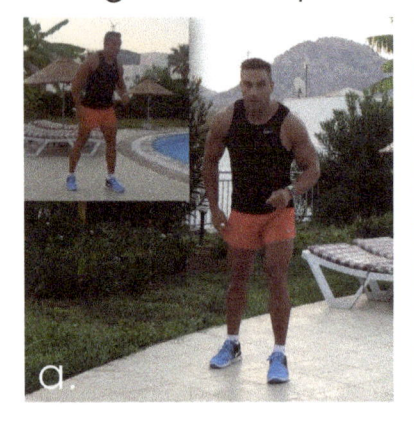

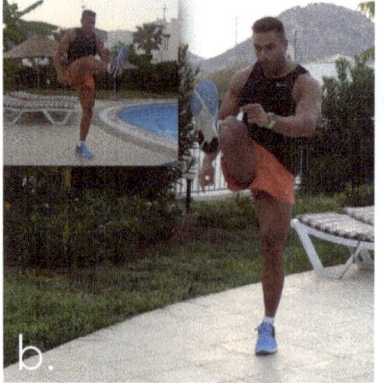

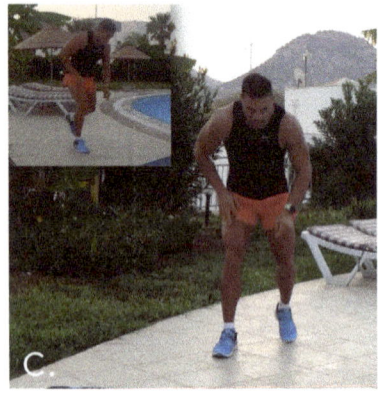

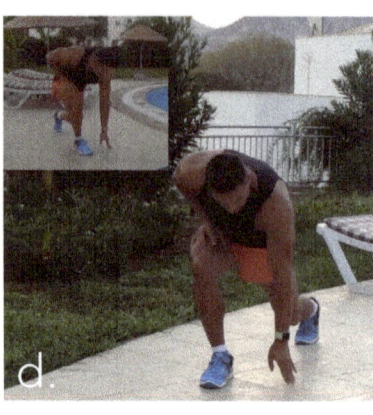

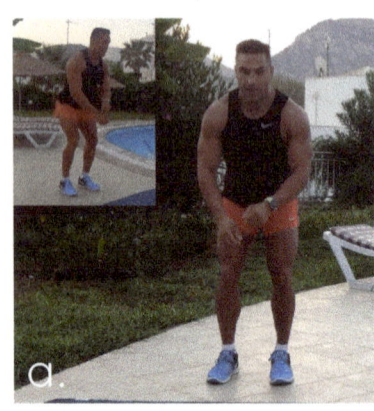

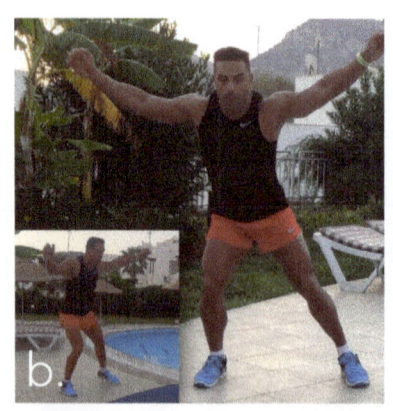

4. Reverse Crunches with Knee Flexion

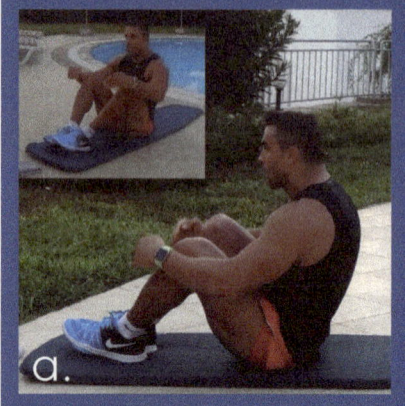

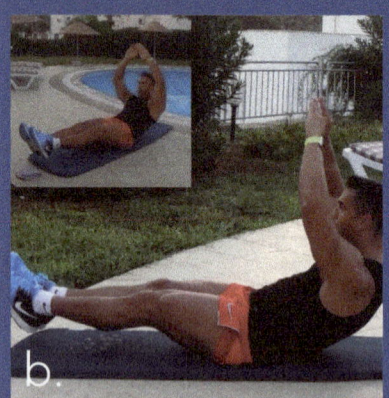

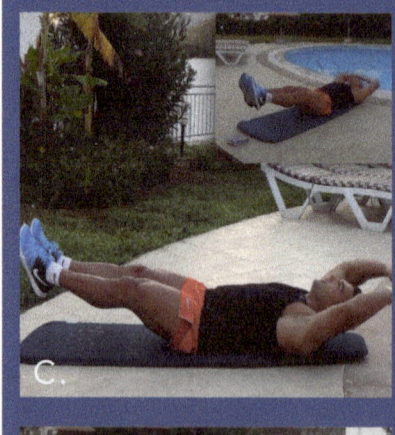

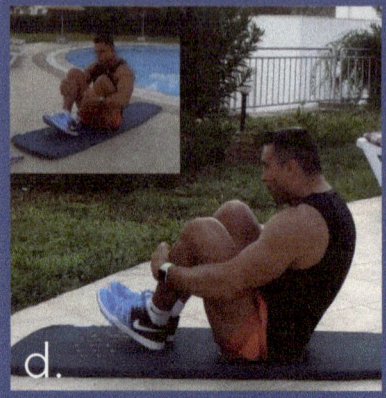

5. Side Tap, Side Laterals

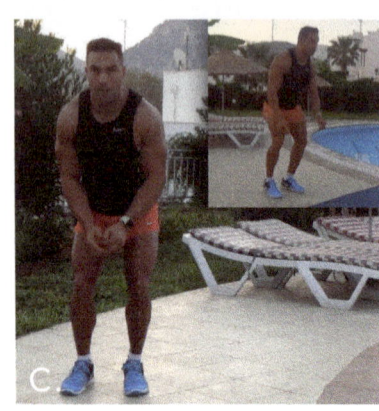

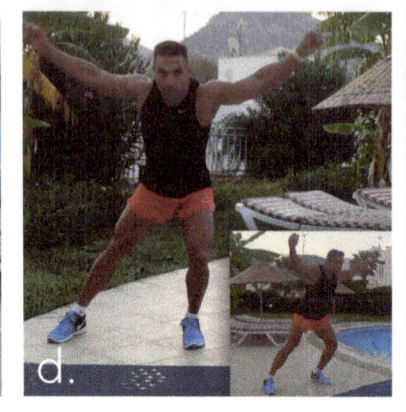

6. Burpees and Forward Lunges

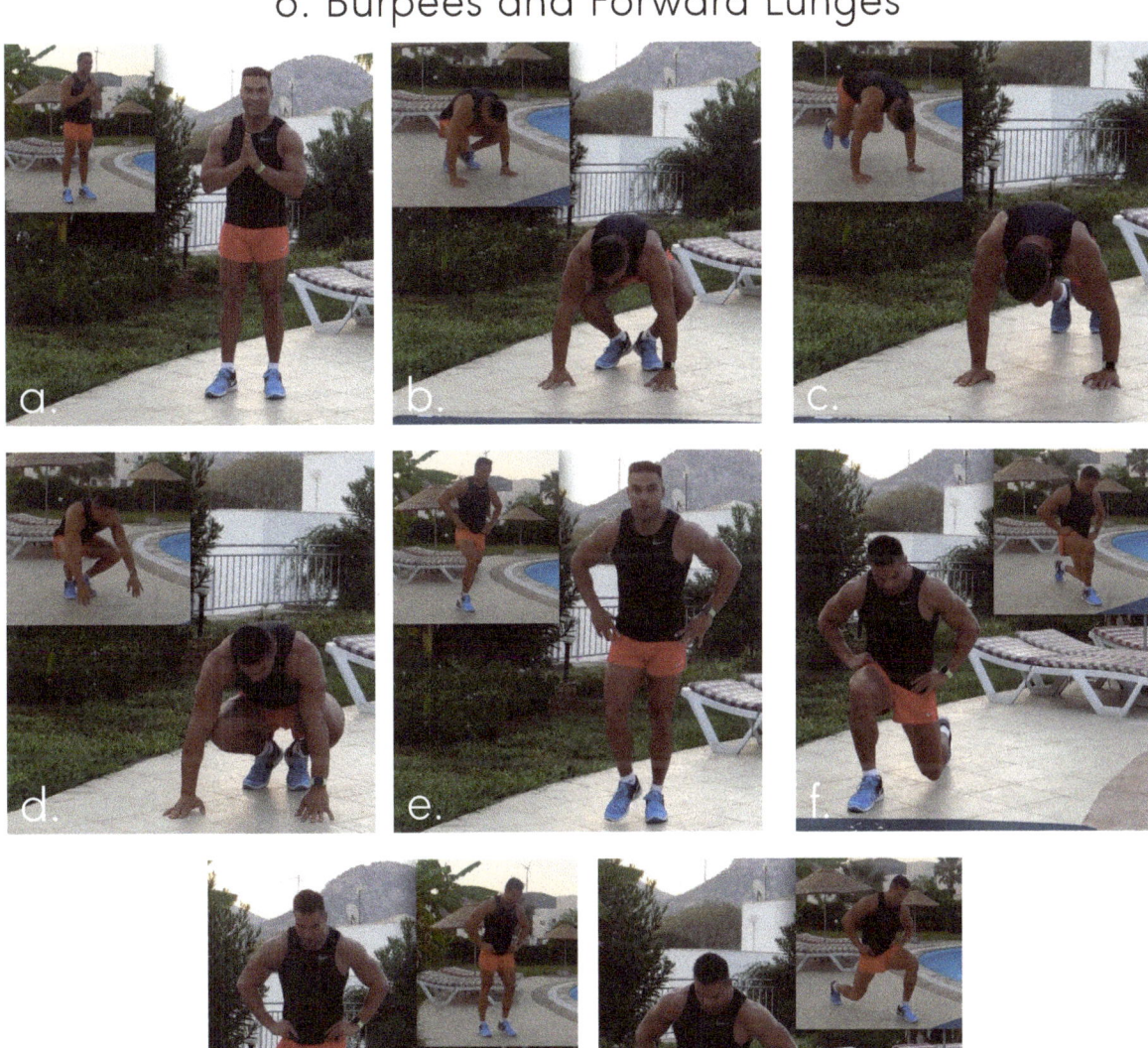

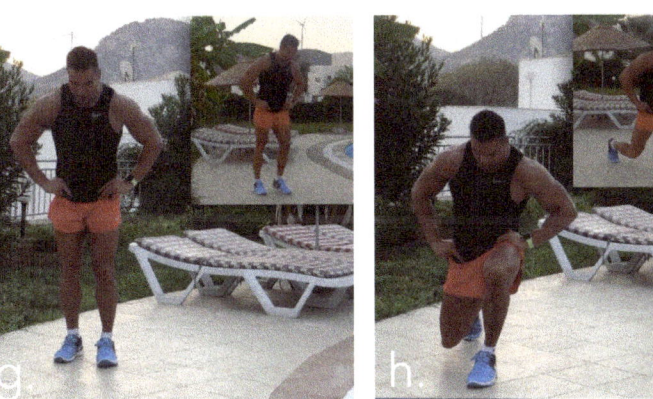

DAY 35 OFF

WEEK 5 PROGRESS JOURNAL

Use these pages to set your intentions at the start of the week and record and reflect on your progress at the end of the week. Alternatively, use a special notebook for this purpose.

PART 1: INTENTIONS/PLANNING

My starting weight this week: _____

My starting waist measurement: _____

My goal weight at the end of this week: _____

My goal waist measurement at the end of this week: _____

Any other goals for the week (e.g. no alcohol during the week and no more than 14 units during the weekend or going to bed early weekdays and sleep minimum 7 hours etc.)

_____

_____

Which days are going to be tricky this week and why? (E.g. client dinner on Thursday which involves drinking alcohol)

_____

How will I deal with this? _____

_____

Any other notes/thoughts:

PART 2: RECORD/REFLECTIONS

At the end of this week how many goals did I achieve? _____

How many did I come close to? _____

How am I feeling about my progress? _____

Which goals did I not reach? _____

Why was that? Family commitments, too much work and no time, not motivated enough? Can I define exactly what hindered my progress? Can I take action on that next week?

What actions can I take next week to improve on this?

What were my wins this week? (e.g. weight loss, mileage run etc?)

I've achieved

Give marks out of 10 for progress this week

8.9 WEEK 6 PROGRAMME AND JOURNAL PAGES

This is another gym-heavy week. I hope you'll do your best to fit these in. Remember, they're not randomly selected exercises but part of a careful progressive programme so do try to stick to the plan. Home workouts this week last for 20 minutes each. Start with Part 1 of your journal, as usual.

Here's a summary of your Week 6 programme:

Day 36	Upper Body Weight Training P2(b)
Day 37	Lower Body Weight Training P2(b)
Day 38	Home Workout 13
Day 39	Upper Body Weight Training P2(a)
Day 40	Lower Body Weight Training P2(a)
Day 41	Home Workout 14
Day 42	OFF

Now tackle your day-by-day exercises on the following pages.

DAY 36
UPPER BODY WEIGHT TRAINING PROGRAMME 2(B)

This is the same as the workout you did on Day 25. The tempo for each repetition should be 1 second up, 1 second down (or vice versa).

1. Barbell Shoulder Press — 4 sets x 12 repetitions
2. Dumbbell Side Laterals — 4 sets x 12 reps
3. Cable Front Raise — 3 sets x 12 reps
4. EZ Barbell Biceps Curl — 3 sets x 12 reps
5. Dumbbell Inclined Biceps Curl — 3 sets x 12 reps
6. Standing EZ Bar Triceps Extension — 3 sets x 12 reps
7. Dumbbell One Arm Triceps Kick — 3 sets x 12 reps each side
8. Cycling in the Air — 3 sets x 30 secs
9. Dead Bug — 3 sets x 15 reps each side

1. Barbell Shoulder Press

2. Dumbbells Side Laterals

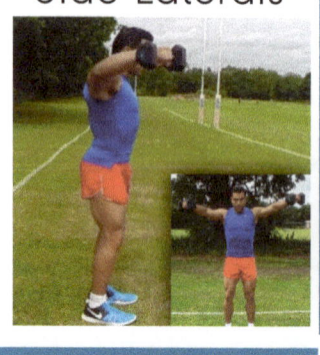

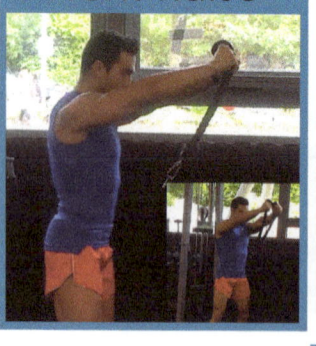

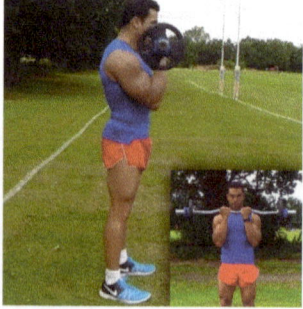

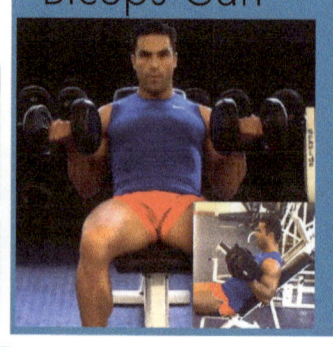

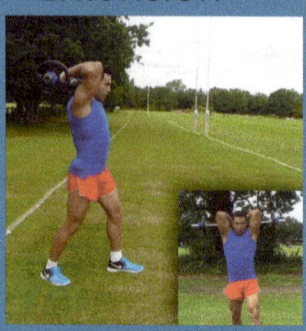

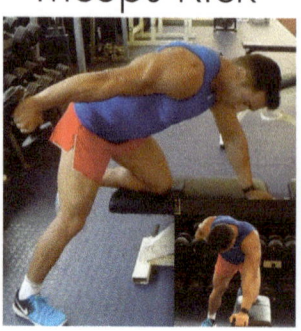

3. Cable Front Raise

4. EZ Barbell Biceps Curl

5. Dumbbell Inclined Biceps Curl

6. Standing EZ Bar Triceps Extension

7. Dumbbell One Arm Triceps Kick

8. Cycling in the Air

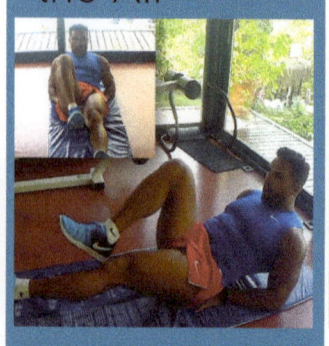

9. Dead Bug

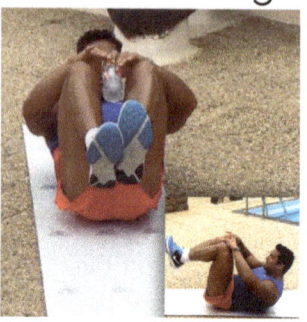

208 | GOKAY KURTULDUM

DAY 37
LOWER BODY WEIGHT TRAINING PROGRAMME 2(B)

This is the same as the workout you did on Day 26. The tempo for each repetition should be 1 second up, 1 second down (or vice versa).

1. Leg Extension — 3 sets x 15 repetitions
2. TRX Squat Jumps — 3 sets x 15 reps
3. Leg Curl — 3 sets x 15 reps
4. Split Squats — 3 sets x 15 reps each side
5. Abdominal Crunches with Raised Arms — 3 sets x 30 reps
6. Abs Scissors Heel Taps — 3 sets x 20 reps each side
7. Oblique Crunches — 3 sets x 30 reps each side
8. Plank Weight Rotation — 3 sets x 10 each direction

1. Leg Extension

2. TRX Squat Jumps

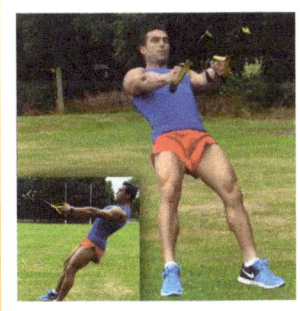

3. Leg Curl

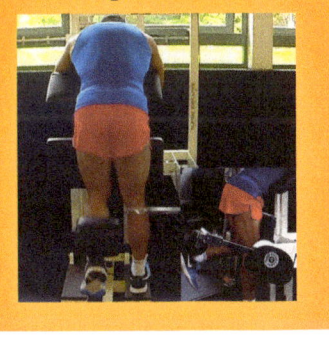

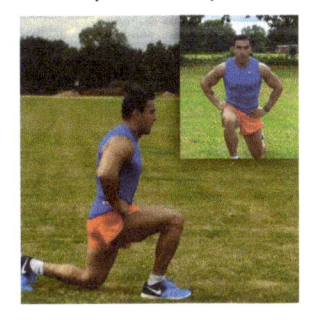

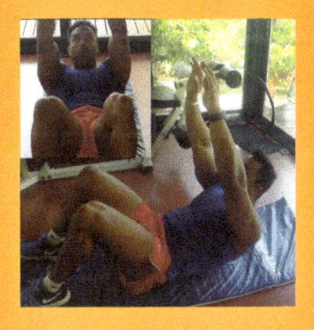

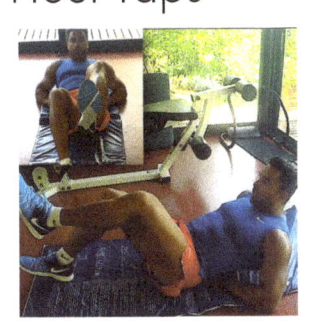

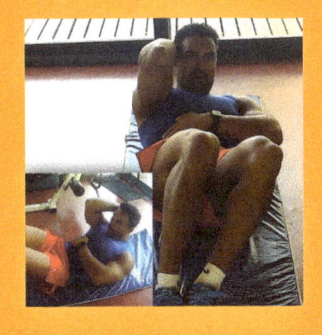

4. Split Squats

5. Abdominal Crunches with Raised Arms

6. Abs Scissors Heel Taps

7. Oblique Crunches

8. Plank Weight Rotation

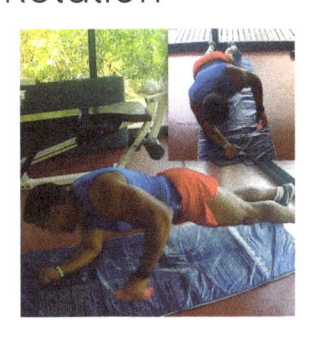

GET FIT, STAY FIT | 209

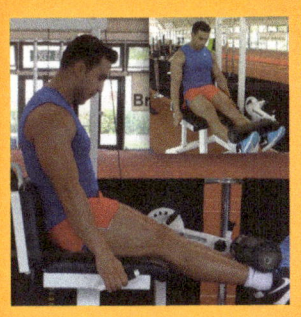

DAY 38
HOME WORKOUT 13

Today, each exercise lasts for 30 seconds and the rest time between sets is 20 seconds. Just to let you know, you'll need a chair, step or a bench for this one. Do 4 sets.

1. Press-ups/Star Jumps — 30 secs on, 20 secs off
2. Low Kick Dance — 30 secs on, 20 secs off
3. Squat Side Jumps — 30 secs on, 20 secs off
4. Triceps Dips — 30 secs on, 20 secs off
5. Single Leg Hops — 15 secs on each leg, 20 secs off
6. Lying Flying — 30 secs on, 20 secs off

1. Press-ups/Star Jumps

a.
b.
c.
d.
e.

2. Low Kick Dance

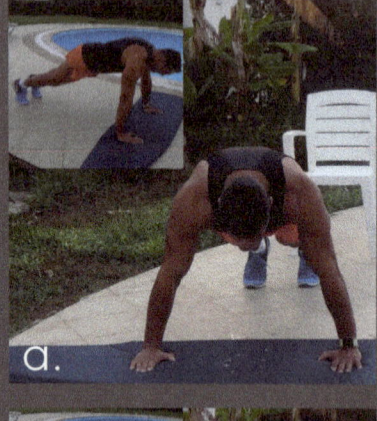

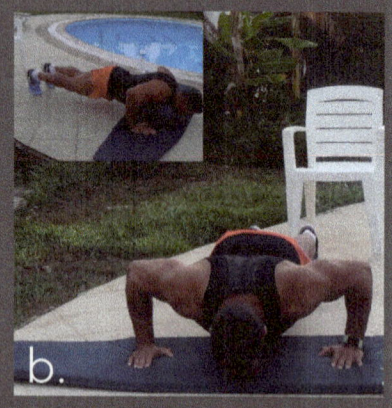

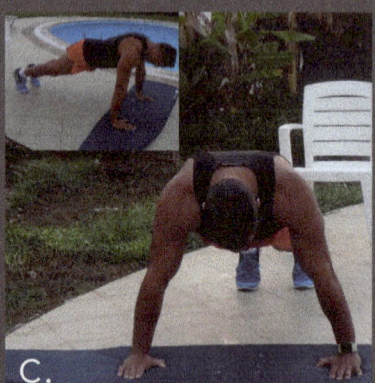

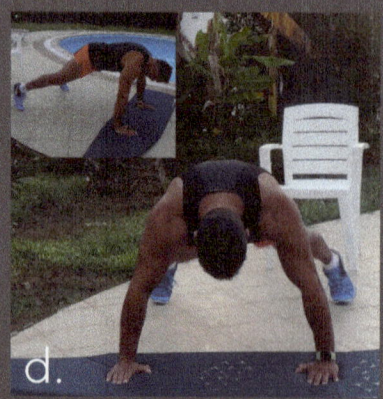

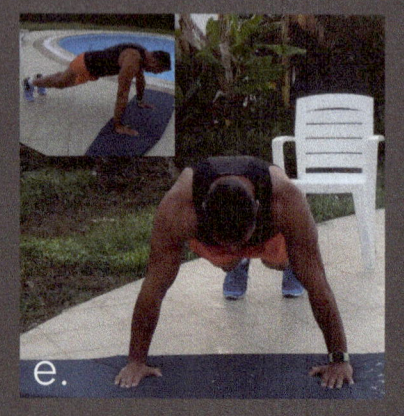

a.
b.
c.

210 | GOKAY KURTULDUM

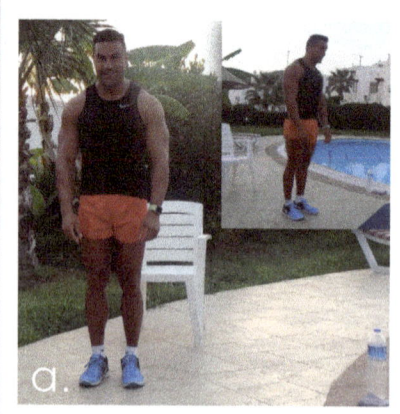

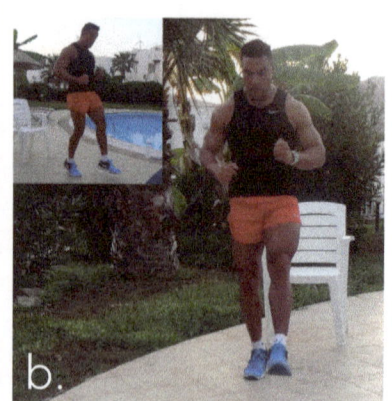

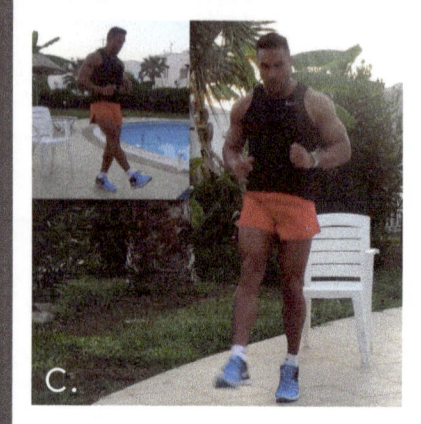

3. Squat Side Jumps

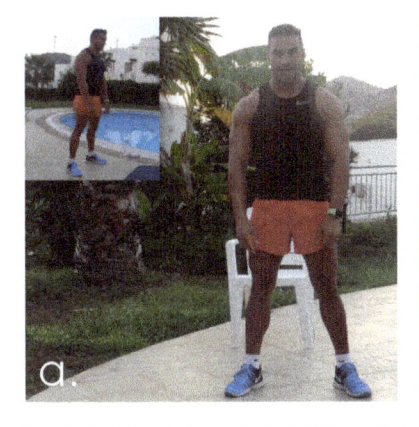

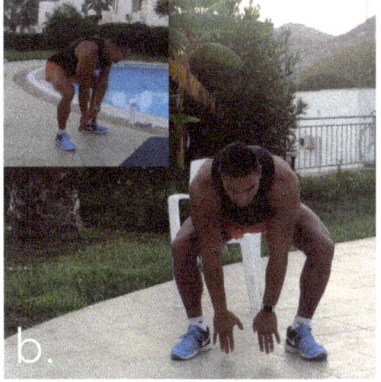

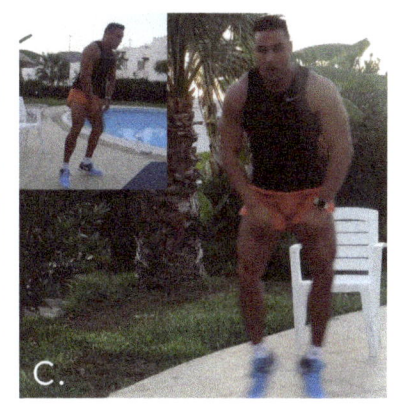

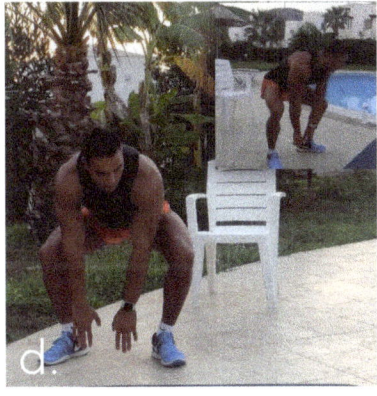

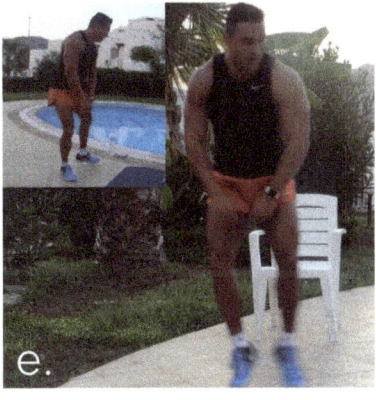

a.
b.
c.
d.
e.

4. Triceps Dips

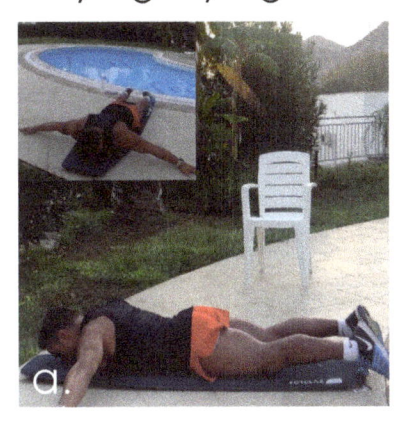

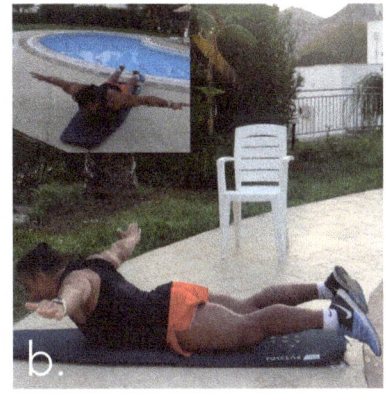

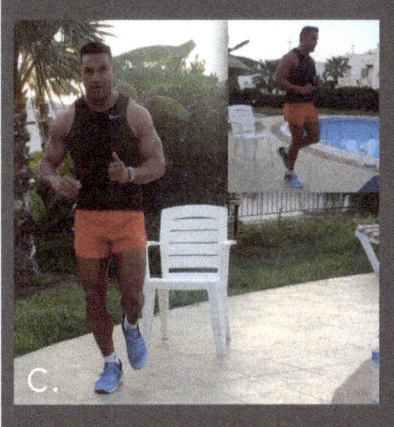

a.
b.

5. Single Leg Hops

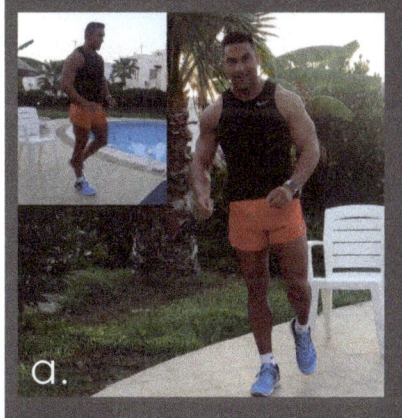

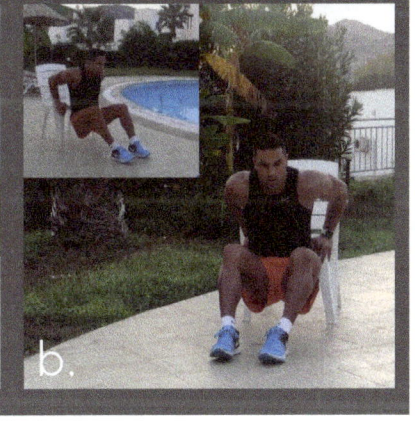

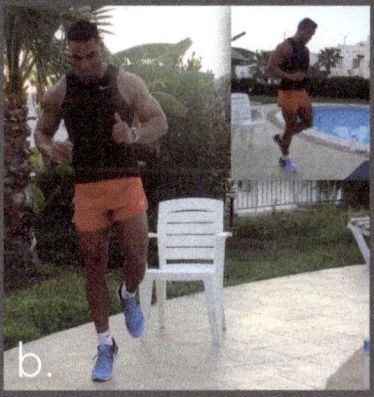

a.
b.
c.

6. Lying Flying

a.
b.

GET FIT, STAY FIT | 211

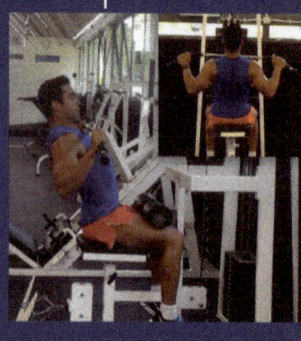

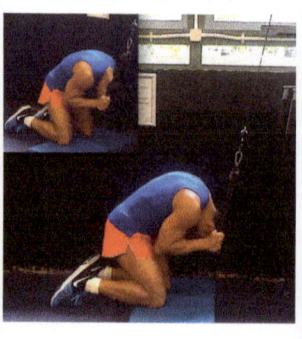

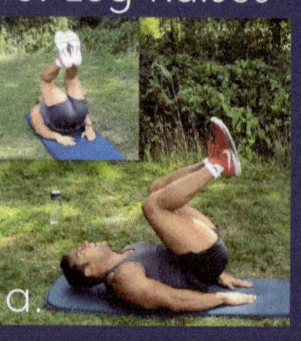

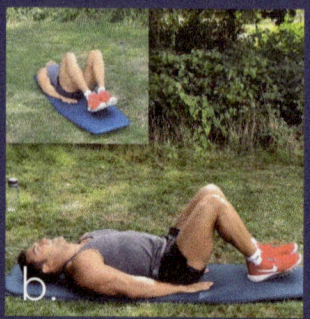

DAY 39
UPPER BODY WEIGHT TRAINING PROGRAMME 2(A)

This is the same as the workout you did on Day 30 and Day 22. The tempo for each repetition should be 1 second up, 1 second down (or vice versa).

1. Inclined Barbell Bench Press — 4 sets x 12 repetitions
2. Dumbbells Chest Fly — 4 sets x 12 reps
3. Dumbbells Inclined Bench Press — 4 sets x 12 reps
4. Dumbbell One Arm Rowing — 4 sets x 12 reps
5. Cable Reverse Fly (Back Extension) — 4 sets x 12 reps
6. Lat Pull Down Wide Overhand Grip — 4 sets x 12 reps
7. Cable Crunches — 4 sets x 25 reps
8. Leg Raises — 4 sets x 25 reps

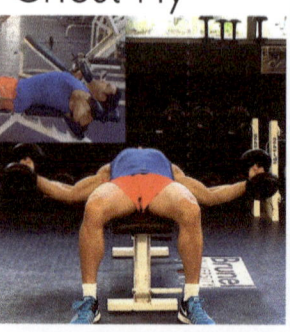

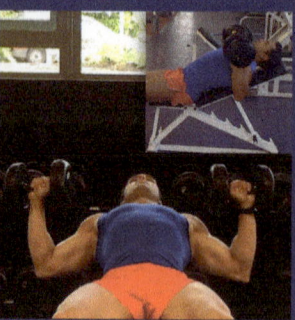

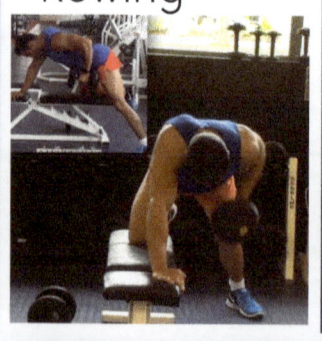

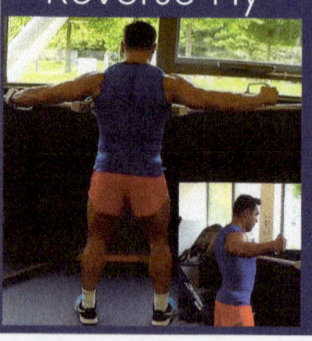

1. Inclined Barbell Bench Press
2. Dumbbells Chest Fly
3. Dumbbells Inclined Bench Press
4. Dumbbell One Arm Rowing
5. Cable Reverse Fly
6. Lat Pull Down Wide Overhand Grip
7. Cable Crunches
8. Leg Raises

DAY 40
LOWER BODY WEIGHT TRAINING PROGRAMME 2(A)

This is the same as the workout you did on Day 32 and Day 23. The tempo for each repetition should be 1 second up, 1 second down (or vice versa). There are 7 exercises only so you will do 4 sets of leg exercises and 3 sets of core.

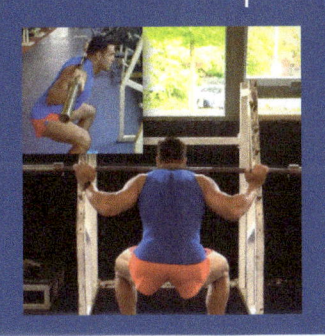

1.	Barbell Squats	4 sets x 12 repetitions
2.	Side Lunges	4 sets x 15 reps each side
3.	Barbell Deadlift	4 sets x 12 reps
4.	Oblique (Russian) Twist	3 sets x 20 reps each side
5.	Plank	3 sets x 45 secs
6.	Oblique Crunches	3 sets x 25 reps each side
7.	Slow Release Sit-ups	3 sets x 20 reps

1. Barbell Squats

2. Side Lunges

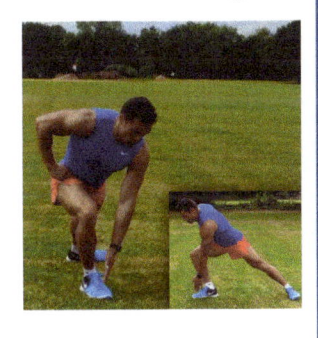

3. Barbell Deadlift

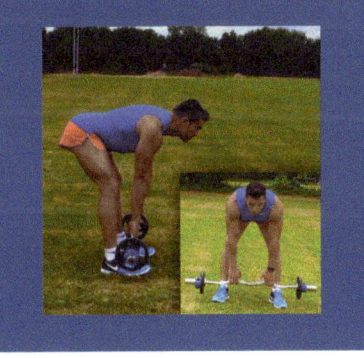

4. Oblique (Russian) Twist

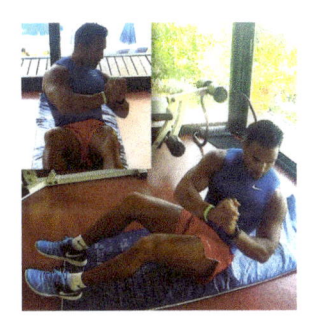

5. Plank

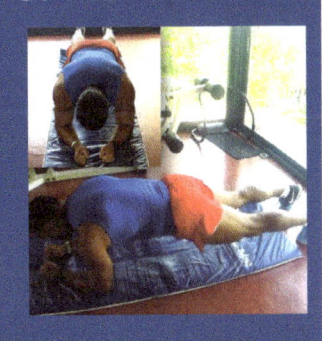

6. Oblique Crunches

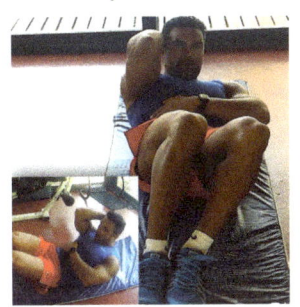

7. Slow Release Sit-ups

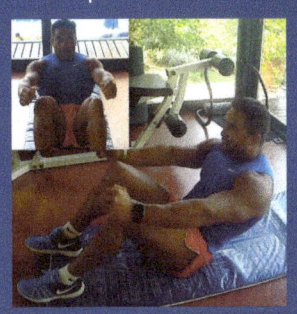

GET FIT, STAY FIT | 213

DAY 41
HOME WORKOUT 14

Today's workout contains 6 exercises, performed in a descending pyramid. So you will start with 50 seconds on, 10 seconds off. Then 40 seconds on, 10 seconds off. For each set you will reduce the number of seconds by 10. Set 5 will be for 10 seconds on, 10 seconds off.

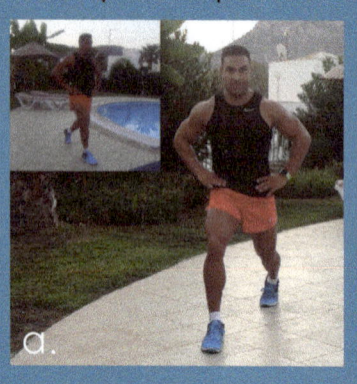

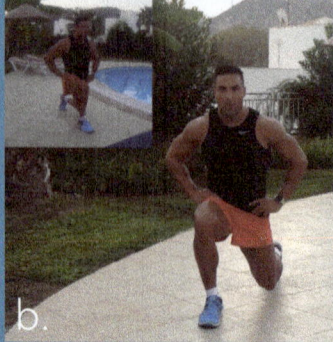

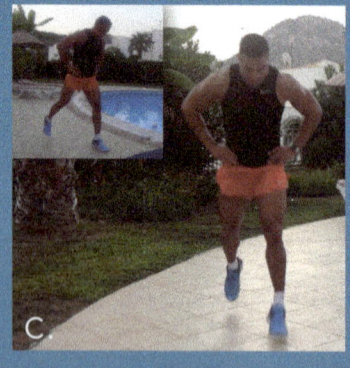

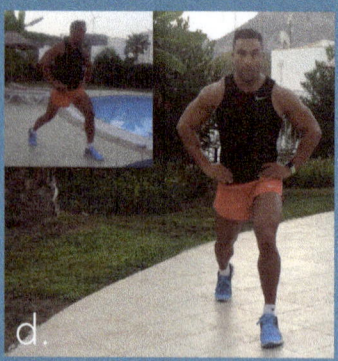

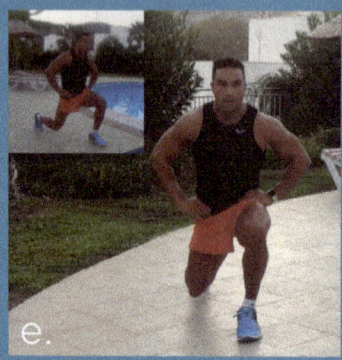

Set 1: each exercise for 50 secs
Set 2: each exercise for 40 secs
Set 3: each exercise for 30 secs
Set 4: each exercise for 20 secs
Set 5: each exercise for 10 secs

The exercises are:

1. 5 Split Squats and Jumps to Alternate Foot
2. Diagonal Toe Touch Crunches
3. Clap under Thighs/Squat Jumps
4. Plank
5. Press-ups to Sides
6. Leg Oblique Side Drops

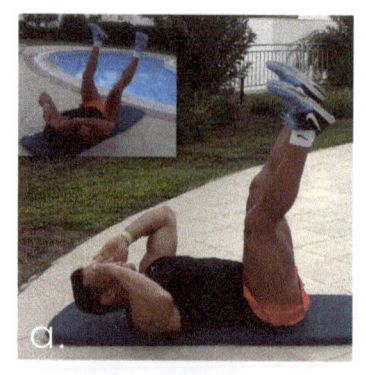

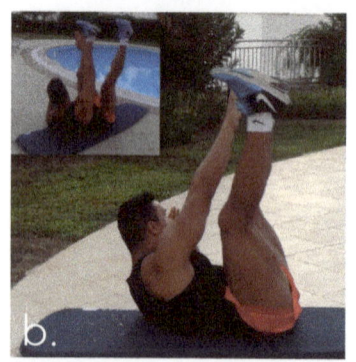

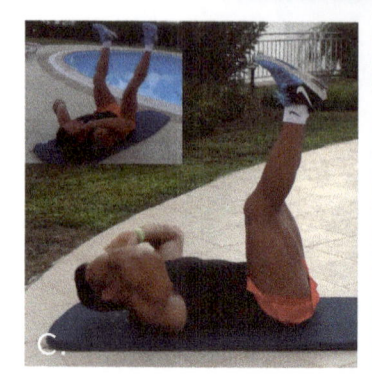

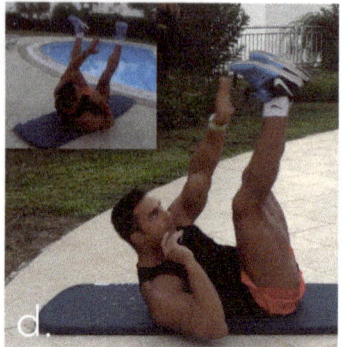

1. 5 Split Squats and Jumps

2. Diagonal Toe Touch Crunches

214 | GOKAY KURTULDUM

3. Clap under Thighs/Squat Jumps

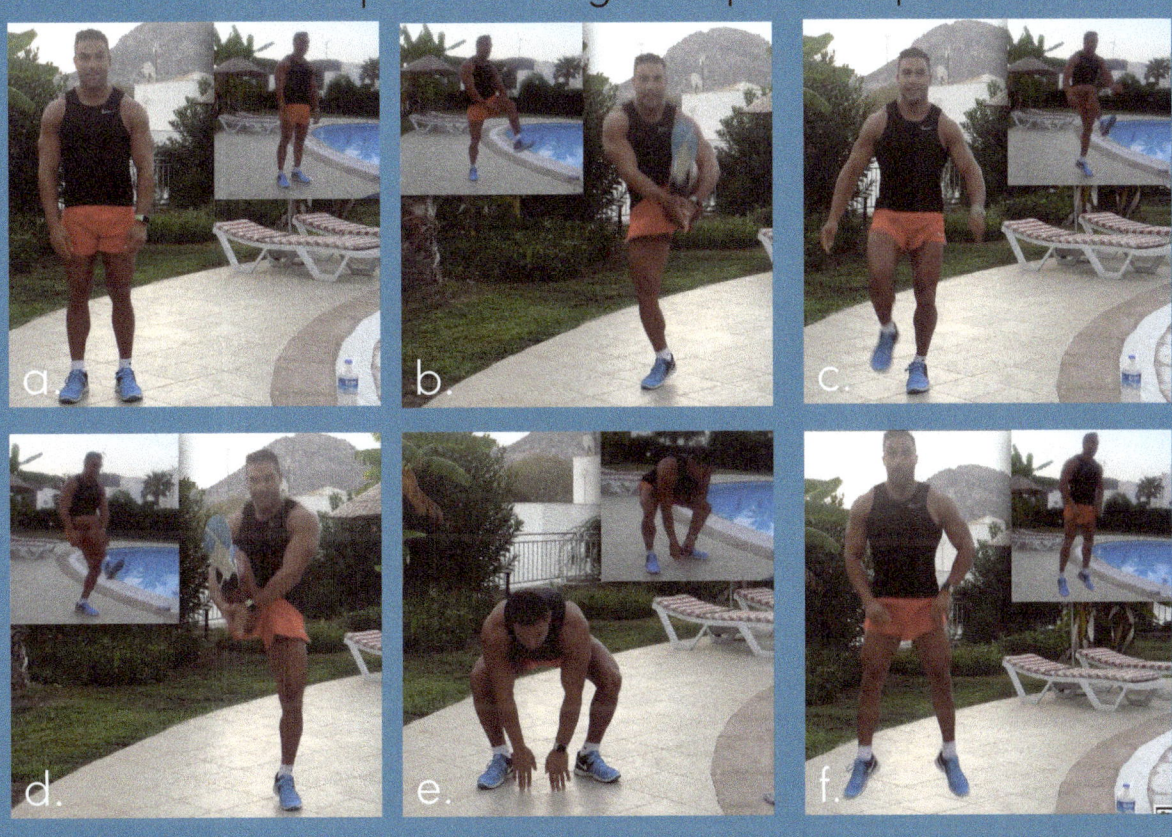

4. Plank

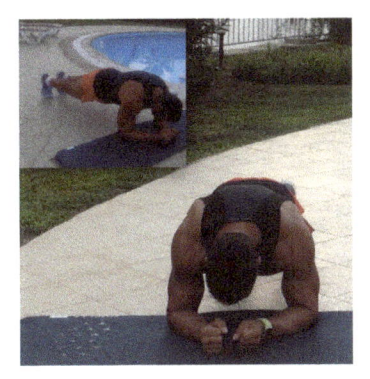

5. Press-ups to Sides

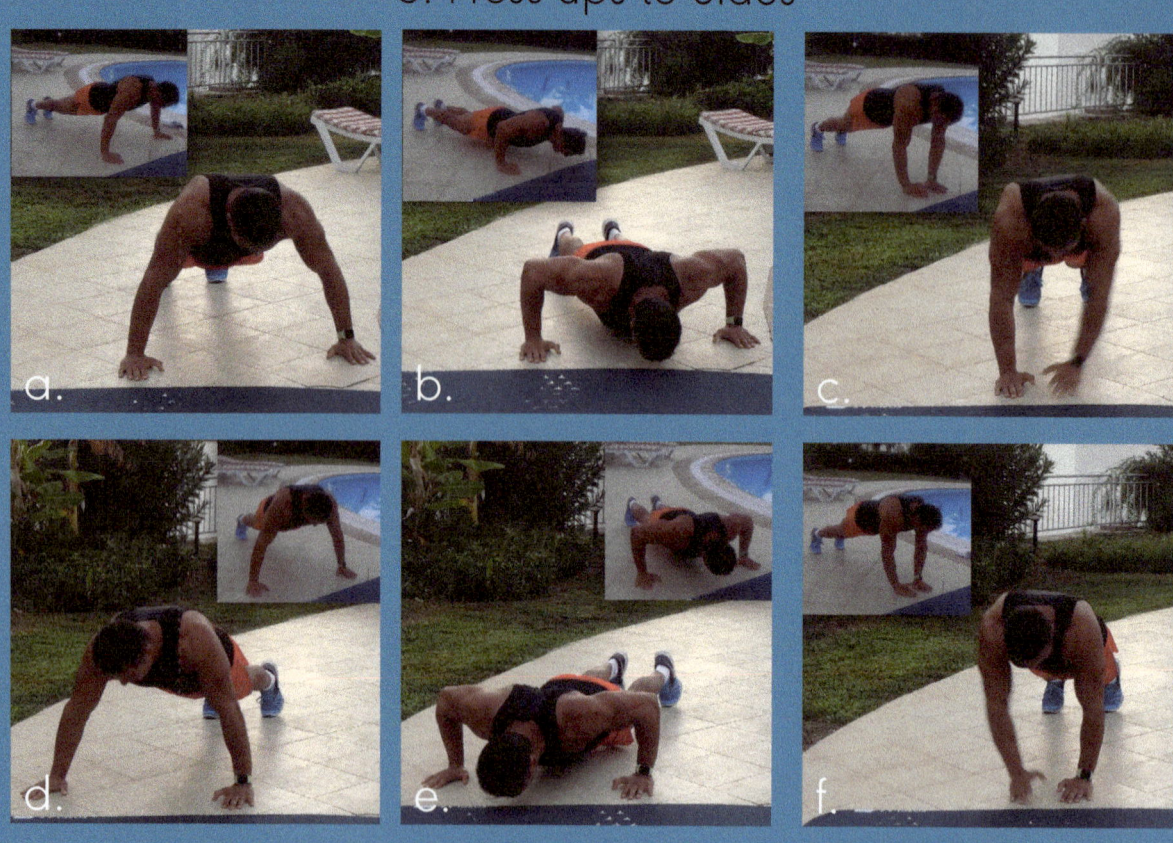

a.

b.

c.

d.

e.

f.

6. Leg Oblique Side Drops

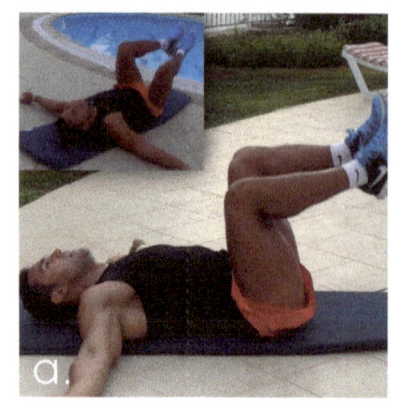

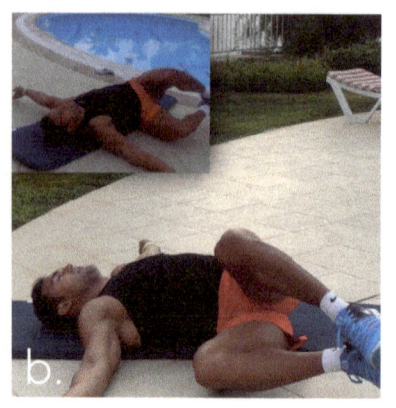

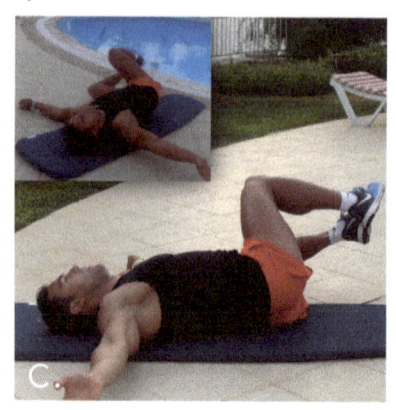

a.

b.

c.

DAY 42 OFF

WEEK 6 PROGRESS JOURNAL

Use these pages to set your intentions at the start of the week and record and reflect on your progress at the end of the week. Alternatively, use a special notebook for this purpose.

PART 1: INTENTIONS/PLANNING

My starting weight this week: _____

My starting waist measurement: _____

My goal weight at the end of this week: _____

My goal waist measurement at the end of this week: _____

Any other goals for the week (e.g. no alcohol during the week and no more than 14 units during the weekend or going to bed early weekdays and sleep minimum 7 hours etc.)

_____

_____

Which days are going to be tricky this week and why? (E.g. client dinner on Thursday which involves drinking alcohol)

_____

How will I deal with this? _____

_____

GET FIT, STAY FIT | 217

Any other notes/thoughts:

PART 2: RECORD/REFLECTIONS

At the end of this week how many goals did I achieve?

How many did I come close to?

How am I feeling about my progress?

Which goals did I not reach?

Why was that? Family commitments, too much work and no time, not motivated enough? Can I define exactly what hindered my progress? Can I take action on that next week?

What actions can I take next week to improve on this?

What were my wins this week? (e.g. weight loss, mileage run etc?)

I've achieved

Give marks out of 10 for progress this week

8.10 WEEK 7 PROGRAMME AND JOURNAL PAGES

You'll be visiting the gym only twice this week, and you'll have four 20-minute home workouts. Start with your journal as usual.

Here's a summary of your Week 7 programme:

Day 43	Home Workout 15
Day 44	Upper Body Weight Training P2(b)
Day 45	Home Workout 11
Day 46	Lower Body Weight Training P2(b)
Day 47	Home Workout 12
Day 48	Home Workout 13
Day 49	OFF

Now it's time to do the day-by-day exercises on the following pages.

DAY 43
HOME WORKOUT 15

Today, you'll have 5 exercises. I call this workout style 'add one every time'. Each exercise is for 30 seconds with 20 seconds' rest in between. Here are the set structures and the exercises: as you can see, there is a mix of cardio, strength and core exercises.

Set 1: You will do Exercise 1
Set 2: Exercises 1 and 2
Set 3: Exercises 1, 2 and 3
Set 4: Exercises 1, 2, 3 and 4
Set 5: Exercises 1, 2, 3, 4 and 5
Set 6: You will drop Exercise 1, so Exercises 2, 3, 4 and 5
Set 7: You will drop Exercise 1 and 2, so you will do Exercises 3, 4 and 5
Set 8: Exercises 4 and 5
Set 9: Exercise 5

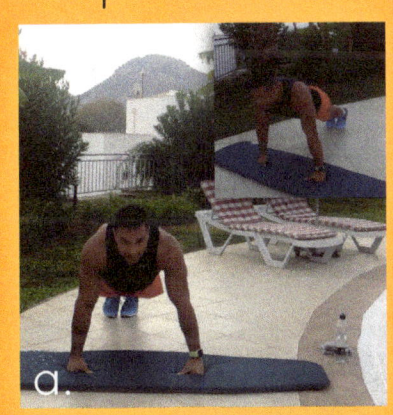

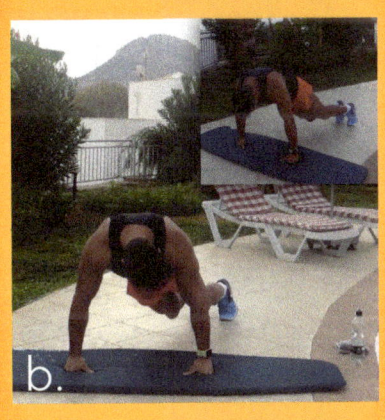

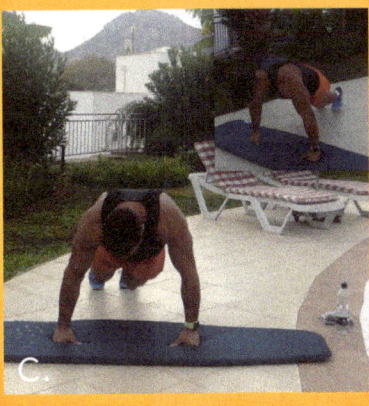

1. Horizontal Side Jumps
2. Leg Raises
3. Press-ups and Diagonal Touch
4. Heel Touches
5. Jumping Lunges

1. Horizontal Side Jumps

a.
b.
c.

2. Leg Raises

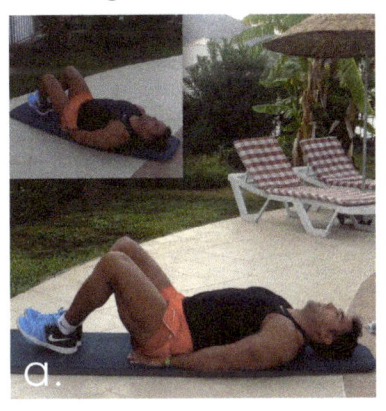

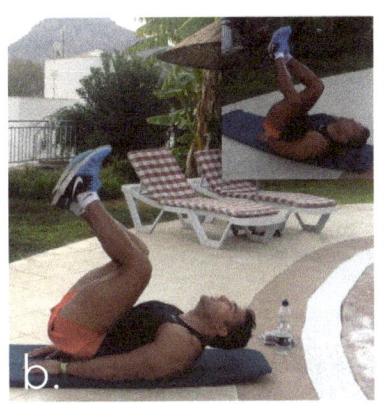

a.
b.

GET FIT, STAY FIT | 221

3. Press-ups and Diagonal Touch

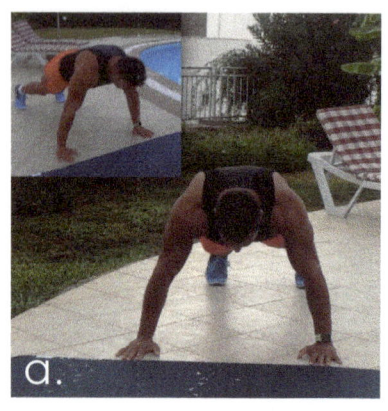

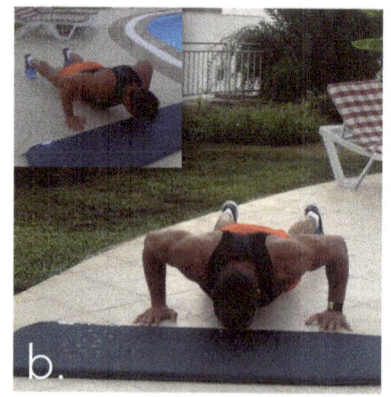

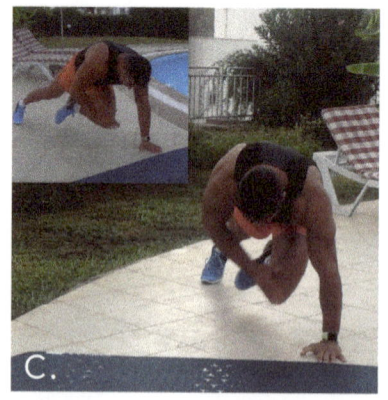

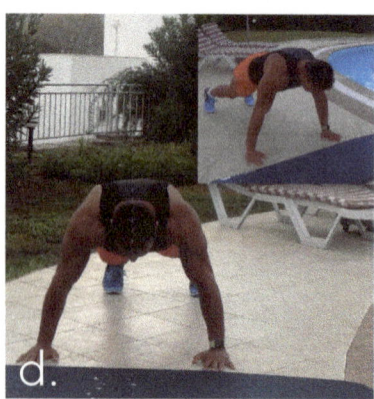

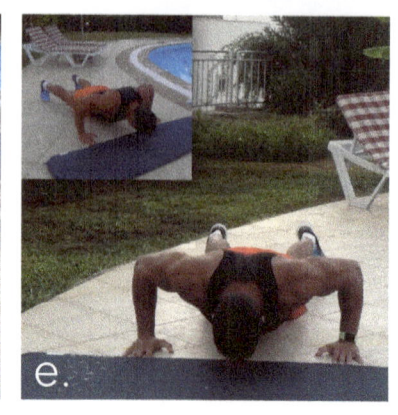

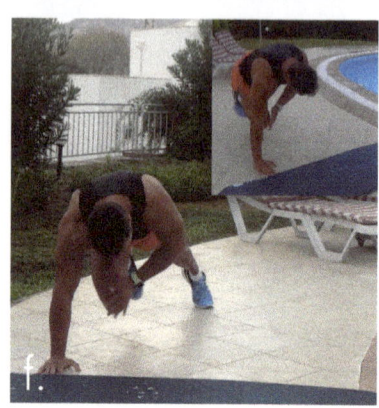

a.   b.   c.
d.   e.   f.

4. Heel Touches

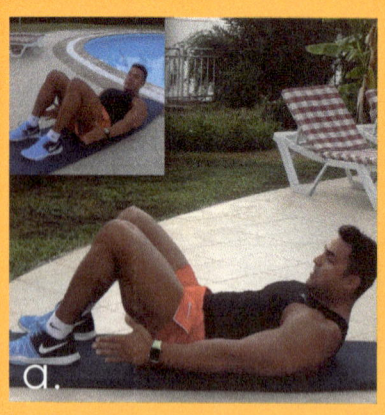

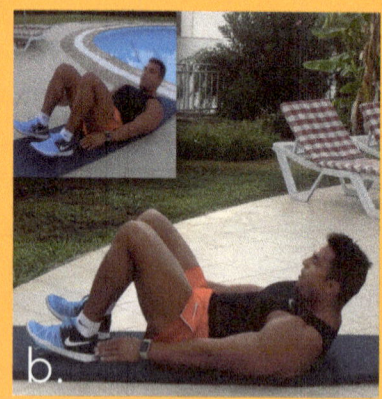

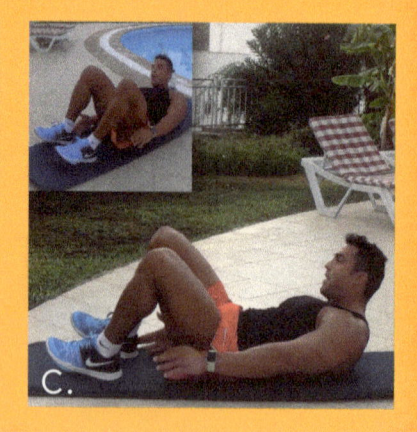

a.   b.   c.

5. Jumping Lunges

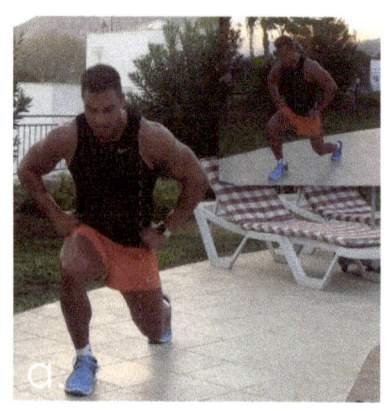

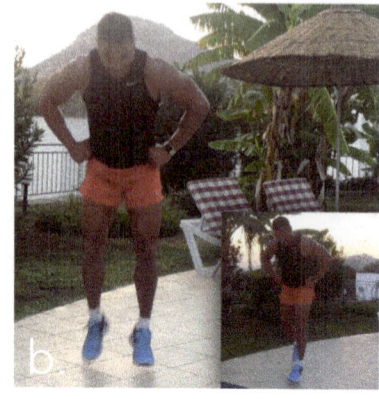

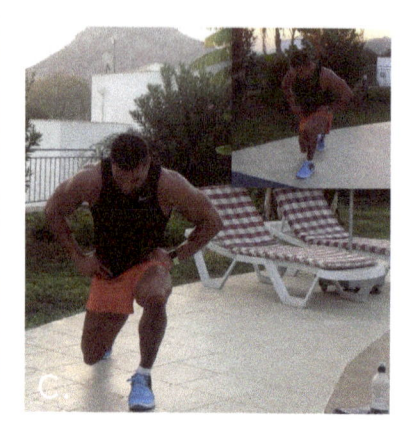

a.   b.   c.

222 | GOKAY KURTULDUM

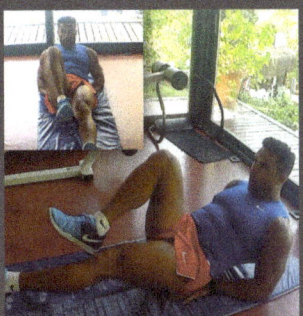

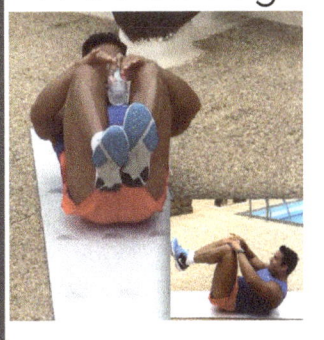

DAY 44
UPPER BODY WEIGHT TRAINING PROGRAMME 2(B)

This is the same as the workout you did on Day 36 and Day 25. The tempo for each repetition should be 1 second up, 1 second down (or vice versa).

1.	Barbell Shoulder Press	4 sets x 12 repetitions
2.	Dumbbell Side Laterals	4 sets x 12 reps
3.	Cable Front Raise	4 sets x 12 reps
4.	EZ Barbell Biceps Curl	4 sets x 12 reps
5.	Dumbbell Inclined Biceps Curl	4 sets x 12 reps
6.	Standing EZ Bar Triceps Extension	4 sets x 12 reps
7.	Dumbbell One Arm Triceps Kick	4 sets x 12 reps each side
8.	Cycling in the Air	3 sets x 30 secs
9.	Dead Bug	3 sets x 15 reps each side

1. Barbell Shoulder Press
2. Dumbbells Side Laterals
3. Cable Front Raise
4. EZ Barbell Biceps Curl
5. Dumbbell Inclined Biceps Curl
6. Standing EZ Bar Triceps Extension
7. Dumbbell One Arm Triceps Kick
8. Cycling in the Air
9. Dead Bug

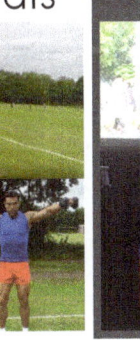

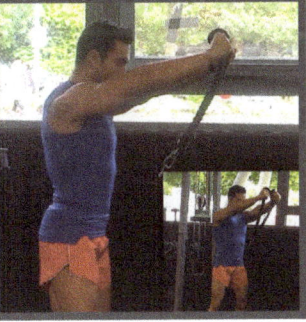

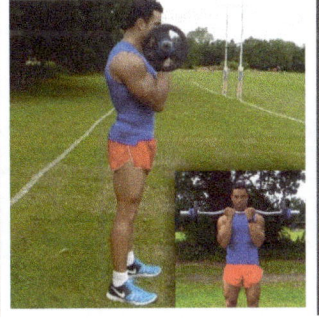

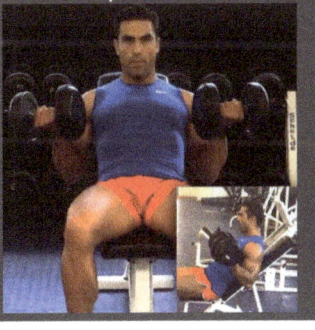

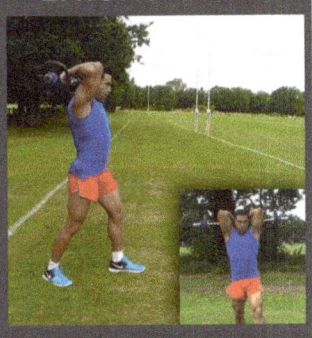

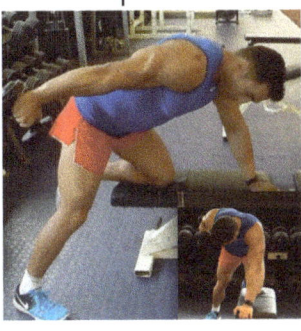

DAY 45
HOME WORKOUT 11

This is the same as the workout you did on Day 33. Today's workout contains 6 exercises performed in a descending pyramid. For Set 1, each exercise will be for 50 seconds, Set 2 is 40 seconds, Set 3 is 30 seconds, all the way down to 10 seconds each in 5 sets. The rest time between each exercise is 10 seconds. Here are the set structures and exercises:

Set 1: each exercise for 50 secs
Set 2: each exercise for 40 secs
Set 3: each exercise for 30 secs
Set 4: each exercise for 20 secs
Set 5: each exercise for 10 secs

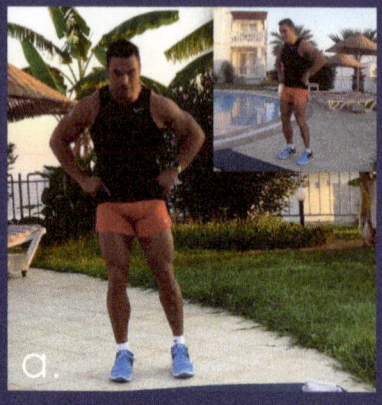

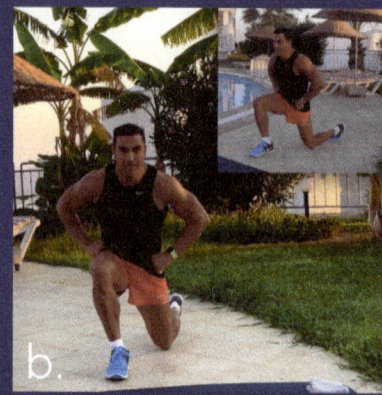

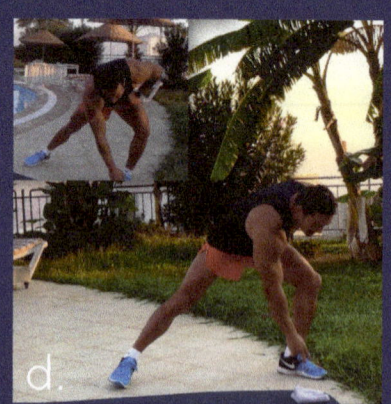

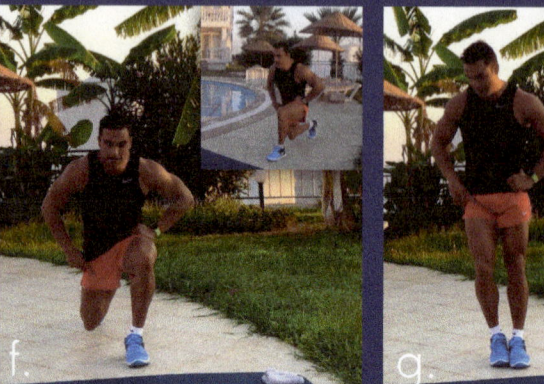

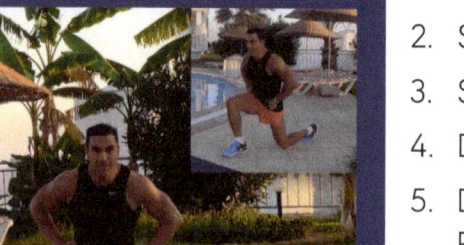

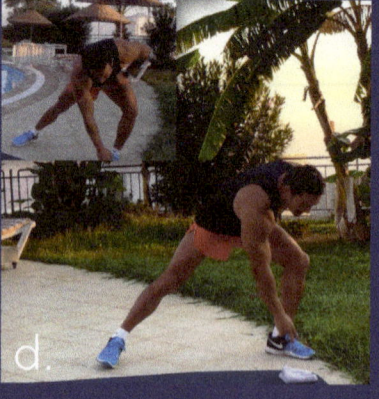

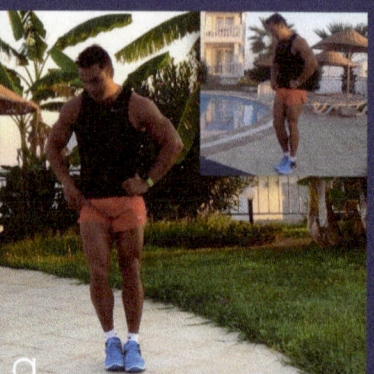

These are the exercises:

1. Lunge Back and Side
2. Squat Thrust to Sides
3. Scissors
4. Duck Squats
5. Dynamic Plank to Press-ups with a Jump
6. Knee Hits

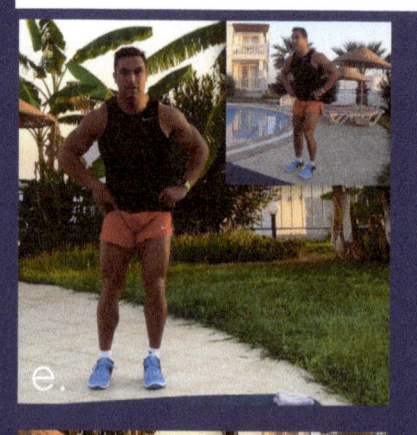

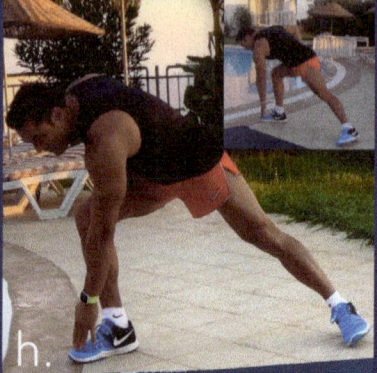

1. Lunge Back and Side

a.
b.
c.
d.
e.
f.
g.
h.

224 | GOKAY KURTULDUM

2. Squat Thrust to Sides

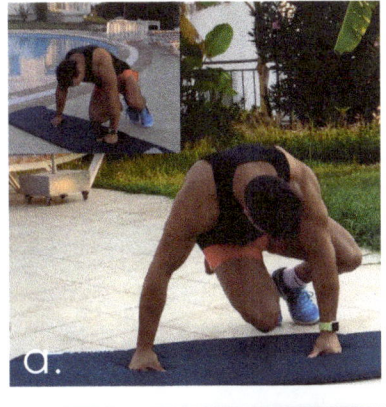

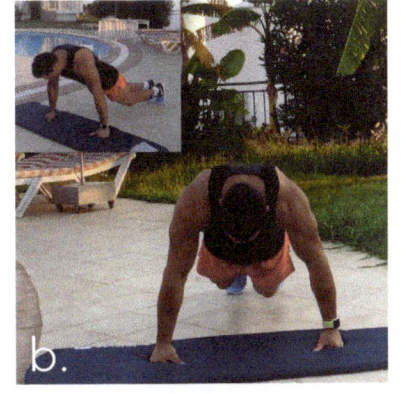

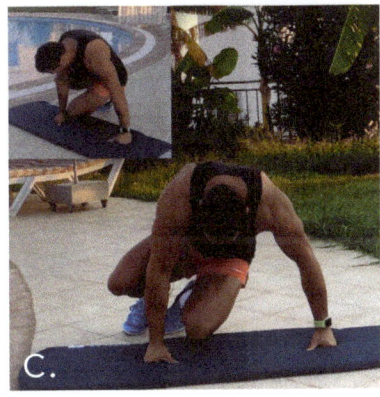

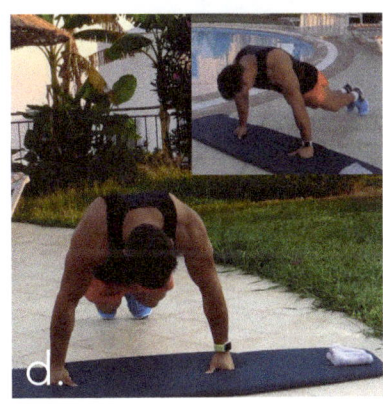

a.
b.
c.
d.

3. Scissors

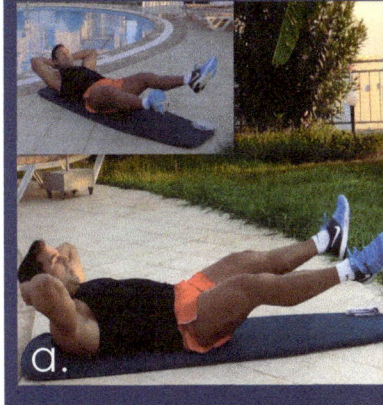

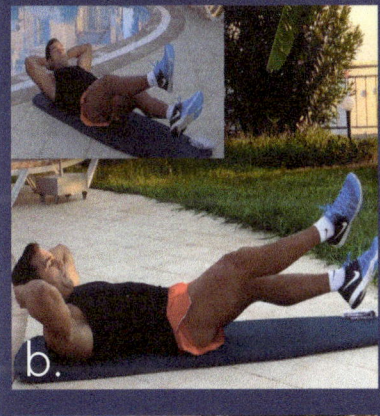

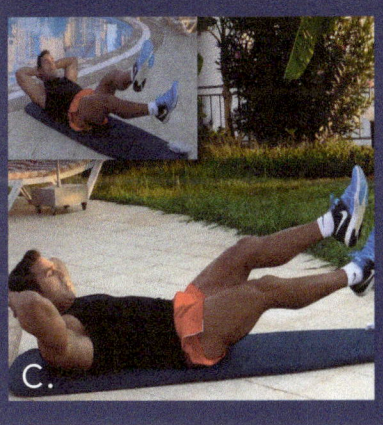

a.
b.
c.

4. Duck Squats

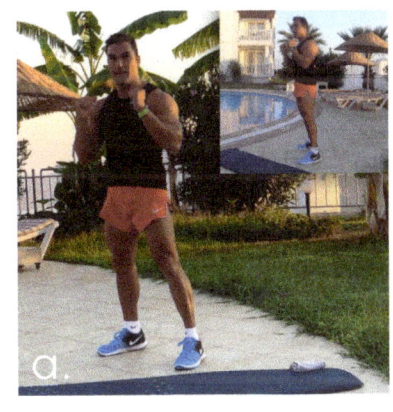

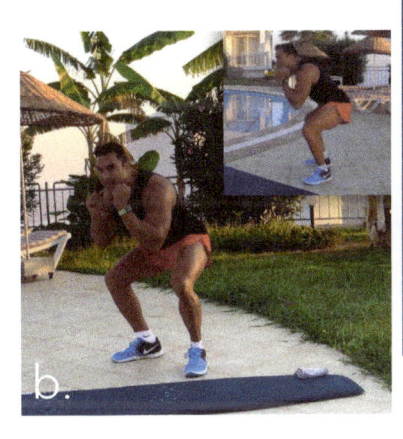

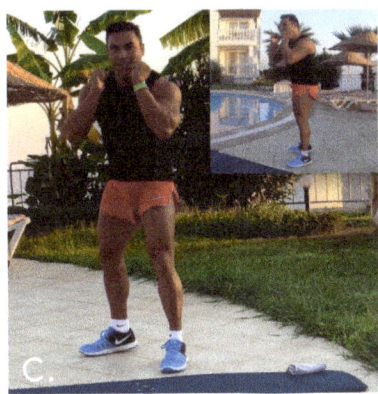

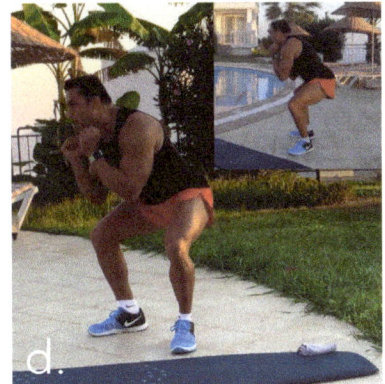

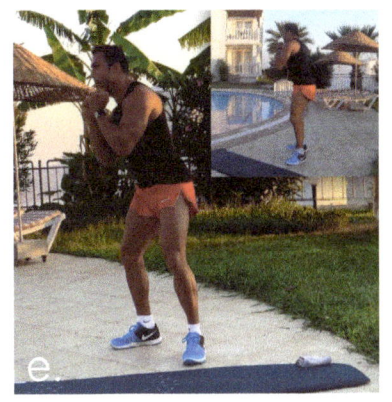

a.
b.
c.
d.
e.

GET FIT, STAY FIT | 225

5. Dynamic Plank to Press-ups with a Jump

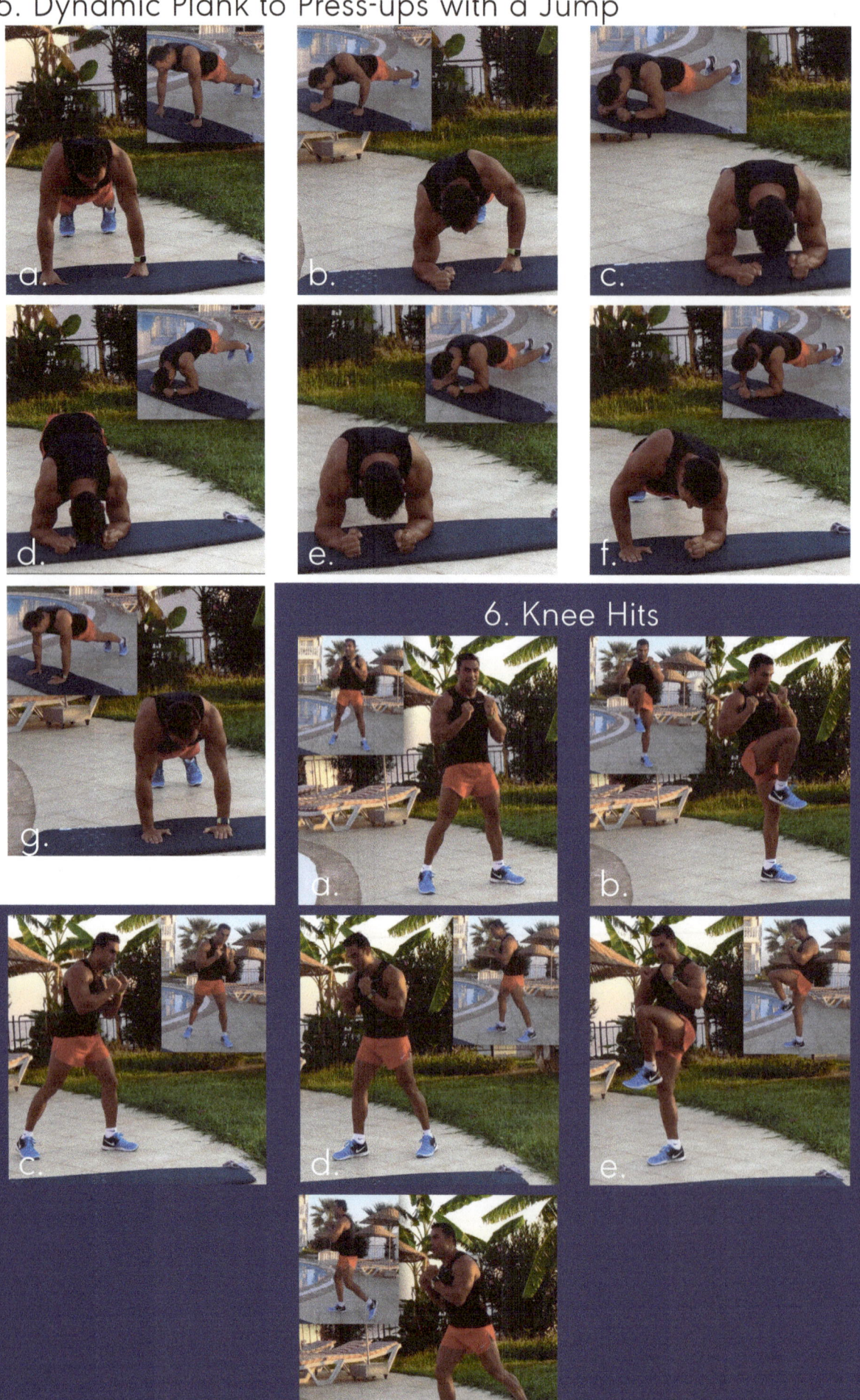

6. Knee Hits

226 | GOKAY KURTULDUM

DAY 46
LOWER BODY WEIGHT TRAINING PROGRAMME 2(B)

This is the same as the workout you did on Day 37 and Day 26. The tempo for each repetition should be 1 second up, 1 second down (or vice versa).

1.	Leg Extension	4 sets x 15 repetitions
2.	TRX Squat Jumps	4 sets x 15 reps
3.	Leg Curl	3 sets x 15 reps
4.	Split Squats	3 sets x 15 reps each side
5.	Abdominal Crunches with Raised Arms	3 sets x 30 reps
6.	Abs Scissors Heel Taps	3 sets x 20 reps each side
7.	Oblique Crunches	3 sets x 30 reps each side
8.	Plank Weight Rotation	3 sets x 10 each direction

1. Leg Extension

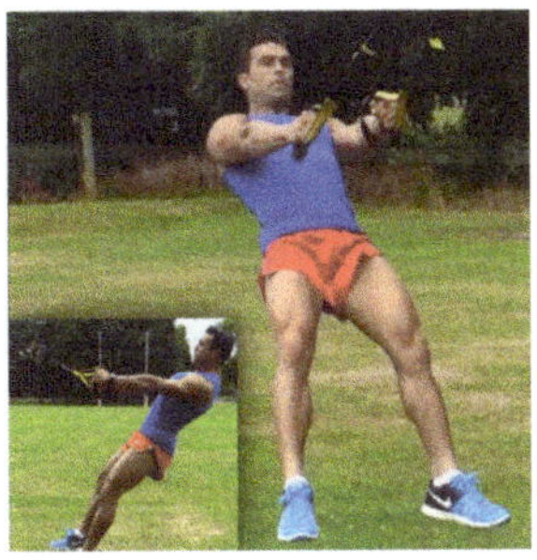

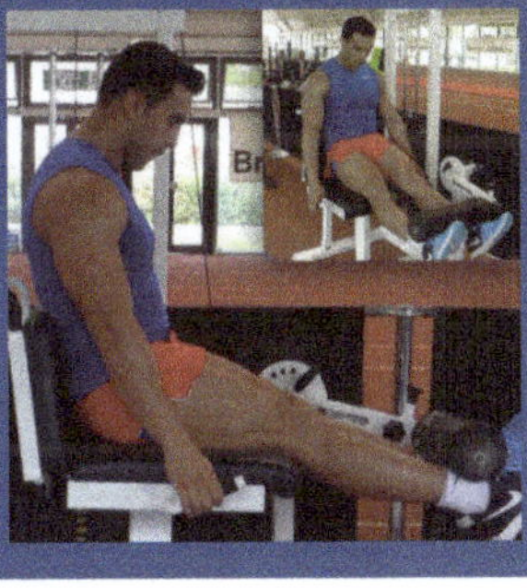

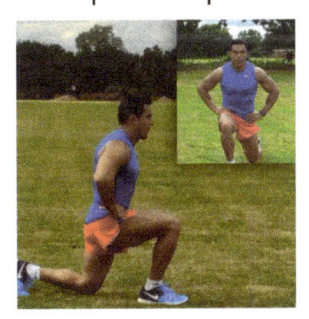

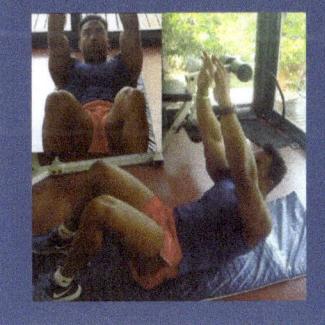

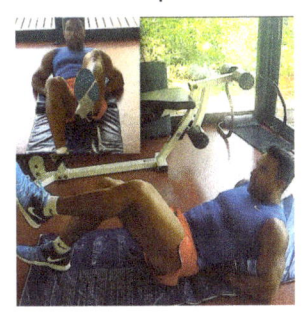

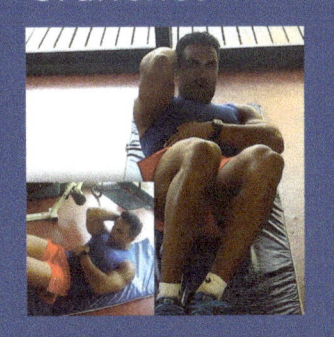

2. TRX Squat Jumps

3. Leg Curl

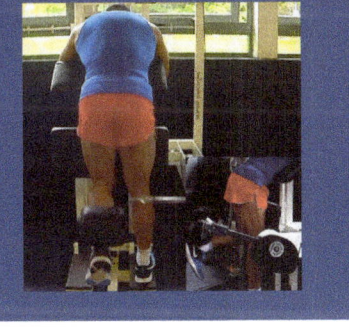

4. Split Squats

5. Abdominal Crunches with Raised Arms

6. Abs Scissors Heel Taps

7. Oblique Crunches

8. Plank Weight Rotation

GET FIT, STAY FIT | 227

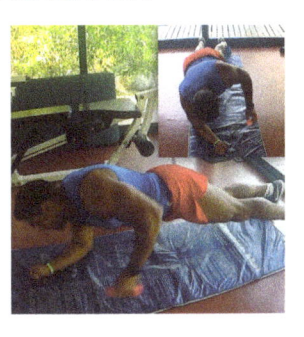

DAY 47
HOME WORKOUT 12

This is the same as the workout you did on Day 34. There are 6 exercises. Each exercise lasts for 40 seconds and the rest time between sets is 10 seconds only! Do 4 sets.

1. Skiing Torso Rotation — 40 secs on, 10 secs off
2. Squats Increasing Claps — 40 secs on, 10 secs off
3. Leg Kick, Tap with Opposite Hand — 40 secs on, 10 secs off
4. Reverse Crunches with Knee Flexion — 40 secs on, 10 secs off
5. Side Tap, Side Laterals — 40 secs on, 10 secs off
6. Burpees and Forward Lunges — 40 secs on, 10 secs off

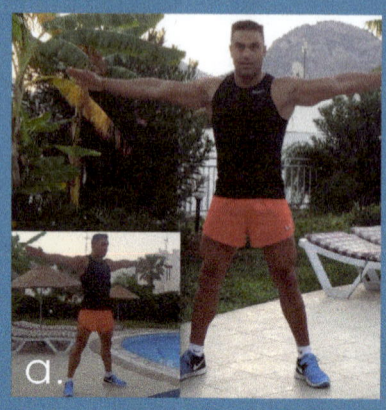

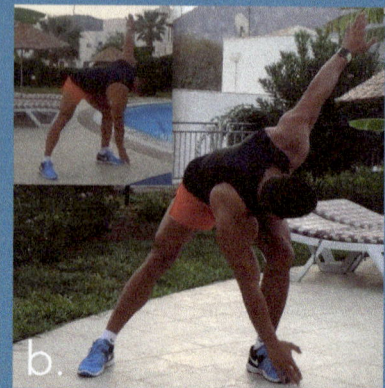

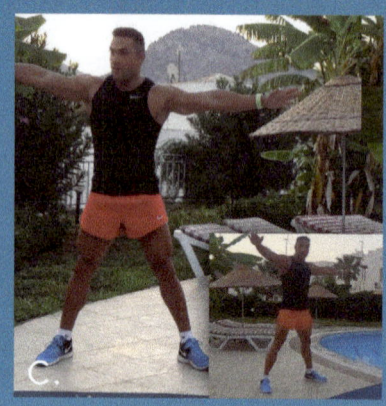

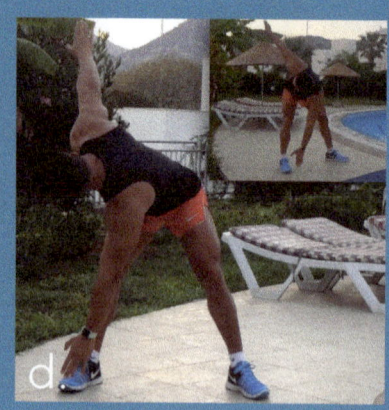

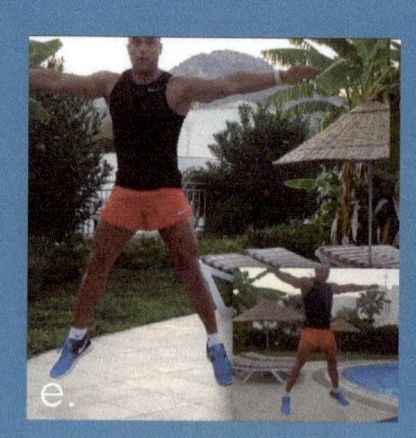

1. Skiing Torso Rotation

2. Squats Increasing Claps

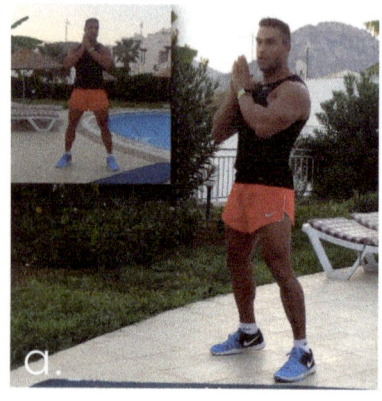

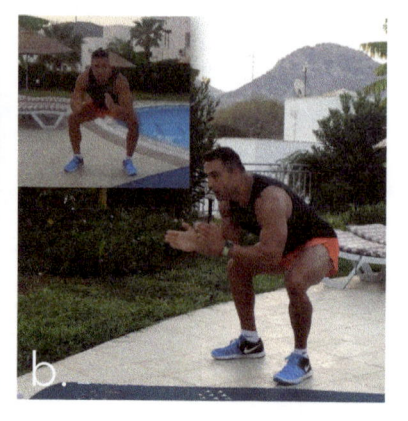

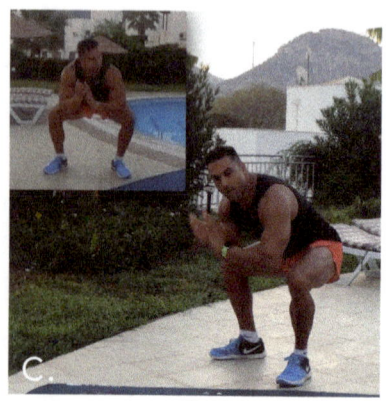

228 | GOKAY KURTULDUM

3. Leg Kick, Tap with Opposite Hand

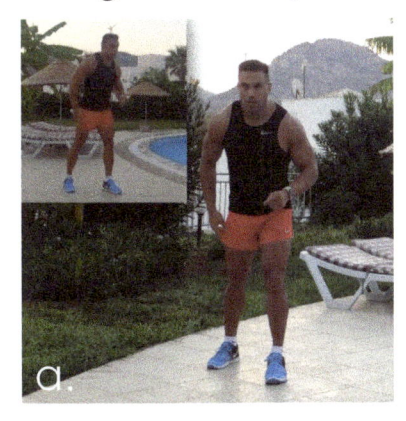

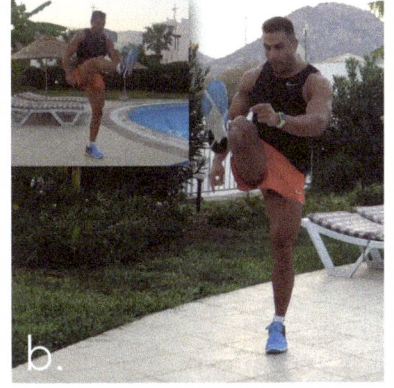

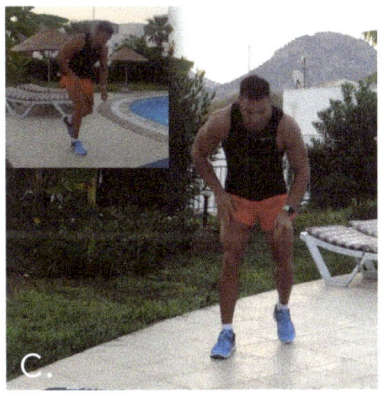

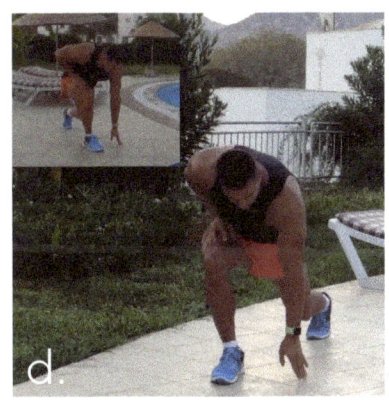

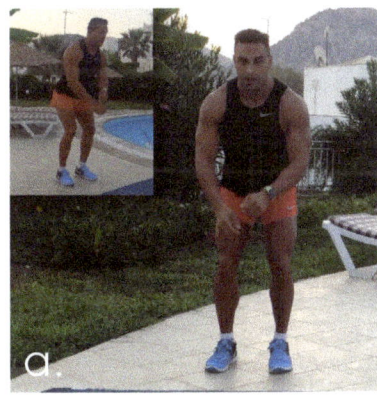

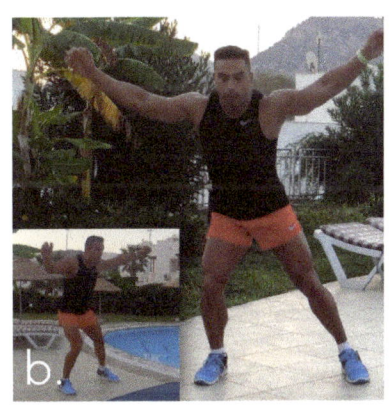

a.
b.
c.
d.

4. Reverse Crunches with Knee Flexion

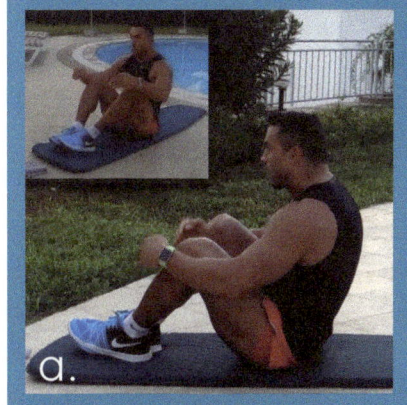

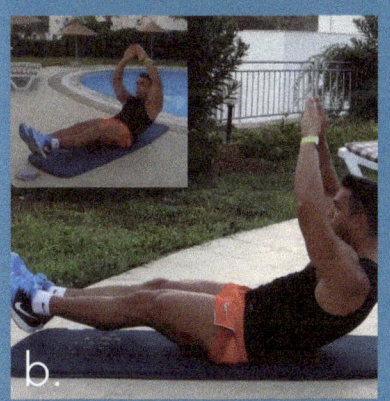

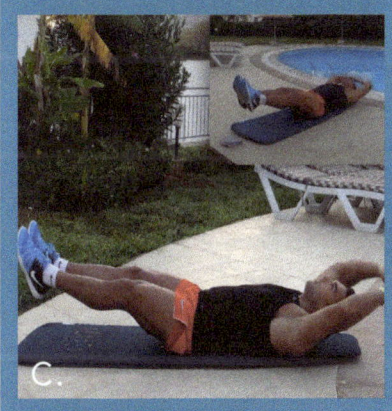

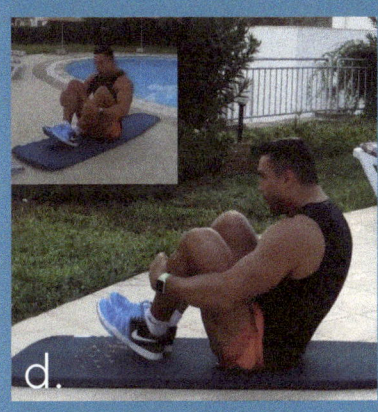

a.
b.
c.
d.

5. Side Tap, Side Laterals

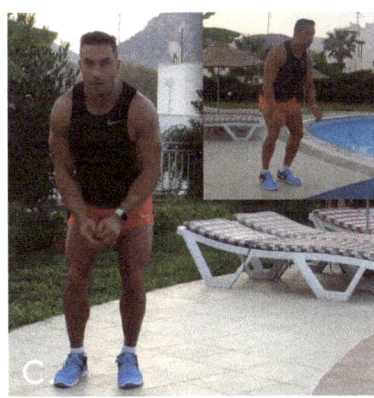

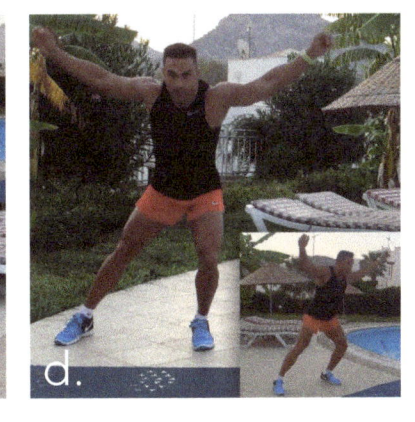

a.
b.
c.
d.

GET FIT, STAY FIT | 229

6. Burpees and Forward Lunges

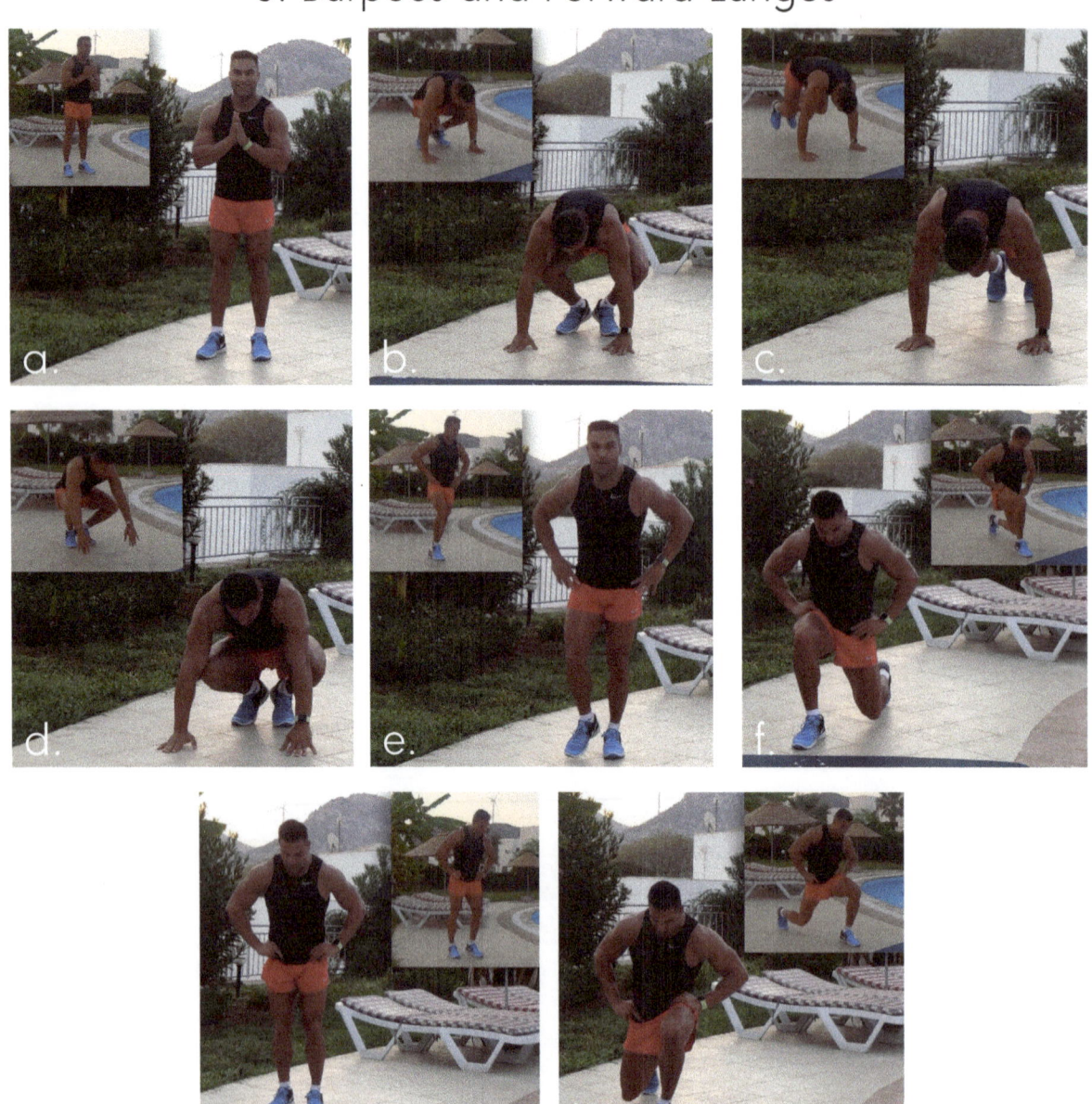

DAY 48
HOME WORKOUT 13

Today you'll repeat the workout you did on Day 38. There are 6 exercises. Each exercise lasts for 30 seconds and the rest time between sets is 20 seconds. Just to remind you, you'll need a chair, step or a bench for this one.

1. Press-ups/Star Jumps — 30 secs on, 20 secs off
2. Low Kick Dance — 30 secs on, 20 secs off
3. Squat Side Jumps — 30 secs on, 20 secs off
4. Triceps Dips — 30 secs on, 20 secs off
5. Single Leg Hops — 15 secs on each leg, 20 secs off
6. Lying Flying — 30 secs on, 20 secs off

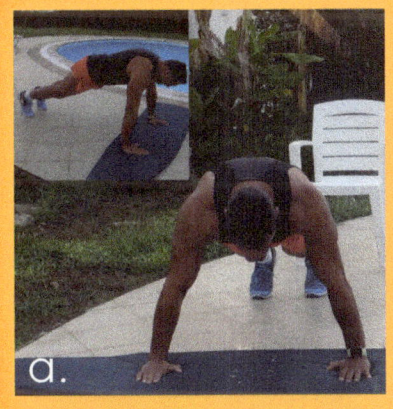

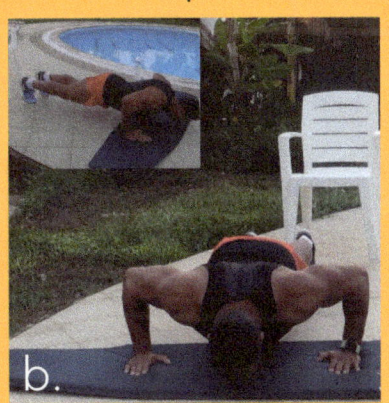

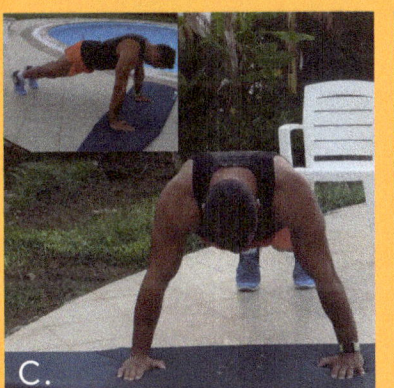

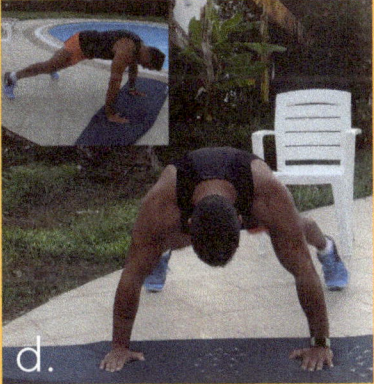

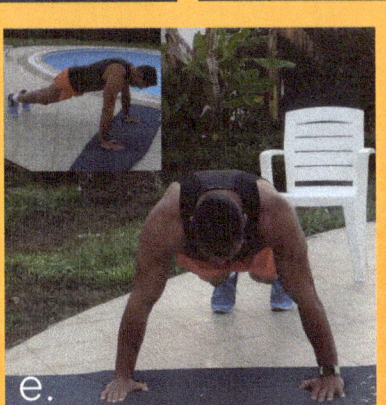

1. Press-ups/Star Jumps

2. Low Kick Dance

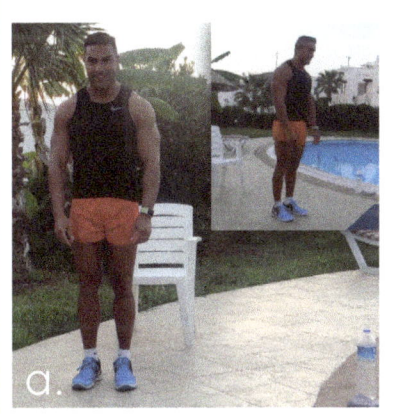

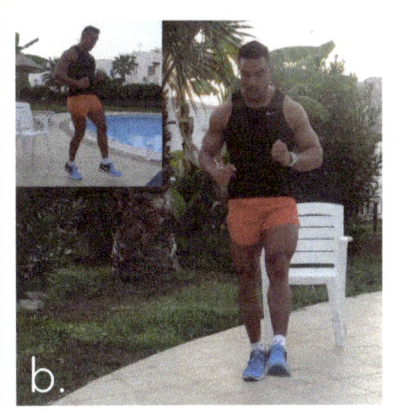

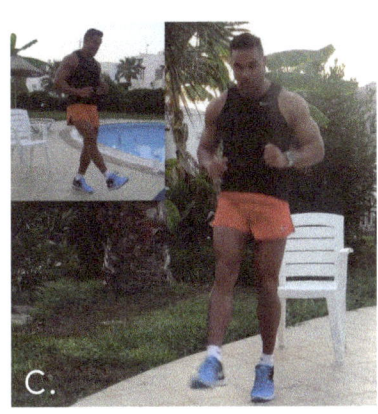

GET FIT, STAY FIT | 231

3. Squat Side Jumps

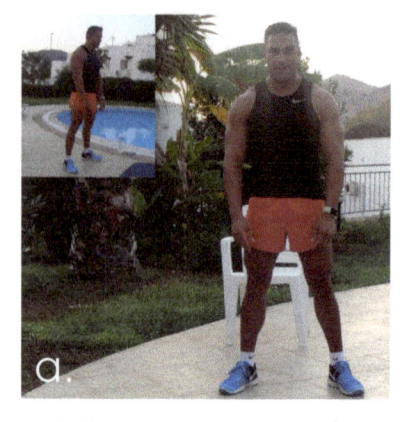

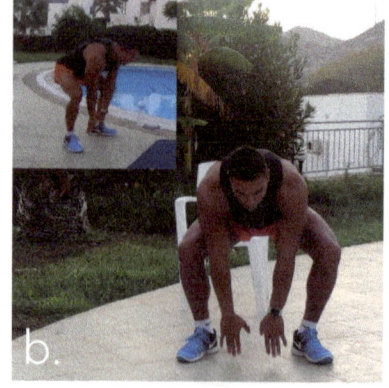

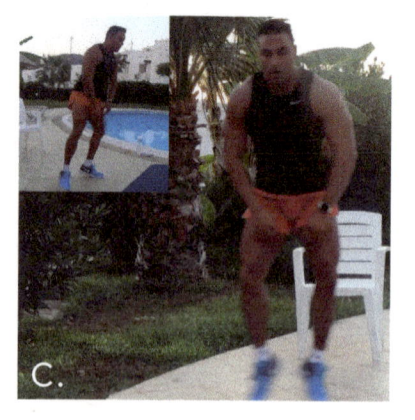

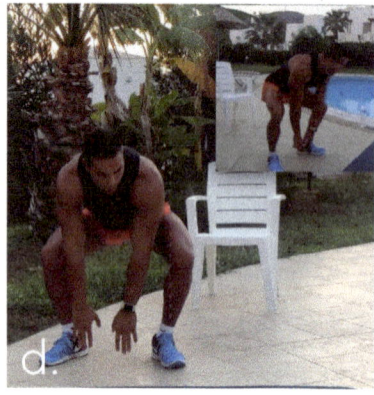

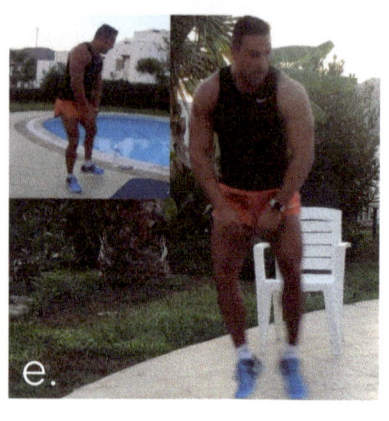

a.
b.
c.
d.
e.

4. Triceps Dips

a.
b.

5. Single Leg Hops

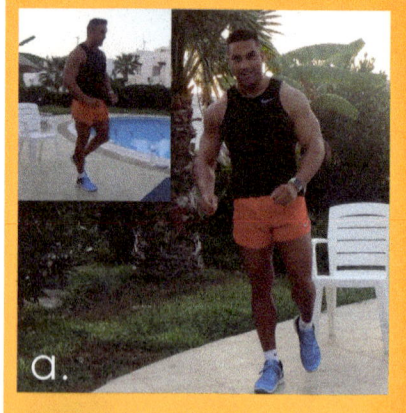

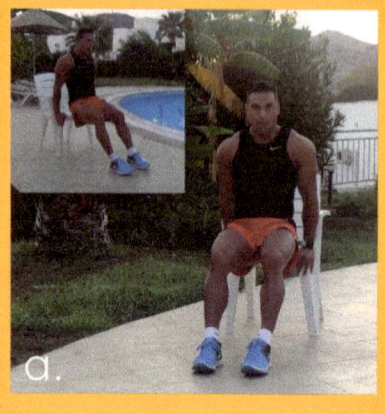

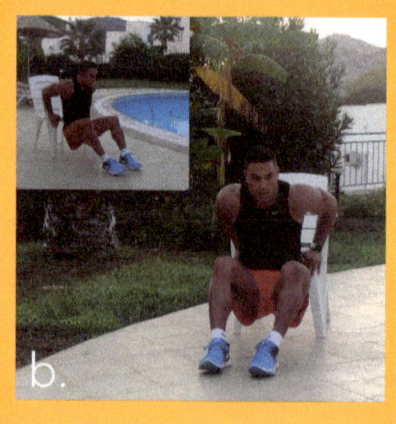

a.
b.
c.

6. Lying Flying

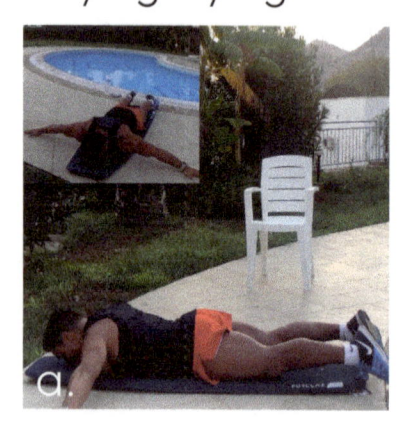

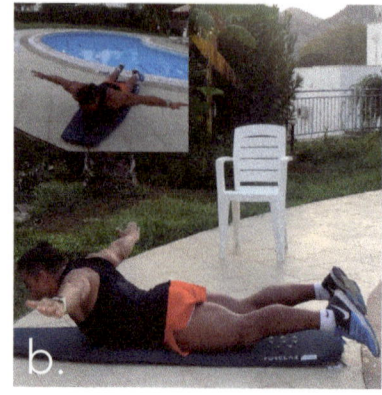

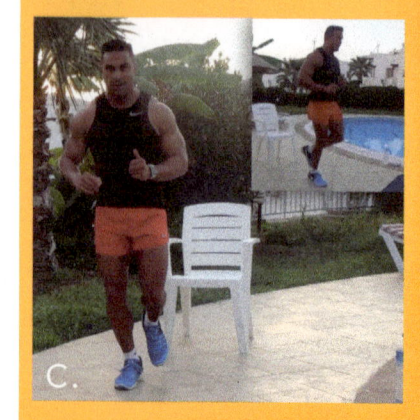

a.
b.

232 | GOKAY KURTULDUM

DAY 49 OFF

WEEK 7 PROGRESS JOURNAL

Use these pages to set your intentions at the start of the week and record and reflect on your progress at the end of the week. Alternatively, use a special notebook for this purpose.

PART 1: INTENTIONS/PLANNING

My starting weight this week: _____

My starting waist measurement: _____

My goal weight at the end of this week: _____

My goal waist measurement at the end of this week: _____

Any other goals for the week (e.g. no alcohol during the week and no more than 14 units during the weekend or going to bed early weekdays and sleep minimum 7 hours etc.)

_____

_____

Which days are going to be tricky this week and why? (E.g. client dinner on Thursday which involves drinking alcohol)

_____

How will I deal with this? _____

_____

Any other notes/thoughts:

PART 2: RECORD/REFLECTIONS

At the end of this week how many goals did I achieve?

How many did I come close to?

How am I feeling about my progress?

Which goals did I not reach?

Why was that? Family commitments, too much work and no time, not motivated enough? Can I define exactly what hindered my progress? Can I take action on that next week?

What actions can I take next week to improve on this?

What were my wins this week? (e.g. weight loss, mileage run etc?)

I've achieved

Give marks out of 10 for progress this week

8.11 WEEK 8 PROGRAMME AND JOURNAL PAGES

This is another gym-heavy week, with only two home workouts, each 20 minutes long. Start with the planning section of your last journal pages. You're nearly there! Hang on in there and stay committed!

Here's a summary of your Week 8 programme:

Day 50	Upper Body Weight Training P2(a)
Day 51	Lower Body Weight Training P2(a)
Day 52	Home Workout 14
Day 53	Upper Body Weight Training P2(b)
Day 54	Lower Body Weight Training P2(b)
Day 55	OFF
Day 56	Home Workout 15

Now it's time for the last week of your 8 week plan! Work through the programme on the following pages.

DAY 50
UPPER BODY WEIGHT TRAINING PROGRAMME 2(A)

This is the same as the workout you did on Day 39, Day 30 and Day 22. The tempo for each repetition should be 1 second up, 1 second down (or vice versa).

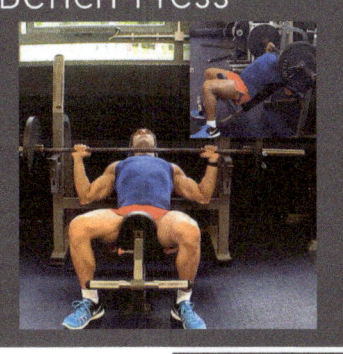

1. Inclined Barbell Bench Press — 4 sets x 12 repetitions
2. Dumbbells Chest Fly — 4 sets x 12 reps
3. Dumbbells Inclined Bench Press — 4 sets x 12 reps
4. Dumbbell One Arm Rowing — 4 sets x 12 reps
5. Cable Reverse Fly (Back Extension) — 4 sets x 12 reps
6. Lat Pull Down Wide Overhand Grip — 4 sets x 12 reps
7. Cable Crunches — 4 sets x 25 reps
8. Leg Raises — 4 sets x 25 reps

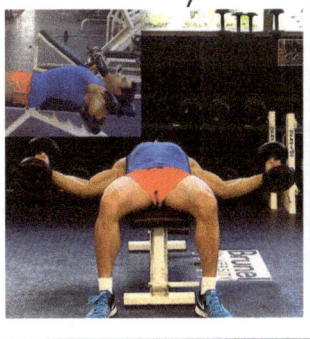

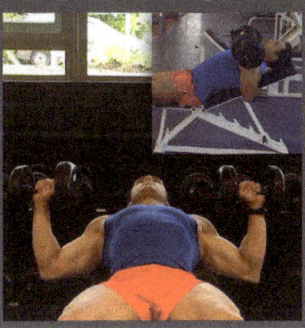

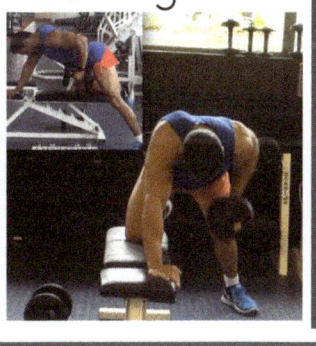

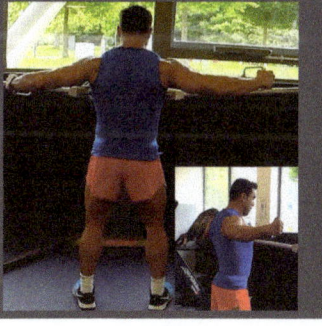

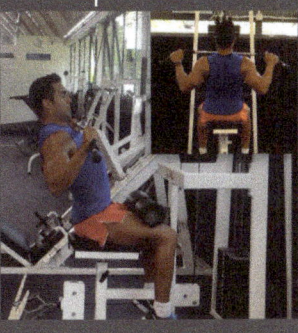

1. Inclined Barbell Bench Press

2. Dumbbells Chest Fly

3. Dumbbells Inclined Bench Press

4. Dumbbell One Arm Rowing

5. Cable Reverse Fly

6. Lat Pull Down Wide Overhand Grip

7. Cable Crunches

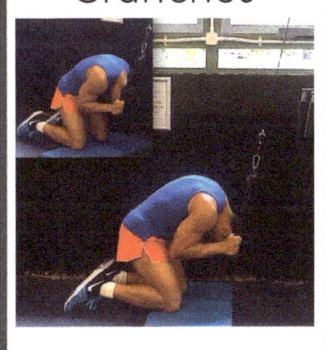

8. Leg Raises

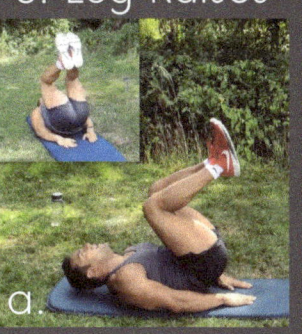

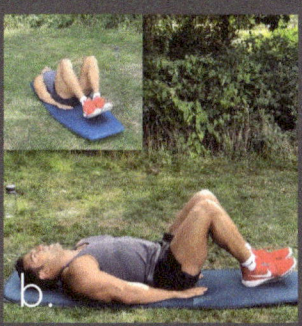

a.   b.

GET FIT, STAY FIT

DAY 51
LOWER BODY WEIGHT TRAINING PROGRAMME 2(A)

This is the same as the workout you did on Day 40, Day 32 and Day 23. The tempo for each repetition should be 1 second up, 1 second down (or vice versa). There are 7 exercises only so you will do 4 sets of leg exercises and 3 sets of core.

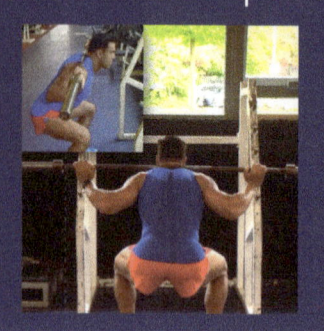

1. Barbell Squats — 4 sets x 12 repetitions
2. Side Lunges — 4 sets x 15 reps each side
3. Barbell Deadlift — 4 sets x 12 reps
4. Oblique (Russian) Twist — 3 sets x 20 reps each side
5. Plank — 3 sets x 45 secs
6. Oblique Crunches — 3 sets x 25 reps each side
7. Slow Release Sit-ups — 3 sets x 20 reps

1. Barbell Squats

2. Side Lunges

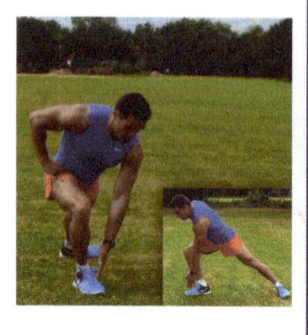

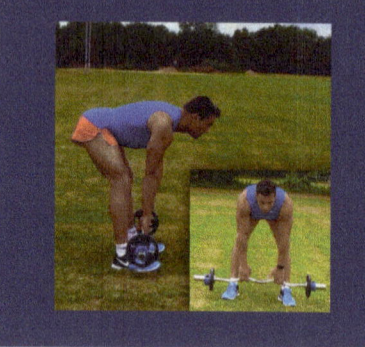

3. Barbell Deadlift

4. Oblique (Russian) Twist

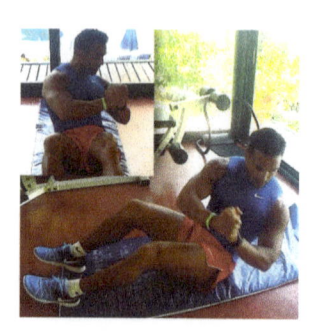

5. Plank

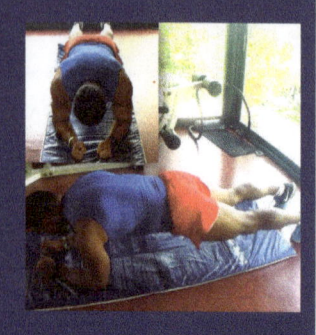

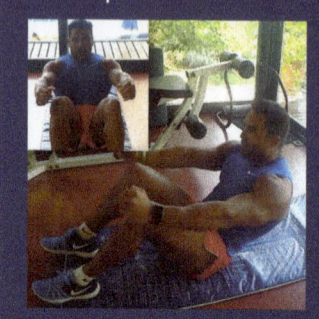

6. Oblique Crunches

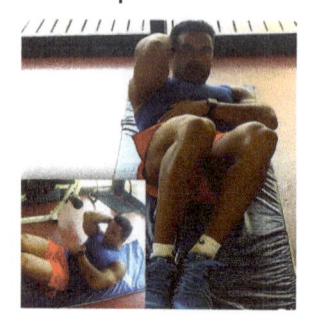

7. Slow Release Sit-ups

DAY 52
HOME WORKOUT 14

Today you'll repeat the workout you did on Day 41.

As before, there are 6 exercises, forming a descending pyramid. So you will start with 50 seconds on, 10 seconds off. Then 40 seconds on, 10 seconds off. For each set you'll reduce the seconds by 10. Set 5 will be for 10 seconds on, 10 seconds off. Here are the set structures and the exercises:

Set 1: each exercise for 50 secs
Set 2: each exercise for 40 secs
Set 3: each exercise for 30 secs
Set 4: each exercise for 20 secs
Set 5: each exercise for 10 secs

The exercises are:
1. 5 Split Squats and Jumps to Alternate Foot
2. Diagonal Toe Touch Crunches
3. Clap under Thighs/Squat Jumps
4. Plank
5. Press-ups to Sides
6. Leg Oblique Side Drops

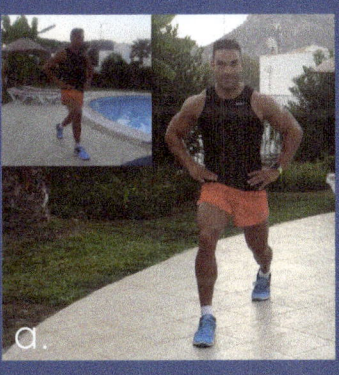

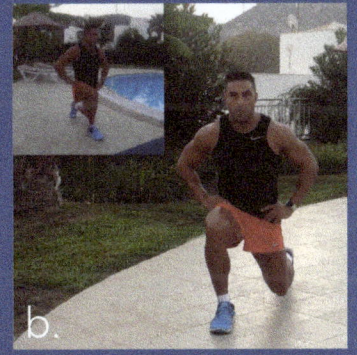

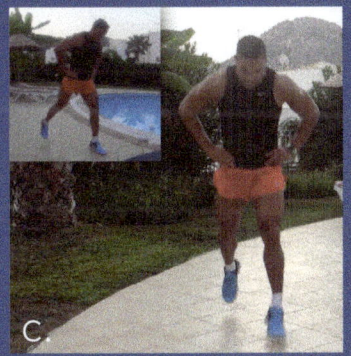

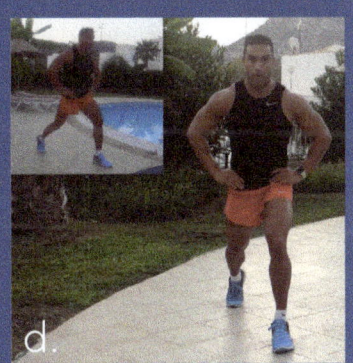

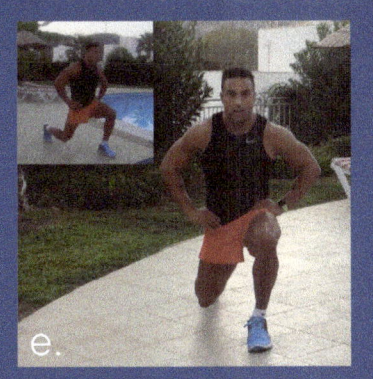

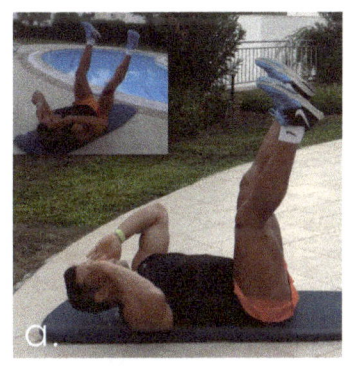

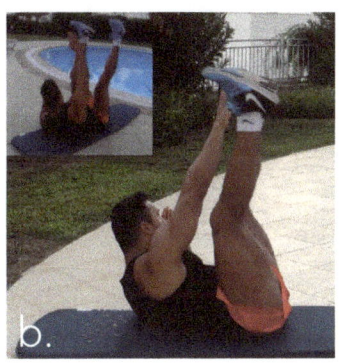

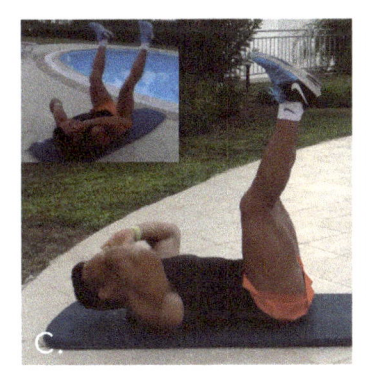

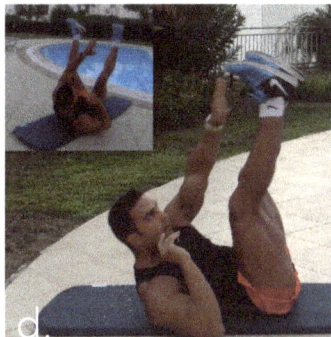

1. 5 Split Squats and Jumps

a.
b.
c.
d.
e.

2. Diagonal Toe Touch Crunches

a.
b.
c.
d.

3. Clap under Thighs/Squat Jumps

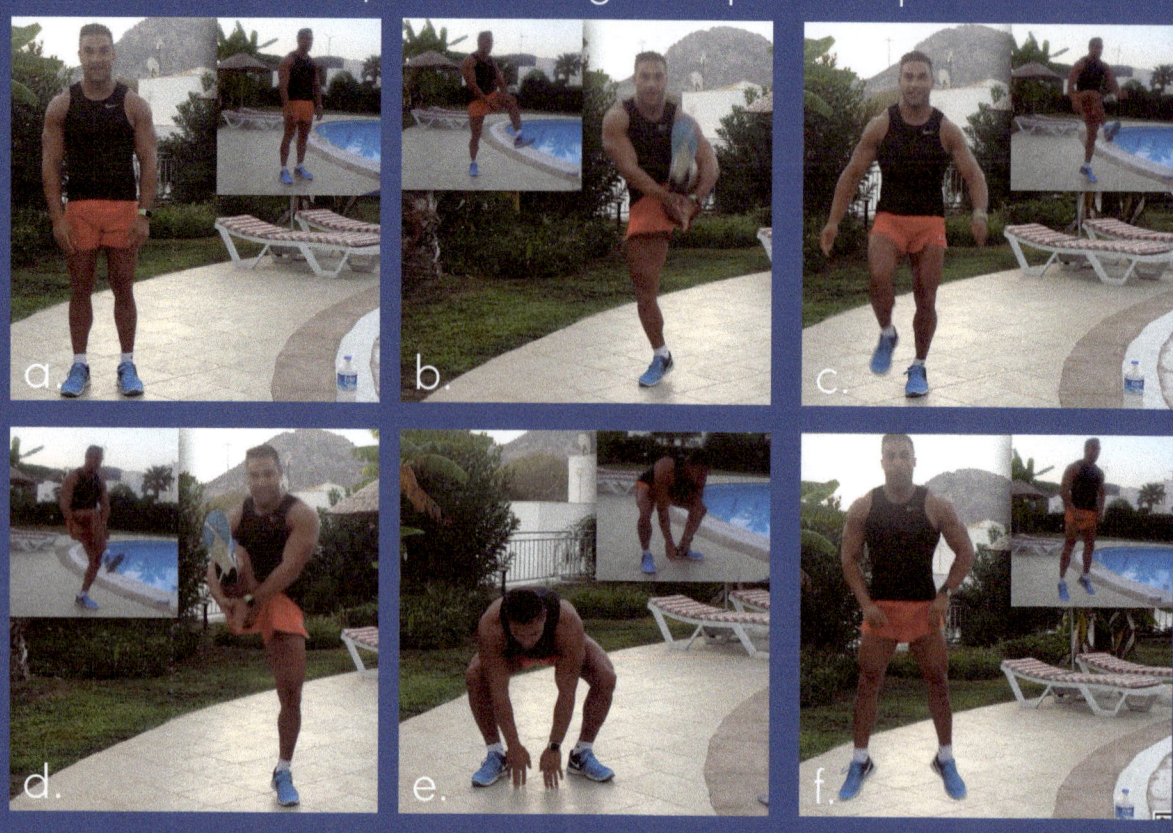

a.
b.
c.
d.
e.
f.

4. Plank

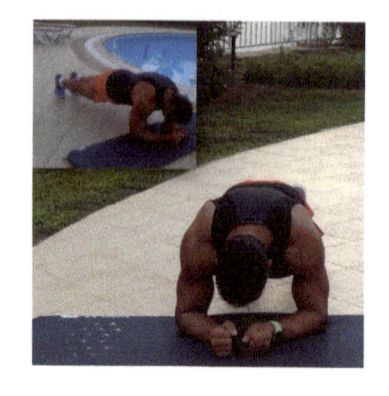

5. Press-ups to Sides

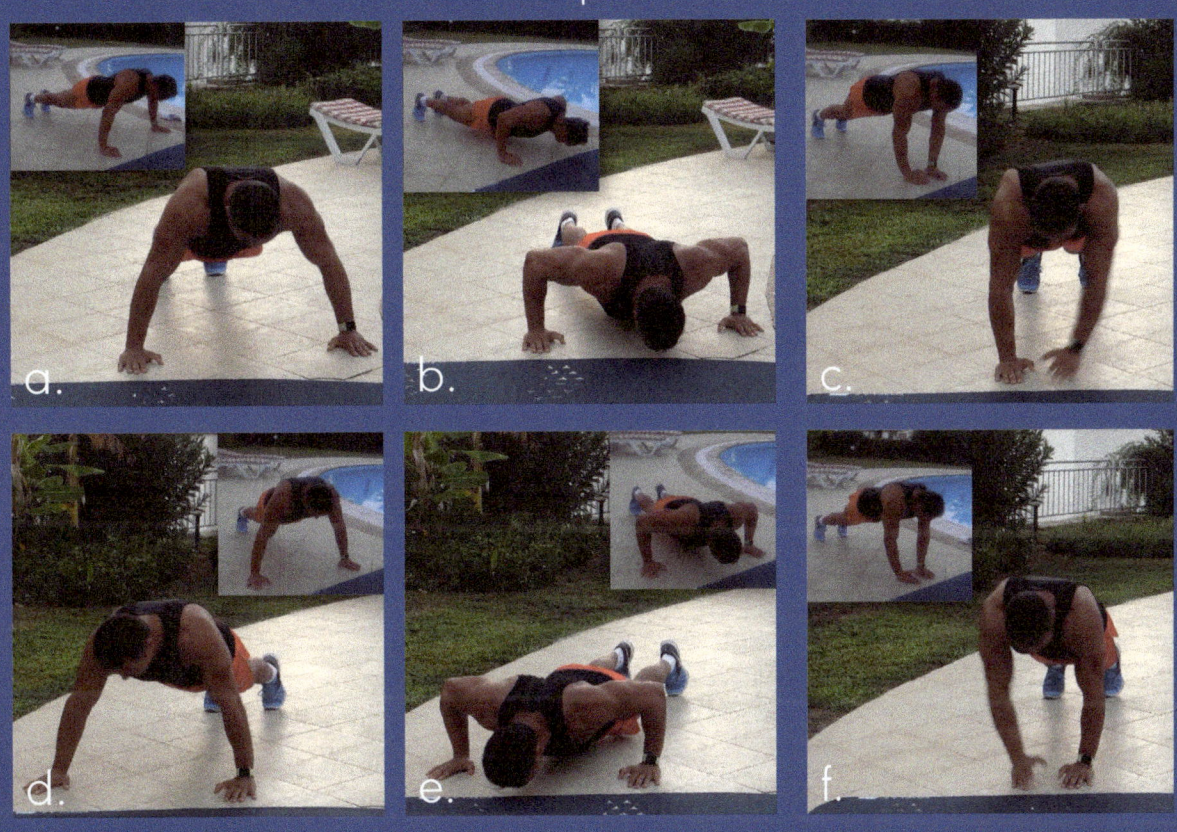

a. b. c.
d. e. f.

6. Leg Oblique Side Drops

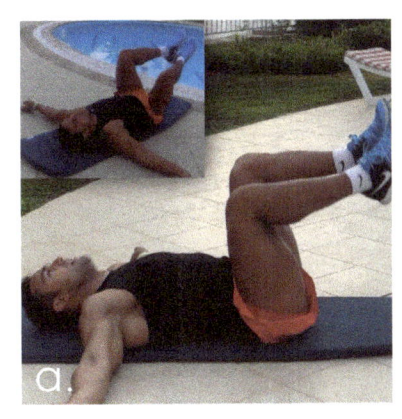

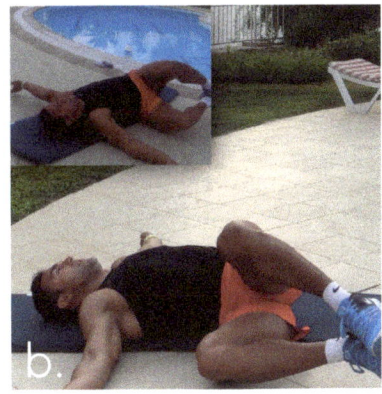

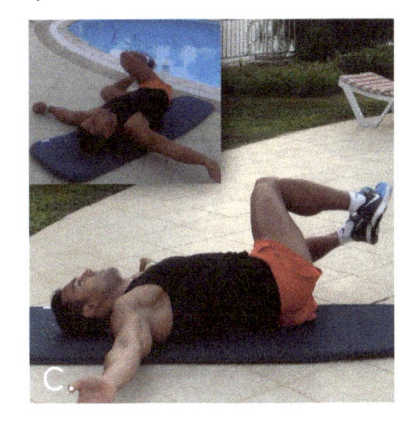

a. b. c.

GET FIT, STAY FIT | 241

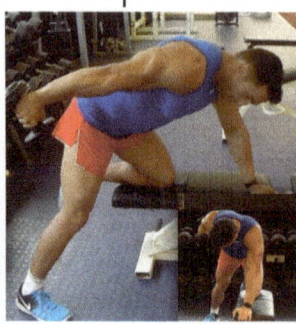

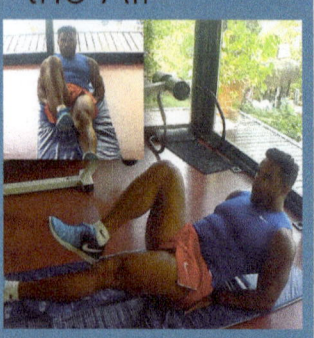

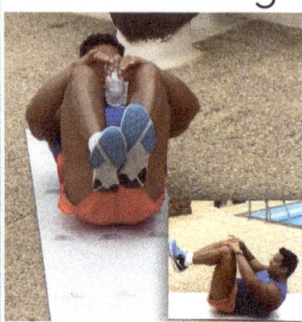

DAY 53
UPPER BODY WEIGHT TRAINING PROGRAMME 2(B)

This is the same as the workout you did on Day 44, Day 36 and Day 25. The tempo for each repetition should be 1 second up, 1 second down (or vice versa).

1. Barbell Shoulder Press — 4 sets x 12 repetitions
2. Dumbbell Side Laterals — 4 sets x 12 reps
3. Cable Front Raise — 4 sets x 12 reps
4. EZ Barbell Biceps Curl — 4 sets x 12 reps
5. Dumbbell Inclined Biceps Curl — 4 sets x 12 reps
6. Standing EZ Bar Triceps Extension — 4 sets x 12 reps
7. Dumbbell One Arm Triceps Kick — 4 sets x 12 reps each side
8. Cycling in the Air — 3 sets x 30 secs
9. Dead Bug — 3 sets x 15 reps each side

1. Barbell Shoulder Press
2. Dumbbells Side Laterals
3. Cable Front Raise
4. EZ Barbell Biceps Curl
5. Dumbbell Inclined Biceps Curl
6. Standing EZ Bar Triceps Extension
7. Dumbbell One Arm Triceps Kick
8. Cycling in the Air
9. Dead Bug

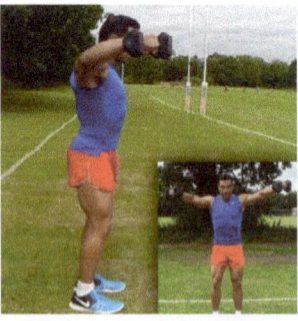

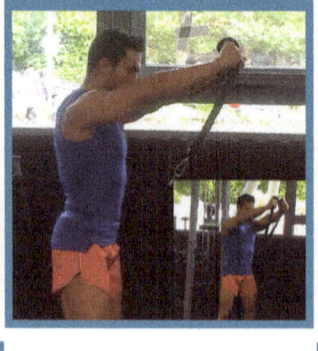

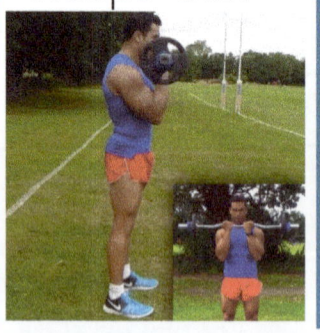

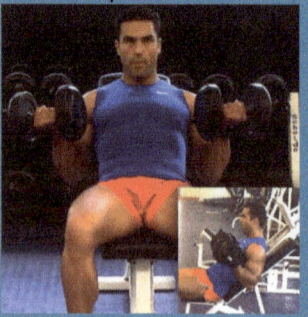

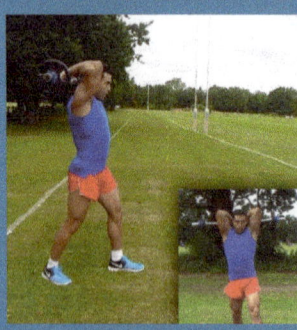

DAY 54
LOWER BODY WEIGHT TRAINING PROGRAMME 2(B)

This is the same as the workout you did on Day 46, Day 37 and Day 26. The tempo for each repetition should be 1 second up, 1 second down (or vice versa).

1.	Leg Extension	4 sets x 15 repetitions
2.	TRX Squat Jumps	4 sets x 15 reps
3.	Leg Curl	3 sets x 15 reps
4.	Split Squats	3 sets x 15 reps each side
5.	Abdominal Crunches with Raised Arms	3 sets x 30 reps
6.	Abs Scissors Heel Taps	3 sets x 20 reps each side
7.	Oblique Crunches	3 sets x 30 reps each side
8.	Plank Weight Rotation	3 sets x 10 each direction

1. Leg Extension

2. TRX Squat Jumps

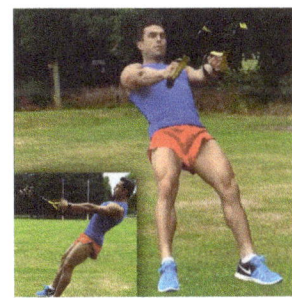

3. Leg Curl

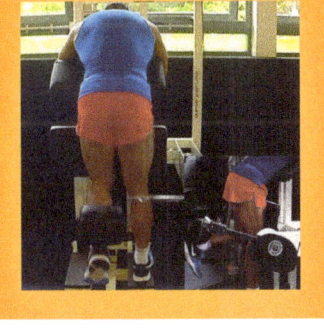

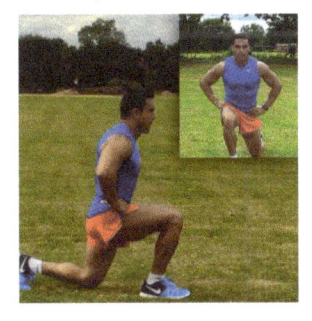

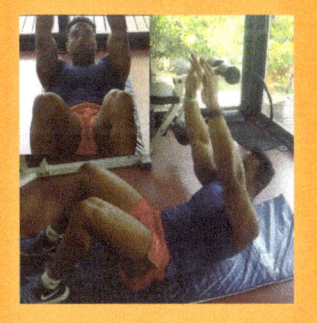

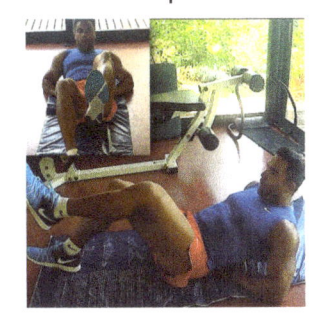

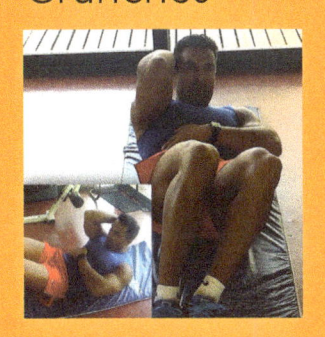

4. Split Squats

5. Abdominal Crunches with Raised Arms

6. Abs Scissors Heel Taps

7. Oblique Crunches

8. Plank Weight Rotation

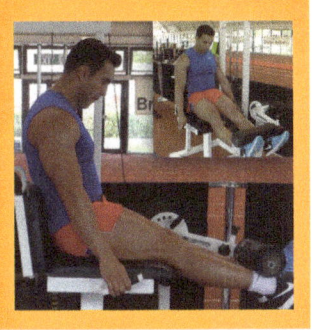

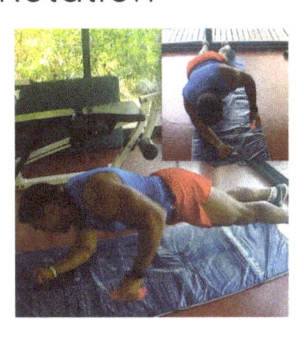

DAY 55 OFF

DAY 56
HOME WORKOUT 15

Today is your last day. Congratulations for being on track! You must be so proud of yourself. You'll be repeating the workout you did on Day 43 today.

There are 5 exercises. I call this workout style 'add one every time'. Each exercise is for 30 seconds with 20 seconds' rest in between.

Here are the set structures and exercises: as you can see, there is a mix of cardio, strength and core exercises.

Set 1: You will do Exercise 1
Set 2: Exercises 1 and 2
Set 3: Exercises 1, 2 and 3
Set 4: Exercises 1, 2, 3 and 4
Set 5: Exercises 1, 2, 3, 4 and 5
Set 6: You will drop Exercise 1, so Exercises 2, 3, 4 and 5
Set 7: You will drop Exercise 1 and 2, so you will do Exercises 3, 4 and 5
Set 8: Exercises 4 and 5
Set 9: Exercise 5

1. Horizontal Side Jumps
2. Leg Raises
3. Press-ups and Diagonal Touch
4. Heel Touches
5. Jumping Lunges

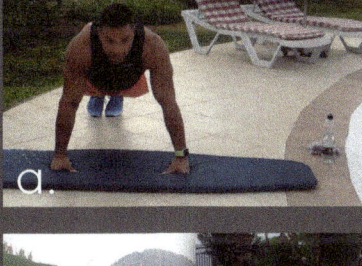

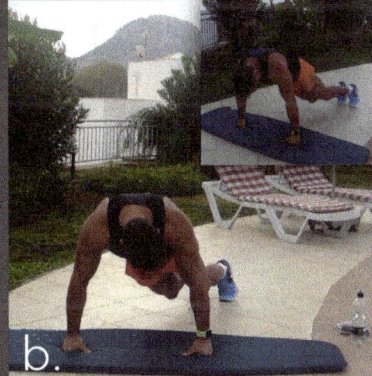

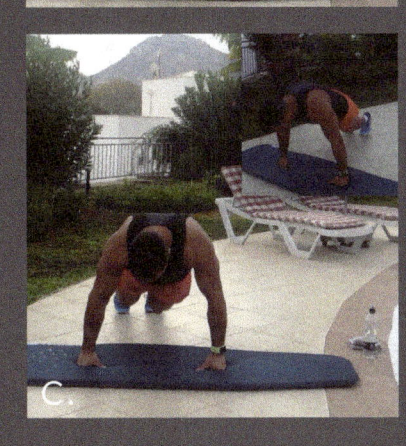

1. Horizontal Side Jumps

2. Leg Raises

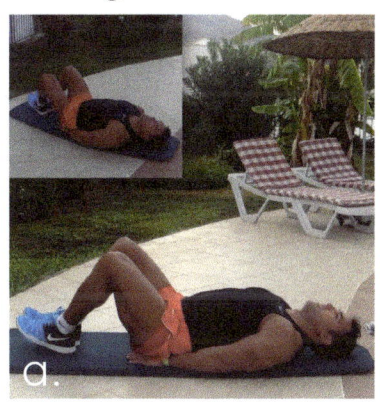

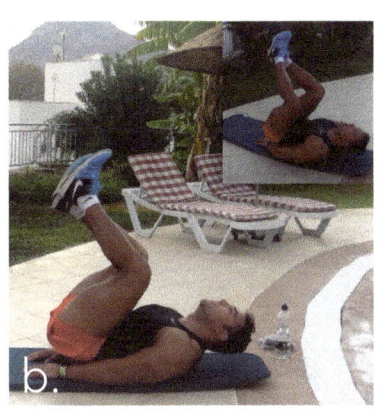

GET FIT, STAY FIT | 245

3. Press-ups and Diagonal Touch

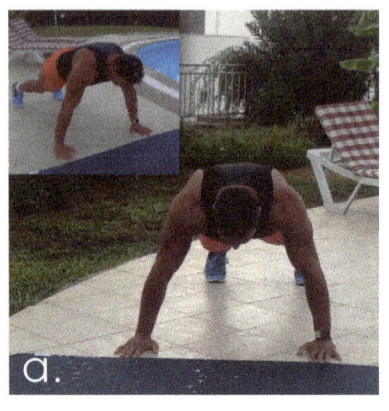

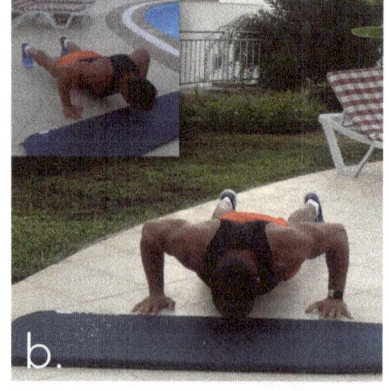

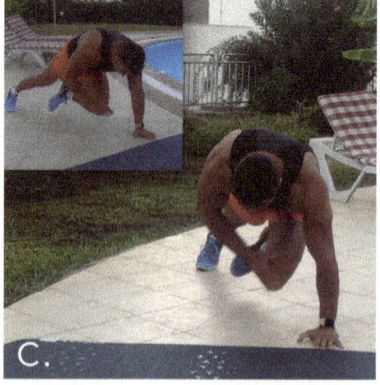

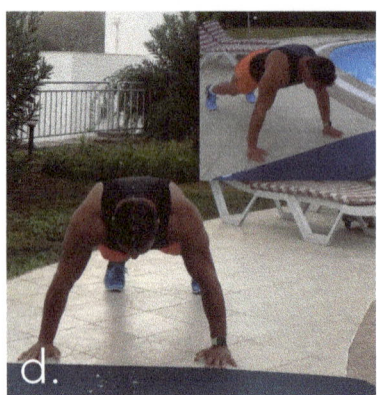

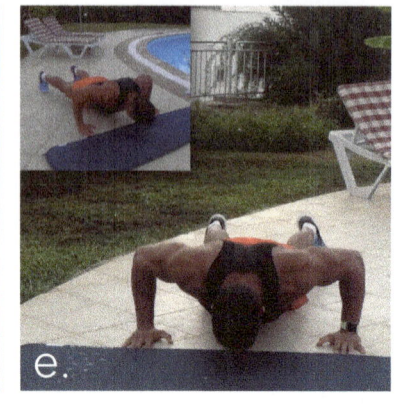

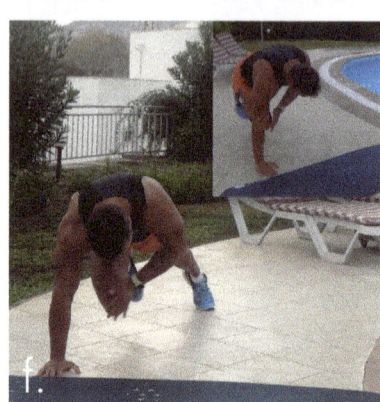

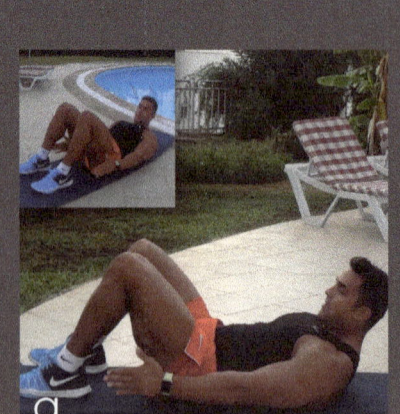

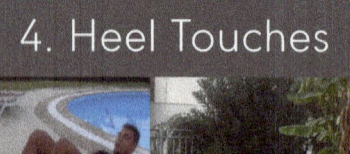

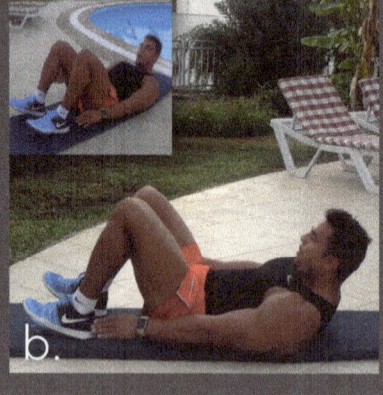

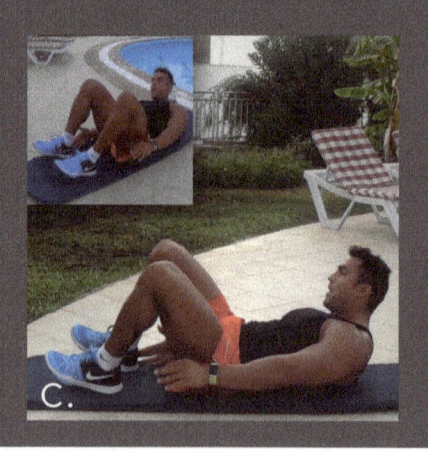

4. Heel Touches

5. Jumping Lunges

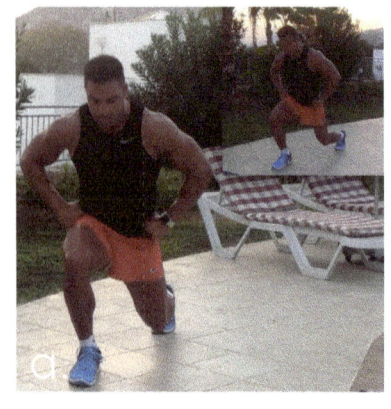

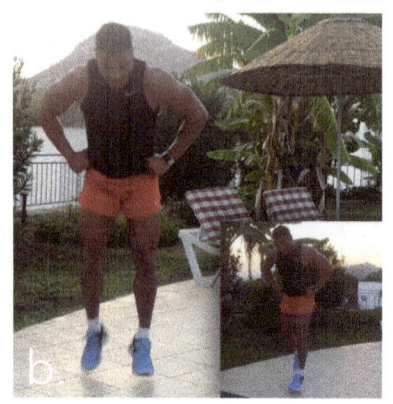

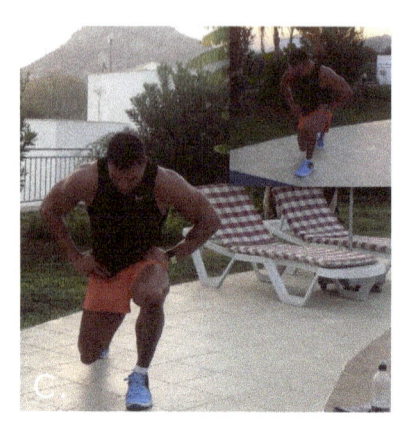

WEEK 8 PROGRESS JOURNAL

Use these pages to set your intentions at the start of the week and record and reflect on your progress at the end of the week. Alternatively, use a special notebook for this purpose.

PART 1: INTENTIONS/PLANNING

My starting weight this week: _____

My starting waist measurement: _____

My goal weight at the end of this week: _____

My goal waist measurement at the end of this week: _____

Any other goals for the week (e.g. no alcohol during the week and no more than 14 units during the weekend or going to bed early weekdays and sleep minimum 7 hours etc.)

_____

_____

Which days are going to be tricky this week and why? (E.g. client dinner on Thursday which involves drinking alcohol)

_____

_____

How will I deal with this? _____

_____

_____

GET FIT, STAY FIT | 247

Any other notes/thoughts:

PART 2: RECORD/REFLECTIONS

At the end of this week how many goals did I achieve?

How many did I come close to?

How am I feeling about my progress?

Which goals did I not reach?

Why was that? Family commitments, too much work and no time, not motivated enough? Can I define exactly what hindered my progress? Can I take action on that next week?

What actions can I take next week to improve on this?

What were my wins this week? (e.g. weight loss, mileage run etc?)

I've achieved

Give marks out of 10 for progress this week

PART FIVE

CHAPTER 9: OPTIMISE YOUR EXERCISE

You now have your full exercise programme laid out for you and you can check in the Resources section in Chapter 11 every time you need the specific instructions for any particular exercise. Job done, eh?

Well, no, not really. It's important to factor in other actions that benefit your body and I also think we need to consider variety, so in this section we will look at different exercise routines you might want to explore during or after the main programme. We'll look at the importance of keeping your body flexible and mobile through stretching. Finally, we'll see how important sleep is to your overall sense of wellbeing. What you're learning in this book, I hope, is that fitness is a holistic process and when all the elements – strength, mobility, nutrition, mental attitude and rest – are working together in balance, you really feel the difference.

9.1 SWITCH IT UP: DIFFERENT TYPES OF TRAINING METHODS

Let's get into some detail on the various kinds of training available to you. For example, I'm sure you've heard of circuit training as one type of training technique. Circuit training is not the only way to get fit though. So I'd like to talk about some of the other training methods.

Here are some examples:

Drop Sets

Negatives

Super Sets

Giant Sets

Super Slow Sets

Forced Reps

Pre-Exhaust

Post-Exhaust

German Volume Training

Wave Training

Pyramid Training

HIIT

Fartlek Training

Circuit Training ... have I missed anything?!

Before I start, I'd like to say I love almost all of these training methods and if you were training in person with me we'd be using some of these techniques in your training programme anyway.

Let's take a look at each in turn (and by the way, you're now familiar with terms like 'Bicep Curl' or 'Cable Fly' but if you need reminding, refer to the specific exercise instructions in Chapter 11)

Drop Sets: this is a great technique that works well with many exercises. You lift a weight until you can't do it anymore, and once you can no longer lift it, you drop the weight a little bit (10-20%) and carry on until the next failure, then again drop the weight. Repeat this 3 or 4 times. I can almost feel the burn right now while writing these lines!

Negatives: this is also called eccentric training. It is the action of lengthening your muscle under load, i.e. lowering the dumbbell back down during a Bicep Curl. It is very useful for those who want to improve their Chin-ups. You can imagine how hard it would be to pull your entire bodyweight up to a chin-up bar; however, you could lower yourself from the top position much more easily. This method is also used for rehabilitation. I think elderly people would also benefit from this eccentric training method for various muscles, as it puts less stress on the heart and lungs.

Super Sets: these are two exercises back to back without a rest in between. You could either work the same muscle groups (e.g. Chest Press followed by Cable Fly) or opposing (antagonist) muscles (e.g. Chest Press followed by Lat Pull Down). This is useful for definition/toning up and will also raise your heart rate more than an ordinary set due to the total duration of both sets. Another advantage is that you complete your workout more quickly.

Giant Sets: This is an advanced and pretty hard workout as you do 4 exercises back to back on the same muscle group without any rest in between. It's great if you haven't got much time as you complete the workout quickly as in Super Sets (even quicker) but those muscles really burn hard! (e.g. Squats, Lunge Walks, Split Squats and Side Lunges)

Super Slow Sets: A great technique to work with light weights. I do this in 4/3 ratio for big muscle groups and in 3/2 ratio for small muscle groups. So if you are doing the Barbell Bench Press, you lower the weight for 4 seconds really slowly, then lift it up for 3 seconds. This slow movement makes the exercise much harder even if the weight you are using is much lighter than your normal weight for that exercise.

Forced Reps: This can't be done alone. You might have seen gym buddies 'spotting' each other? 'Spotting' means supporting someone as they lift the weight, thus allowing them to safely push more than they would normally be able to. It's mainly about your presence, even if you don't actually help them physically. Most of the time it's a psychological encouragement. Even if you help a bit physically, you are most likely lifting just 5% of the total weight so that you allow the person to complete the set safely.

This is exactly what Forced Reps mean. The most common example is on Bench Press. You start doing your repetitions while your buddy stands behind you. Towards the end (last 2-3 reps) they give you a hand to lift the weight. Having said that, they take no more than 10% of the total weight. So if someone is trying to do a Bicep Curl while spotting your Chest Presses, there is something wrong. Spotting should be a tiny bit of help; as I said, often just your buddy's presence is enough psychologically.

Pre-Exhaust: This is a technique that starts with an isolation* exercise followed by a compound** exercise. Let me explain. If you are working on your chest, you start with Cable or Dumbbells Chest Fly then do your Bench Press afterwards. By doing this, you warm up your muscles perfectly to perform your main compound exercise such as the Barbell Bench Press. You might not be able to lift as much as your normal weight due to the pre-exhaust exercise, but this technique does reduce the risk of injury.

*Isolation Exercises are the movements you carry out by moving one joint only: e.g. Dumbbells Chest Fly moves your shoulder joint.

**Compound Exercises are the movements you perform by moving multiple joints: e.g. Press-ups or Bench Presses move your shoulder and elbow joints.

Post-Exhaust: This is the opposite to Pre-Exhaust Training. You start with your main exercise, such as Squats followed by Leg Curls. The benefit of this training is it helps to overload the muscle for an extra 30 seconds (during your second isolation exercise) which increases your endurance. It is also a great way of breaking out of a plateau as you shock your muscles!

German Volume Training: I must say this German technique is as good as their BMWs! It is a great way of increasing the volume of your training. You do 10 sets of 10 repetitions of the same exercise. It might sound boring but it is very effective for improving your strength and muscle mass. This training is done for compound exercises such as Chest Press, Barbell Rowing, Squats and Shoulder Press. You pick a weight that you can lift for 20 repetitions. Then you use that weight for 10 sets of 10 repetitions with 60-90 seconds of rest in between. Towards the end you might struggle to complete 10 repetitions but do as many as you can without reducing the weight. After completing the 10 sets, you do 2-3 sets of an isolation exercise for each muscle group. Make sure you rest that muscle for 4-5 days afterwards.

Wave Training: This is similar to German Volume Training, but you increase and decrease the weight in every set. Start with 8 repetitions of a reasonably heavy weight, then increase the weight about 5-10% and do 5 repetitions, increase it again 5-10% and do 3 repetitions. After that you decrease the weight about 5-10% from what you lifted on your first set (of 8 repetitions) and do 10 repetitions. Decrease again and do 12 repetitions. You repeat these 5 sets twice (10 sets in total). Rest time in between sets is 60-90 seconds. After 10 sets, you do 2-3 sets of 10-12 repetitions of an isolation exercise. E.g. Bench Press

8 repetitions of 50 kg

5 repetitions of 52.5-55kg

3 repetitions of 55-60 kg

10 repetitions of 42.5-45 kg

12 repetitions of 40-42.5 kg

Pyramid Training: This is similar to Wave Training. There is no set repetition or weight you use here. It's very effective for increasing your strength and pushing yourself to your limit. You can follow a descending or ascending pyramid, or both in the same workout. Start with a relatively low weight and do high repetitions, rest a bit (30-60 seconds) then increase the weight and decrease the repetitions for each set. After 3-4 sets, increase the repetitions and decrease the weight.

HIIT: HIIT is a form of cardiovascular exercise; as I mentioned earlier, HIIT stands for High Intensity Interval Training. It basically works like this: you push yourself nearly to your maximum heart rate for anywhere from 10 seconds to a few minutes, then cool down for a few minutes with a less intense exercise or pause before increasing the pace again and repeating for a few cycles. For safety's sake it is important to know what the maximum heart rate for your age should be (see Chapter 7.11). Because it's intense, it's a time-efficient form of exercise. You might do a short period of high intensity exercise such as star jumps, burpees, or fast springs, followed by either a short rest or low intensity exercise. The ratios of high to low can vary. When you begin you could do a 1:2 ratio, which means you do the high intensity exercise for 30 seconds, then the low intensity recovery exercise for 60 seconds. You are doubling your recovery time. If you opt for a 1:1 ratio, with the exercise and recovery time the same, this is a bit harder. For experienced people, the ratio can be 3:1: 90 seconds on, 30 seconds off.

Fartlek Training: This is a technique mainly used for running. It is a Swedish term which means you play with the speed. You change your pace throughout your run, alternating between fast runs and slow jogs. Fartleks are more unstructured; you randomly increase the fast pace and don't have to stick at any particular pace for a specific time. The best example is going for a jog and doing sprint runs between the benches or lampposts around a park. You can experiment with it and every workout can be different.

Circuit Training: One of the most common and well-known exercise techniques. It saves you a lot of time and ticks many boxes such as cardio and strength, with a variety of options, so it is not as boring as the treadmill. You throw a bunch of exercises together and give yourself a certain time or number of repetitions to complete each one with a certain length of break in between, or no break if you want to make it harder. Choosing suitable exercises is important here as they need to flow well together, with actions that complement each other. That's what differentiates a circuit class designed by a good trainer from one designed by a bad one!

9.2 BODY MOBILITY: 5 STRETCHES YOU SHOULD BE DOING ON A DAILY BASIS

Why is stretching so important? Even though we keep hearing about it, we are generally inclined to skip it at the end of our training sessions. (See also Chapter 7.13)

Stretching relieves the tension in your muscles, increases joint mobility, reduces the risk of injury and helps you achieve your fitness goals. Tight muscles will prevent you from carrying out the full range of movement in your exercises.

There are two types of stretching. One is called **dynamic** stretching, which is better prior to exercising. You basically move in and out of the pose. You move through a challenging but comfortable range of motion repeatedly, around 8-10 times. The other one is **static** stretching, where you hold your position for a set amount of time, ideally at least 30 seconds.

Let's talk about these useful stretches. The good news is you can do these almost anywhere and at any time.

1a) Static Hamstring Stretch

If you sit a lot due to your work (or if you are a Netflix addict!), you will get tight hamstrings, so this stretch is crucial.

There are a few options here. One is to bend down towards your feet and hold that relatively uncomfortable position for 30 seconds with your legs straight. Towards the end, it should feel easier as hopefully your hamstrings are lengthening. However, if you don't repeat this regularly, they will revert to their tight state. So the more you do it, the more flexible you will get. I don't mean 30 minutes a day for 7 days a week! Short amounts of time but often will give you the results you want.

1b) Dynamic Hamstring Stretch

Stand tall and stretch your arms in front of you. Step your left foot forward and swinging your leg up, try to kick your hand. Swing your foot back and repeat this, 15-20 times per leg.

2a) Static Quadriceps Stretch

I had to add this. If you do any type of strength training exercises for your legs, you must do the quadriceps stretch as well. All those squats, lunges, leg presses and leg extension exercises are great for giving you nice, toned legs but make sure you stretch these big muscles before they get too tight and you risk pulling your kneecap or giving yourself knee pain.

Stand on one foot, bend the other leg back and reach behind you to lift the foot towards your hip. Make sure you keep your knees together and push your hips forward, keeping your chest straight.

2b) Dynamic Quadriceps Stretch

Alternatively, you can perform this dynamic stretch: start in a standing position. Take a small controlled step forward and grab your back foot from behind, hold it there for 2 seconds and let it go, taking another step forward with that foot; this time grab your other foot from behind and repeat this by walking small steps forward.

3) Gluteus Stretch

I love this one. I sometimes do this when I am on the Underground! Sit down, put one leg on top of the other one, parallel to the floor, and lean forwards. That instant stretch in your bum somehow makes you feel like you are doing a good thing!

4) Static Lower Back Stretch

Another one of those 'makes you feel good' stretches. Lie on your back. Bend your knees up. Keep your arms out. Lower your knees to one side as far as you are able. Once you complete your time, swap sides. You can hold this for longer to really feel the stretch.

5) Pecs Stretch

If you spend a long time at your desk in front of a computer, or if you do loads of bench presses, you might have 'upper cross syndrome'. You'll recognise this posture when people have their shoulders forward and down. It also makes you look shorter. To stretch this chest muscle, place your left forearm vertically on a door frame and step the left foot forward by 45-50 cm, bending the leg. Lean forwards until you feel the stretch and stay there for 30 seconds. If you don't feel it much, twist your upper body away from your forearm to increase the stretch. Repeat on the right side.

There are many other stretches you might benefit from, but let's keep it simple and quick. I don't want to overwhelm you with possibilities! These are the key ones to help mobilise your body and keep it supple.

9.3 BODY HARMONY THROUGH SLEEP

Most of us take a good night's sleep for granted. Most of us are unaware how a lack of sleep can affect our performance at work, our behaviour, relationships, home life and our bodies.

The American Society of Clinical Investigation's 1968 study 'Growth Hormone Secretion during Sleep' says that the human growth hormone is secreted during sleep. So it is critical to have quality sleep to refresh ourselves, rebuild cells and muscle tissue and, ultimately, grow.

When you've had poor sleep, it's almost like having a hangover. It might present many challenges and a lot of people in the UK suffer from some sort of sleep disorder.

With technology such as Fitbits and Apple watches we are now able to track our sleeping patterns and give more attention to this important area.

There is also a ring that you can wear called the 'Oura' ring, which is the first consumer-available wearable technology that gives circadian alignment guidance.

More information can be found at: https://ouraring.com/circadian-rhythms-bedtime

Here are some tips to help direct you towards a better night's sleep.

BEFORE SLEEP

Preparing yourself to get the best quality of sleep is crucial, yet this aspect is almost always overlooked.

- Set your mobile phone to notify you when it is time to start getting ready for bed
- Stay away from foods containing caffeine for at least 4 hours prior to bedtime (try decaffeinated coffee). I can however drink a double espresso and sleep within minutes, so this doesn't apply to everyone!
- Avoid big meals late at night
- Avoid alcohol before bed
- 2 hours before bedtime, stop doing anything that would stimulate your mind and body, so no late workouts or studying. Again, this is not for everyone. I personally know a few people who work out at 8 p.m. and go to bed before 10 p.m. with no issue!
- An hour before bed switch off electronic devices and anything that might emit blue light and switch your phone to flight mode. Blue light inhibits the sleep hormone melatonin, which signals to us that it is time to rest. We stay artificially alert, our circadian rhythms disrupted and this has a knock-on effect the next day as we are groggy and tired
- Dim the lights in your room
- Task Dump – write down any tasks, worries or ideas on a pad next to the bed so that you do not toss and turn in bed thinking about them (I do this very often)

DURING SLEEPING-HOURS

- Ensure the room is as dark as possible
- Use an eye-mask if needed
- Make sure your room is cool enough as a high room temperature might make you sweat and have disturbed sleep

WAKING UP

- The best tip for people who have trouble getting going in the mornings is to simply wake up and get moving. Go out as soon as possible as fresh air will definitely revive you
- When your alarm goes off, immediately open your curtains and blinds to let the sun in (if you are lucky enough to have sun where you are!)
- Sunlight is our body's natural alarm clock. The sooner you expose yourself to it, the sooner you will be awake

USE A SLEEP TRACKER

Similar to using a workout app, I also like using an app to track my sleep, though I must admit I don't wake up *every* morning and check how many hours I slept and what the quality of it was and how much deep sleep I had.

What I do is to monitor my sleeping trend over a period of time. Currently I am using an app called 'Autosleep'. It is very detailed and it gives you a hell of a lot of data! I have linked it with my Apple watch so that it monitors my heart rate during my sleep as well as the depth and quality of my sleep-phases. See http://autosleep.tantsissa.com

Then weekly or monthly you can check if you are getting enough sleep and if the quality of your sleep is satisfactory. If not, take action. Can you see why I am monitoring all kinds of data, from calories consumed to daily steps or sleep? Without knowing how well or badly you are doing, it is very hard to take action to improve any of these aspects. Measuring and monitoring is a crucial part of the initial process and when it comes to maintaining what we've achieved, as we'll see in the next section.

CHAPTER 10:
YOU'VE GOT FIT – NOW STAY FIT

10.1 MONITOR AND MAINTAIN FOR SUSTAINED FITNESS SUCCESS

In this section, let's start by celebrating all you've achieved so far! I hope you've enjoyed rediscovering your fitness. You have shown commitment and you've been rewarded with improved energy, a more toned body and greater health all round. It's a good idea to pause now and look back at your earliest journal entries or the introductory section of this book where I asked you to think about the weight-gain and energy-drain you might be experiencing at this stage of your life. Do you see the contrast?

Now, having worked so hard over the past couple of months, the last thing you want to do is let all you've achieved fade and fall away. So in this section I'll give you advice on maintaining the fitness level you've reached. (You can even go further, beyond consolidation to further improvement too, of course!) And if you find you need another fitness boost in the future, you know you can choose to come here and revisit this guidance, or, indeed, work through the whole book again if you really need to follow the entire process once more. What's important is that this programme is always available to you, always there to encourage and guide you.

In my opinion, this phase is much easier than what you have had to do so far. All you need to do is to maintain what you've achieved. Well, that's easy to say, of course! But you might be wondering, just *how*, precisely, you're going to maintain your new shape and level of fitness.

Well, that's what this chapter is all about!

10.2 THE THREE PATHS

When it comes to losing weight, to get the results you desire you have three potential pathways to follow:

1) The Fast-Track Path

2) The Slow but Steady Path

3) The Combined Path

1) THE FAST-TRACK PATH

You must have heard of crash diets. They are criticised heavily in public and by many experts, but it may be worth considering the positives. If, for example, you are someone who has 3 stone (18kg) to lose, your willpower is limited and your lifestyle is hectic, then attending a fitness camp and losing the first 2 stone in 8-12 weeks might be a good idea, as that first tough stage is over and done with. You've had support (because supervision is crucial with this approach) and you are already in the maintenance mode. You are lighter and hopefully healthier, plus everything in daily life is much easier as you are also much more energetic.

However, one of the downsides of the fast-track method is that you are more likely to injure yourself. If you've had a sedentary lifestyle, especially after 40, your brain may think you are still in your 20s, but not your body, sadly. To be able to get quick results, you are more likely to be starving yourself, doing extra hard workouts and finding your mood is all over the place. Starving yourself limits the nutrition you need especially during your recovery and workout times. Extra hard workouts put you at risk of pulling a muscle or developing joint-related injuries/illnesses.

Another downside is that you might end up yoyo-dieting. So you lose the weight, get fit, then stop; everything goes back to how it was before – if not worse. Then you start all over again. Nightmare, huh? And not very healthy either.

Don't get me wrong: if you are ready for it mentally and physically, extra hard short burst workouts are excellent. They save time and you feel great afterwards. But not if you are coming from a fully sedentary life and if you are overweight. You can of course build up to the tough stuff.

2) THE SLOW BUT STEADY PATH

This is the most popular one with all the fitness gurus. You must have heard how people advise making small but significant changes: introduce one exercise a week, walk a bit further, cut down on your wine a bit, eat fewer snacks, swap your flat white for a black Americano… All of this I agree with, to a certain degree. You are less likely to injure yourself, your mood won't be so changeable, you won't suffer from having to make tricky decisions at work lunches.

However, how long can you last with these small changes? Your mind will be expecting quick results and the changes you make may require more time than you expect. This is a perfectly practical method if all the conditions are fixed. What I mean is that, when you cut down some of your extra calories and increase your activity a little bit, you will be creating a deficit of around 1000 calories a week. The problem begins when your mind thinks you have done very well all week so it will tempt you to eat that rich dinner or take-away or drink another bottle of wine during that weekend dinner party. (We humans love our rewards!) Then by Monday you are back to square one!

3) THE COMBINED METHOD PATH

This is my favourite method by far, and the one that creates the most sustained effect. You follow the initial fast-track phase, then the slow but steady method.

The important factor here is to increase the intensity of your workouts *gradually*. You allow yourself 2-3 weeks to build up to those high intensity workouts, exactly as I have designed for you in this book.

So the ideal programme is this:

Build-up Period

Fast-Track Period

Slow but Steady Period

Reassessment

Mind you, if you are relatively active already and only have 3-5 kg to lose this approach is not for you, as you are already somewhere in the middle of this process. So you could decide where you are at and take it from there. For example, if you only have 5kg excess weight, you might only need to follow the Slow but Steady Method.

If we look at method 3 you can see how it applies to where you are now: that staying fit has involved a blend of fast-track activities and the patience to stick with the programme for 8 weeks – and beyond.

10.3 REASSESS FOR SUCCESS

When you are in the maintenance phase, one of the most important factors for you will be regular reassessment, not just of your weight but of your overall performance.

You will need to carry on weighing yourself regularly, measuring yourself with a tape measure and evaluating present versus past performance, such as comparing your 5k or 10k run times with your peak performance.

Let's say during your fast-track phase, you get better and better at running or cycling. Your 5k run (or it could be cycling, swimming, rowing – any cardio exercise) typically took about 27 minutes. You managed to lose the weight you wanted to lose and now you are in the Slow but Steady Phase. So you are not killing yourself but still doing your regular but perhaps less intense workouts, plus your diet is less strict but you are in control of it. After a few months, if you realise that your 5k run is taking 30 minutes, then you need to do a week or two of the Fast-Track phase, as you've probably put some weight on and your cardio fitness level is decreasing. This is much easier than letting everything go and having to start again from scratch a few months down the line.

So make a note to yourself to reassess where you are at regular intervals. This is absolutely key and before you know it, it will become part of your normal lifestyle. This is actually how many fitness experts live, including me. We all have a life. We are all invited to parties! We all fall off the wagon.

The more you actively monitor yourself, the better you'll get at it. So, instead of vaguely thinking 'I must weigh myself/time myself some time', take out your diary and enter in specific dates when you will assess your status. You are, in effect, creating a repeat booking appointment with your own wellbeing and your long-term health. You are committing yourself to maintaining your best self.

Part of this commitment is the ability to troubleshoot. When you get to where you'd like to be in terms of fitness and wellbeing, things may indeed go off track due to work trips, big lunches or client entertainment, but all you need to do is to reassess yourself before it is too late. If you've realised you've put 2 kg on, don't let another 2kg pile up. After all, losing that initial 2kg will only take you a week or so. But when the weight accumulates, it will be a much greater challenge to summon up that will-power all over again. Remember the different people I mentioned in Chapter 4? You need to be a 'Reliable', not a 'Boomerang'. The main difference between these two categories may lie in the fact that 'Reliables' reassess themselves on a regular basis, knowing this is the foundation of a lasting healthy lifestyle.

10.4 FINAL TIPS TO KEEP YOU ON-TRACK

HEALTHY EATING HABITS

- Remember to see this as a lifestyle change, not just a temporary change of diet and activity levels

- Remember the 'calories in/calories out' equation when considering how much exercise you incorporate into your new life
- Seek out natural carbohydrates, those you find in vegetables and salad
- Check the sugar content – especially those hidden sugars! – in everything you eat
- Try to have at least 5 servings of fruit and vegetables every day
- Use your imagination! Diets often fail when we are bored, so keep experimenting with new flavour combinations
- Don't limit yourself: eat a wide variety of food, as long as you keep the proportions of fat, protein and carbohydrates balanced
- Keep a daily record of what you eat because you want to eat consciously from now on

MAKE TIME FOR YOURSELF

One of the most important yet often underestimated things we can do for ourselves is simply to make time for ourselves. This is particularly true if you're a high-performing professional. You know how focused and happy you are after that relaxing Sunday morning walk, but you still put it at the bottom of your to do list. It's time to change that!

Go for a walk, sit and listen to some music or a podcast, do some stretching or deep breathing exercises or something that you love doing but never find the time for. Do it regularly. Make these part of your life. Not once or twice a year. Any of these activities will definitely give you a moment to restore yourself and recover from the pressures around you.

GET CONNECTED

In today's world, it's way more easy to get connected than it's ever been. We have Facebook to find our old friends, WhatsApp to reach out to them for free and create a group where we hang out with other people in less than 30 seconds. Studies of the oldest people in the world have revealed that close friendships are a main contributor to a long happy life. Isolation creates both mental and physical illness faster than almost anything else. It's proven that connecting with friends or joining any kind of social or spiritual group reduces stress and boosts happiness.

GET CREATIVE

I must be one of the least creative people in the world. I'm crap at drawing, singing or handicrafts. But creativity doesn't have to be a traditional activity. I've realised shooting a video and editing it, writing this book or drafting a blog post gives me the same amount of happiness that I would get from drawing if I were an artist.

Expressing yourself isn't just an artistic outlet: it is a way of finding out who you are. So explore your options: join a dance club, take an evening class in art or cookery. When you feel fulfilled as a creative artist the renewed energy you feel will spill over into the other parts of your life, and will help you continue to make healthy choices for your life, in a holistic way.

GIVE SUPPORT

You must have heard this. The more you give, the more you receive.

Getting involved with helping others can lift your spirits and restore a sense of meaning and purpose to your life. You don't need to give people financial support, necessarily. Giving your time to listen to a friend or advising someone will help you create a healthier emotional life.

However you decide to proceed, be creative and experiment with what works for *you*.

10.5 THE END - AND THE BEGINNING!

We are finally at the end of your Get Fit, Stay Fit programme and journal. I am hoping that you took all the necessary actions and applied all the advice I provided for the different areas of your new healthy lifestyle, from nutrition to rest and of course exercise.

Now you know how to turn your life around - because you've done it! During this journey, you not only improved your fitness, health and wellbeing but also motivated people around you by becoming a good role model for them. You proved to everyone, including yourself, that your mind is strong. Your determination gave you the results you wished for. You stayed the course: well done!

I know from experience that people I've helped have become heroes at work, at home and in their neighbourhood due to their dramatic lifestyle changes.

The success stories I've shared with you in this book were there to show you that you could be one of them. I'd love to hear from you as you complete this journey: let me know how the whole process helped you, with all its ups and downs. I'd love to know where you were at in the beginning, how you took action and how you achieved success in terms of your health and wellbeing.

I understand that from time to time you might get sidetracked and you're not going to be able to stick to every rule in this book. I don't expect you to never have a glass of wine or a bar of chocolate again! We are human and these temptations are all around us every single day. The key thing is, to keep everything in moderation. Obviously the more disciplined you are, the more quickly you will see results and the longer they will last.

For some people, the time needed to achieve the final goal might be longer than 8 weeks. Don't worry about this – the important thing is to keep making progress.

If the unhealthy weight you need to lose is over 10kg, you may need to repeat the last 4 weeks to extend the original 8 week period to 12 weeks. If that's the case, all you need to do is repeat the exercises in Weeks 5 to 8 for another month.

If you need further help, there's online support on my website with different packages available, including tailor-made workout plans using my specially designed fitness app. This comes with a bespoke meal plan to maximise your success and if you sign up for my online app workouts we keep in contact regularly so that I can monitor your progress. Simply, visit www.gokayfitness.com.

I also offer a '20 Workouts in 30 Days' plan which includes most of the video versions of the exercises in the programme in this book. Sign up for this and you'll receive your daily workout videos Monday to Friday for 4 weeks. They gradually get harder every week. They are time-efficient, starting from just 10 minutes a day, building up to 25-minute HIIT workouts.

Remember, the transformation to a healthier, fitter and happier version of yourself starts in your mind first. Be good to yourself and enjoy the whole process. Negative thoughts or temptations will always find us. The trick is to acknowledge them and discover ways of stopping them from derailing us or making us lose faith in our ability to take charge of our personal health on a truly lasting basis.

Whether we ever meet in person or not, I'll be cheering you on as you enjoy your new fitness lifestyle! And if you want to do more see my website for other training options: https://www.gokayfitness.com

PART SIX

CHAPTER 11: RESOURCES

This chapter is your reference section. It's split into three parts. Part **11.1** gives you the detailed list of instructions for the weight-training programmes you'll be doing. Part **11.2** is your resource for the instructions for your home workout exercises. These specific instructions will help you perform them safely and accurately.

The third section, **11.3**, contains a selection of delicious recipes. I have chosen these dishes for their appeal and for their nutritional value. They look great, they taste great – and they'll do you so much good!

11.1 INSTRUCTIONS FOR THE EXERCISES IN THE WEIGHT TRAINING PROGRAMMES

This is your reference guide for the weight training programmes and workouts, showing you how to do each exercise. Check the daily listings in Chapter 8 so that you know exactly which weight training sequence you should be doing. Note that the weight training sequences are designed to be done in the gym, with gym equipment. For your home workouts, use section 11.2.

Make sure you've read Chapter 7 on exercising safely before you begin your programme.

UPPER BODY WEIGHT TRAINING PROGRAMME 1

1) Barbell Chest Press

- Lie on the bench, take hold of the bar, your hands wider than shoulder-width apart
- Squeeze your shoulder-blades together which will put your shoulders in a safer position
- Prepare to inhale as you lower the bar and exhale as you raise it

- Lower the bar, very close to your chest but not touching it
- Raise the bar
- Try to lift the bar straight up and down

2) Cable Chest Fly

- Firstly select the appropriate weight or tension
- Then make sure the handles of the cables are at chest level
- Position yourself in the centre with one foot forward
- Pull your arms forward to meet in front of your chest, keeping your elbows soft
- Release back slowly, extending your arms back as much as possible

3) Lat Pull Down

- Sit, placing your thighs under the pads
- Keep your chest up and back straight
- Take a wide overhand grip of the bar
- Pull the bar down to your chest
- Lean back slightly during this exercise
- Keep your elbows back and shoulder-blades together
- Slowly release the bar back up and repeat

4) Seated Rowing

- Adjust the seat height so that the padded support is on your chest
- Take an overhand grip of the handles
- Pull the handles towards you, bringing your shoulder-blades together
- Bring your elbows as far back as possible and continue rowing

5) Machine Shoulder Press

- Hold the handles so that your arms are at 90 degrees
- Exhale and raise the handles, fully extending your arms
- Lower the handles as much as possible without resting the weights
- Keep your back firmly against the support rest

6) Barbell Biceps Curl

- Hold the bar in an underhand grip, your hands shoulder-width apart
- Curl up, exhale and curl down, inhale
- Be sure to fully straighten your arms at the bottom

7) Cable V-Bar Triceps Extension

- Adjust the weight
- Keep your core tight, knees soft and elbows tucked in
- Take an overhand grip of the V-bar
- Pull down and bring your elbows next to your torso
- This is your starting position
- Extend your arms down to full stretch
- Squeeze your triceps and slowly release up without moving your elbows

8) Plank

- Lie on your front
- Support yourself on your forearms and toes
- Raise your torso up and hold this plank position
- Your body should be as flat as possible so keep your bottom tucked down
- Keep your core engaged
- Keep your pelvis tipped forward and belly button tucked in
- Don't forget to breathe!

LOWER BODY WEIGHT TRAINING PROGRAMME 1

1) Leg Extension

- Adjust the pad so that it rests on top of your foot
- Keep your chest up and begin straightening your legs
- Squeeze your quads at full extension
- Keep control when you lower your feet so the weights don't touch

2) Leg Curl (Some gyms will have machines for seated or lying leg curls instead)

- Stand on the platform, place the pad at the back of your heel

- Curl backward as much as possible and make sure you keep your knee stable
- Now switch legs. Bring your leg slowly down and make sure the weights don't touch each other

3) Leg Press

- Place your feet on the platform, hip-width apart
- Keep your toes in line with your knees
- Release the security handles, bend and straighten your legs by pushing on the platform
- Bring your knees as close to your chest as possible
- Keep the movement controlled and breathe regularly
- Remember to secure the safety handles when you finish

4) Dumbbell Alternating Backward Lunges

- Pick up the dumbbells, keep your chest up and your core engaged, your feet shoulder-width apart
- Step back and lower one knee as much as possible
- Keep your front foot stable and alternate your legs
- Keep your foot, knee and hip in line
- While in the lunging position, keep your chest upright

5) Side Plank

- Lie on your side
- Support yourself on your forearm
- Lift up onto your feet, place one foot on top of the other
- Tuck your tummy in, as you form a side-on triangle to the ground
- Keep a nice straight line
- Switch sides
- Don't forget to breathe

6) Abs Vertical Scissors

- Lie on your back but raise yourself up on your elbows
- Engage your core

- Bend your knees and scissor your legs vertically, while keeping your feet off the ground
- Keep the movement controlled and not too fast

7) Abs Crunches with Hands on Thighs

- Lie down and bend your knees up, feet hip-width apart
- Place your hands on your thighs
- Exhale and curl up towards your knees
- Contract your abs and keep the movement controlled

UPPER BODY WEIGHT TRAINING PROGRAMME 2(A)

1) Inclined Barbell Bench Press

- Hold the bar, with your hands wider than shoulder-width apart
- Inhale when you lower the bar, exhale when you lift it up
- When you lower the bar, keep your forearms vertical

2) Dumbbells Chest Fly

- Pick up the dumbbells and lie on a bench
- Raise the dumbbells above your chest, palms facing each other. This is your starting position
- Open your arms wide, keeping your elbows soft, and lower the dumbbells down as far as you can
- Then bring your arms back together in a controlled movement without letting the dumbbells touch each other

3) Dumbbells Inclined Bench Press

- Pick up the dumbbells and lie on an inclined bench
- Start with your arms at a 90 degree angle
- Raise and straighten your arms, bringing the dumbbells together
- Don't let them touch at the top
- Bring them down as low as possible, keeping your elbows away from your body

4) Dumbbell One Arm Rowing

- Place your right knee on the bench

- Keep your spine neutral, with your left knee soft. Your left foot should be back and out so that your chest is not directly above the bench
- Pick up the dumbbell, raise your hand towards your hip
- Keep your elbow tucked in. The action is similar to starting a lawnmower
- Make sure your elbow goes back, not out, and lower the dumbbell in a controlled movement all the way down
- Change sides (once you've completed your repetitions on one side)

5) Cable Reverse Fly (Back Extension)

- Engage your back muscles throughout this exercise
- Set the weight and stand facing the machine
- Make sure the cable handles are at chest level
- Hold the handles with opposite hands
- Keep your feet shoulder-width apart, elbows soft, and extend your arms out and back
- Contract the muscles between your shoulder-blades

6) Lat Pull Down Wide Overhand Grip

- Sit and place your thighs under the pads
- Keep your chest up and back straight
- Take a wide overhand grip of the bar
- Pull down to your chest
- Lean back slightly during this exercise
- Keep your elbows back and shoulder-blades together
- Slowly release back up and repeat

7) Cable Crunches

- Take a neutral hold of the rope
- Keep a safe distance from the weights
- Kneel down on a mat
- Tuck your elbows in and place your hands next to your ears
- Exhale and crunch down, maintaining this position
- Move only from the waist up

8) Leg Raises

- Lie on your back, place your hands under your bottom
- Keep your feet together and knees soft
- Raise your legs and your bottom and gently lower them back down
- When you lower your legs, make sure you are pulling your belly button towards your spine and keeping your core tight

LOWER BODY WEIGHT TRAINING PROGRAMME 2(A)

1) Barbell Squats

- It is very important to keep your spine neutral and core tight throughout this exercise
- Place the bar on your neck, keep your feet slightly wider than hip-width apart, with your toes pointing out
- Inhale and squat down and exhale on the way up
- Lower your bottom as much as possible, as if you are about to sit on a chair
- Each time when you stand up, squeeze your gluteus

2) Side Lunges

- Keep your feet together, keep your left leg completely straight, while you lunge sideways to the right with your right leg
- Touch your right trainer with your left hand and come back to the starting position
- I like this exercise because you can really feel your inner thigh as well as your right quads, hamstrings and gluteus
- Once you complete your repetitions, use the same technique and lunge to the left
- This time your right leg is completely straight and you feel your right abductors (your right inner thigh muscles)

3) Barbell Deadlift

- Keep your feet wider than shoulder-width apart and toes pointing out
- Hold the bar with arms straight and relaxed
- Keep your spine neutral
- Ensure you breathe in and out during every repetition

4) Oblique (Russian) Twist

- Take up a sitting position on the ground
- Place your feet hip-width apart
- Lean slightly back
- Clasp your hands in front of your chest
- Twist from side to side maintaining the position
- Keep your core stable and feel your obliques
- Try to twist as much as possible

5) Plank

- Lie on your front
- Support yourself on your forearms and toes
- Raise your torso up and hold this plank position
- Your body should be as flat as possible so keep your bottom tucked down
- Keep your core engaged
- Keep your pelvis tipped forward and belly button tucked in

6) Oblique Crunches

- Lie on your back, knees bent and feet together
- Lower your knees slightly to one side
- And with your arm on that side, place it on your obliques
- With your opposite arm place your fist against the side of your head and keep your elbow high
- Crunch straight up, squeezing your obliques
- Keep the movement controlled
- Swap sides, lowering your knees to the other side
- Do not crunch towards your tilted knees. Straight up

7) Slow Release Sit-ups

- Lie on your back on the ground
- Place your feet hip-width apart
- Using your arms to help propel you, rise to a sit-up position
- Hold there for a second and lower back down slowly
- Repeat, keeping your core engaged

UPPER BODY WEIGHT TRAINING PROGRAMME 2(B)

1) Barbell Shoulder Press

- You are going to lower the bar onto your chest
- Hold the bar wide so that your arms are at 90 degrees to your body
- Lower the bar gently just below chin level
- Raise the bar up, fully extending your arms
- Keep your back firmly against the support rest

2) Dumbbell Side Laterals

- Keep your feet hip-width apart, elbows soft
- Holding dumbbells, raise your arms up to ear level, palms facing down
- Remember, engage that core and control your arms on the way down
- Keep breathing

3) Cable Front Raise

- Hold the rope between your legs, palms facing in
- With soft knees and arms straight, pull the rope up to shoulder level
- Keep your core engaged – nice and steady

4) EZ Barbell Biceps Curl

- Take an underhand grip of the EZ bar, your hands shoulder-width apart, palms facing in
- Curl up to chin level, keeping your upper arms supported by tucking them against your torso
- Slowly return to full extension and repeat

5) Dumbbell Inclined Biceps Curl

- Hold the dumbbells in a neutral position, palms facing in
- Curl up and twist your hands so that your palms face up
- Then lower the dumbbells back slowly in a controlled movement
- Let your arms hang completely straight by your sides
- Keep your elbows stable and breathe on each repetition

6) Standing EZ Bar Triceps Extension

- Lower the bar behind your head by keeping your upper arms straight
- Keep your core engaged
- Keep your elbows pointing forward and tucked in
- Feet split apart, well-balanced on the ground
- Lift the bar up with straight arms then lower it back behind your head

7) Dumbbell One Arm Triceps Kick

- Hold the dumbbell with your right hand and place your left knee on the bench
- Stretch your right foot back and out
- Keep your knees soft and back flat
- Raise your right elbow at a 90 degree angle
- Now kick your arm back, but make sure you are not moving your whole arm
- Remember, just from the elbow
- You should really feel this in your triceps!
- Switch sides

8) Cycling in the Air

- Lie on your back but raise yourself up onto your elbows
- Bend your knees and cycle your legs, keeping your core engaged
- Keep the movement controlled and not too fast

9) Dead Bug

- Lie on your back
- Raise your knees up and place a water bottle or small object between them
- Grasp the bottle with your hands and lower your torso back down with your arms behind your head
- Sit up and place the bottle back between your knees and lower yourself back down
- Repeat

LOWER BODY WEIGHT TRAINING PROGRAMME 2(B)

1) Leg Extension

- Adjust the pad so that it rests on top of your foot
- Keep your chest up and begin straightening your legs
- Squeeze your quads at full extension
- Keep control when you lower your feet so the weights don't touch each other

2) TRX Squat Jumps

- Grasp the handles of the TRX straps and lean back, keeping your feet wide
- Squat down to a seated position and jump up
- Keep your arms straight
- Knees, toes and hips are in line

3) Leg Curl (Some gyms will have machines for seated or lying leg curls instead)

- Stand on the platform, place the pad at the back of your heel
- Curl backward as much as possible and make sure you keep your knee stable
- Now switch legs. Bring your leg slowly down and make sure the weights don't touch each other

4) Split Squats

- Ensure that your chest is up, core is engaged and your hip, knee and foot are in line
- Make sure that your front knee doesn't jut out beyond the top of your toe
- The angle between your calves and thighs should be 90 degrees
- Once you complete your repetitions, switch feet and work out the other side

5) Abdominal Crunches with Raised Arms

- Lie down and bend your knees, feet hip-width apart
- Raise your arms above your head
- Exhale and crunch upwards
- Contract your abs and keep the movement controlled

6) Abs Scissor Heel Taps

- Lie on your back but raise yourself up onto your elbows
- Engage your core
- Bend your knees and scissor your legs alternately, tapping your heels on the ground
- Keep the movement controlled and not too fast

7) Oblique Crunches

- Lie on your back, knees bent and feet together
- Lower your knees slightly to one side
- And with your arm on that side, place it on your obliques
- With your opposite arm place your fist against the side of your head and keep your elbow high
- Crunch straight up, squeezing your obliques
- Keep the movement controlled
- Swap sides, lowering your knees to the other side
- Do not crunch towards your tilted knees. Straight up

8) Plank Weight Rotation

- Put a weight or object in front of you
- Lie on your front
- Support yourself on your forearms and toes
- Raise your torso up and hold this plank position
- With one hand pick up the weight in front of you
- Make a semicircle movement and place the weight under your tummy
- With the other hand pick the weight up, then place it back in front of you
- Do this in a clockwise movement then switch to anticlockwise
- Your body should be as flat as possible so keep your bottom tucked down
- Keep your core engaged
- Keep your pelvis tipped forward and belly button tucked in
- Don't forget to breathe!

11.2 INSTRUCTIONS FOR THE EXERCISES IN THE HOME WORKOUTS

Here are the detailed instructions for each of the exercises you'll be performing during your home workouts. Use this section as your go-to resource for mastering the techniques involved in these exercises, or for reminding yourself how to do them later. Whereas the weight training sequences are designed to be done in the gym, with gym equipment, these workouts with no equipment involved can be done at home or even in the park.

HOME WORKOUT 1

1) Squats

- Stand with your feet shoulder-width apart, toes slightly pointing out
- Squat and touch the floor between your feet
- When you squat, stick your bottom out, keep your back flat and your core engaged

2) Horizontal Knees to Chest

- Kneel down and take up a press-up position
- You are going to step forward towards your hands one foot at a time, alternating your feet
- Make sure you keep your core engaged
- And breathe in and out regularly

3) Press-ups

- You can either do this on your feet or on your knees
- Keep your press-up position, hands wide
- Lower your chest as much as possible
- Ideally the angle between your upper arms and forearms should be 90 degrees
- Again make sure you keep that core engaged and breathe in and out on every repetition

4) High Knees

- The easy option is marching on the spot and the hard option is jogging on the spot
- Keep your hands at chest level and raise your knees to touch your hands

HOME WORKOUT 2

1) Good Old Star Jumps!

They remind me of my Air Force training days. A star jump is when you jump to a position with your legs spread wide and your hands touching above your head (you can clap your hands!), before you return to a position with your arms back by your sides and your feet together.

- Star jump your feet and raise your arms up to shoulder level at the same time
- And engage your core throughout the exercise

2) Alternating Backward Lunges

- Standing, keep your feet together, chest up
- Lunge backwards on alternate legs, lowering your back knee as much as possible
- Make sure your toes, knee and hip are in line as you lunge

3) Hooks

- Stand with your feet wider than hip-width apart
- Engage your core
- Twist your upper body and with a clenched fist hit those imaginary pads in front of you, like a sparring boxer
- Your palms should face towards you

4) Side Plank

- Lie on your side
- Raise yourself on your forearm
- You have two options. Option 1 is on your feet, option 2 is on your knees
- Raise your other arm
- Hold this position

HOME WORKOUT 3

1) Oblique Curl Right

- Lie on your back, legs bent

- Keep your feet together and drop your knees a little to the left
- And crunch
- Place your left hand on your right obliques, which is where you should feel the burn!

2) Oblique Curl Left

- Now the other side
- Drop your knees a little to the right
- You can support your head with your left hand
- Place your right hand on your left obliques, which is where you should feel the burn

3) Cycling in the Air

- Lie on your back
- Place your hands palm down on the floor, with your thumbs under your bottom
- Rest your head
- And cycle in the air
- At the same time push your lower back down as much as possible so it doesn't arch

4) Plank

- Take up the plank position on the ground, balancing on your forearms and feet, keeping your core engaged
- Tilt your pelvis forward to activate those core muscles
- If this is too hard, you can do it on your knees

5) Side Touch Shuttles

- You are going to touch the ground to one side, side-shuttle a few steps and then touch the ground again on the other side
- Bend your knees as you touch the ground

HOME WORKOUT 4

1) Side Lunges

- Keep your feet together

- Core engaged
- We are going to the right first
- Lunge sideways and touch your right trainer with your left hand
- Make sure your knee and toes are in line
- Keep your left leg straight
- Next set we will do the other side

2) Horizontal Side Jumps

- Take up a press-up position on the ground
- Feet together, core engaged
- You are going to jump from side to side
- Keep your arms straight under your shoulders as you jump

3) Heel Touches

- Lie on your back
- Keep your head up, legs bent
- You are going to touch your heels, alternating from side to side
- Squeeze your oblique muscles
- This works your abdominals as well as your obliques

4) Leg Kicks

- Stand up and keep your feet apart
- Make fists with your hands and keep them next to your head
- Then kick your back foot up and out
- Change to the other leg after each set

HOME WORKOUT 5

1) Hip Extensions Right

- Start on all fours with knees directly under the hips and elbows below the shoulders
- Keep your right leg straight and extend it by squeezing your right buttock
- Move your leg up and down by engaging and tightening your right gluteus/buttock
- Keep your core engaged

2) Hip Extensions Left

- You can do this on your elbows as well as on your hands
- Keep your left leg straight and extend it by squeezing your left buttock
- Move your leg up and down by engaging and tightening your left gluteus/buttock
- Feel that nice burn in your gluteus

3) Burpees

My favourite! I will show you two alternatives here

- Stand up, jump up, bend down from your knees, put your hands in front of your feet and kick your feet back, drop your chest all the way down and come back up to standing
- Another option is to step back one foot at a time rather than kicking your feet back at the same time, and no jumping when you stand up

4) Leg Raises

This is a great exercise for the lower abdominals

- Lie on your back with your head resting on the mat
- Place your hands palm down on the floor, with your thumbs under your bottom
- Keep your legs bent throughout this exercise
- Raise your feet up in the air, towards your chest and slightly raise your bottom at the same time
- Touch your heels on the ground when you lower your feet back down

HOME WORKOUT 6

1) Squats

- Keep your feet shoulder-width apart, toes slightly pointing out
- Squat and touch the floor
- When you squat, stick your bottom out, keep your back flat and your core engaged

2) Alternating Backward Lunges

- Standing, keep your feet together, chest up

- Lunge backwards on alternate legs, lowering your back knee as much as possible
- Make sure your toes, knee and hip are in line as you lunge

3) Upper Cuts

- This is a cardio exercise
- Keep your feet wider than shoulder-width apart
- Make a fist with both hands at face level
- Squat slightly and throw upper cuts with alternate arms
- Straighten your knees as you come up

4) Lateral Plank Walks

- Start in the plank position
- Engage your core
- Move your feet sideways along the mat in a stepping motion, moving the same arm as leg
- Change direction to sidestep back to the starting position
- Did you feel that nice burn in your abs?!

5) Rhomboid Squeezes

- This is an exercise for your middle back, especially for the muscle between your shoulder-blades
- Lie on your front, open your arms out at right angles to your body
- Raise your chest up and lift your arms as if you are flying
- Make sure you squeeze that muscle between the shoulder-blades
- If you raise your legs, this will also work your gluteus

6) Arm Circles

- This is a very basic but very effective exercise
- Keep your feet shoulder-width apart
- Stretch your arms out parallel to the ground
- Keep your knees soft and rotate your arms forwards as if you are drawing circles with your hands
- After 15 seconds of rotating forward, rotate backwards for another 15 seconds

HOME WORKOUT 7

1) Split Squats Right

- Start with your feet apart, right foot forwards
- Make sure your chest is up, your core engaged and your hips, knees and feet are in line
- Your front knee shouldn't jut out beyond the end of your toes
- As you squat, lower your back knee as much as possible
- Switch feet and work out the other side in the next exercise

2) Split Squats Left

- Keep your left foot forwards
- Core engaged
- The angle between your calves and thighs in these squats should be 90 degrees

3) Dead Bug Parallel Legs

- Lie on your back, your knees up
- You are going to lower your feet one at a time
- Make sure your lower back is pressing into the ground
- You have two options here: you can keep your hands by your torso on the ground, or you can keep your arms raised above your chest

4) Press-ups and Rotate

- Take a press-up position
- Do one press-up, lift one arm up straight and rotate your torso
- Follow your hand with your head to help you rotate better
- Alternate the rotation after each repetition
- You can do this on your knees
- As you rotate lift the knee and straighten the leg on the side that is rotating

5) Slalom Side-hops

- Stand upright, feet together
- This is a cardio exercise
- Hop to the right, then to the left, making sure you only have one foot on the ground at any given time

6) Plank Step In and Out

- The last exercise for this set is another core exercise
- Take up a plank position
- Start with your feet together and step sideways one foot at a time then come back to your starting position
- Right foot out, left foot out, right foot in, left foot in and repeat

HOME WORKOUT 8

1) Good Morning

- Keep your feet wider than shoulder-width apart
- Bend from your hips with soft knees
- Place your hands behind your head
- Bend down, keeping your back flat
- And extend all the way up
- This is really good for your lower back and hamstrings

2) Side Touch Shuttles

- This is a cardio exercise
- Start from one side of your mat
- Sidestep a few times and touch the ground
- Then sidestep back to the other side and touch the ground
- Make sure you bend from your knees

3) Plank with Knee Flexion

- Start in plank position
- Bring one of your knees from the side towards your elbow
- And alternate
- Make sure you squeeze your oblique muscles (they are the ones on each side of your abdominals)

4) Squat and Jump

- Keep your feet shoulder-width apart

- Squat and touch the ground, come back to a standing position then jump up
- Remember, when you squat, stick your bottom out

5) Floor Triceps Dips

- Sit on the ground and keep your feet together in front of you with your legs bent
- Place your hands behind you, leaning back, palms down, fingers facing forwards
- Lift your bottom up as much as possible and triceps dip
- Make sure you bend your elbows as much as possible
- You will have a small range of movement; you need to bend your arms from your elbows each time and straighten them to squeeze your triceps

6) Spotty Dog

- Another cardio exercise
- Start with your feet apart
- One leg back and the opposite arm raised
- As you jump, bring the back leg forwards and the same arm up
- At the same time jump the other leg back and lower the same arm
- Keep your core engaged
- You can also do this exercise keeping your arms on your hips

HOME WORKOUT 9

1) Clams Right

- Lie on your left side with your knees bent in front of you
- Your feet should be in line with your hips
- Keep your body straight
- Roll your hip forwards and place your right hand in front of your torso to support you
- Raise your upper knee, keeping your feet together
- Feel your gluteus and don't twist your hip
- Bring your knee down and repeat

2) Clams Left

- Lie on your right side this time and again with your knees bent in front of you
- Your feet should be in line with your hips
- Keep your body straight
- Roll your hip forwards and place your left hand in front of your torso to support you
- Raise your upper knee, keeping your feet together
- Feel your gluteus and don't twist your hip
- Bring your knee down and repeat

3) Bridge

- Lie on your back, knees bent
- Engage your core and tilt your pelvis forwards
- Lift your bottom up slowly, by keeping your core, hamstrings and gluteus engaged
- To make this more challenging, raise one leg straight out in front of you
- Keep the leg up as you lift your bottom
- You can do 15 seconds raising one leg, then 15 seconds the other

4) Leg Kicks Right

- Kneel on all fours
- Engage your core and keep your back flat
- Bring your right knee in towards your chest and then extend back out and up with a bent knee
- You should feel the burn in your gluteus
- You'll work on the other side next set

5) Leg Kicks Left

- Kneel on all fours
- Engage your core and keep your back flat
- Bring your left knee in towards your chest and then extend back out and up with a bent knee
- You should feel the burn in your gluteus

6) Skydiver

- Lie on your front with your arms by your side, palms facing up
- Raise both your chest and legs and rotate your arms towards your body so your palms are facing down
- Engage your gluteus, lower back and rhomboids (the muscles between your shoulder-blades)

7) Side Leg Kicks Right

- Lie on your left side with your knees bent in front of you
- Your feet should be in line with your hips
- Keep your body straight
- Roll your hip forwards and place your right hand in front of your torso to support you
- Bring your right knee towards your chest, touch your elbow and kick back out
- Your leg should move diagonally

8) Side Leg Kicks Left

- Lie on your right side this time and again with your knees bent in front of you
- Your feet should be in line with your hips
- Keep your body straight
- Roll your hip forwards and place your left hand in front of your torso to support you
- Bring your left knee towards your chest, touch your elbow and kick back out
- Make sure your leg moves diagonally

HOME WORKOUT 10 (PYRAMID)

1) Pyramid press-ups

- Take up a press-up position, hands wide
- Make sure your elbows are at a 90 degree angle as you go down
- Drop that chest as much as possible
- Keep your core engaged and keep breathing during each repetition

2) Pyramid Abs Scissors

- Lie on your back
- Keep your head up, which helps engage your upper abs
- Place your hands behind your head
- Scissor your feet vertically
- Make sure you are engaging your core
- Keep your lower back pressed down as much as possible

3) Pyramid Horizontal Side Jumps

- Take up a press-up position
- Keep your feet together and jump from side to side
- Engage your core. I do this on my fists, but you can also do it on your hands as when you do press-ups
- Keep breathing

HOME WORKOUT 11

1) Lunge Back and Side

- Keep your feet together, core engaged, chest up
- Do a backward lunge followed by a side lunge on your left foot
- Change to your right foot, then keep alternating
- Keep your hands on your hips
- When you do a side lunge touch your foot with your opposite hand

2) Squat Thrust to Sides

- Take up a press-up position either on your hands or on your fists
- Keep your feet together, core engaged
- Jump forward towards your left hand and back to the starting position
- Then jump towards the other hand

3) Scissors

- Lie on your back and scissor your feet up and down
- You can keep your head up if you like

- Feel free to support your head with your hands
- And now try horizontal scissors
- Make sure you press your lower back into the mat and engage that core

4) Duck Squats

- Keep your feet hip-width apart
- Make fists with your hands and hold them up next to your cheeks
- Squat up and down
- Imagine you are drawing a letter U with your nose on an imaginary wall in front of you

5) Dynamic Plank to Press-ups with a Jump

- Start in the plank position
- Push yourself up to a press-up position and jump your feet up. You're on all fours and you jump both feet off the ground for a few inches, keeping your hands on the ground
- Then back down to the plank position again
- Alternate your hands on each repetition
- Left hand up, right hand up, left hand down, right hand down, and jump
- Then right hand up, left hand up, right hand down, left hand down, and jump

6) Knee Hits

- Stand with your feet apart
- Make a fist with your joined hands, in front of your chest
- Imagine there is a kick pad or punchbag in front of you and hit that imaginary pad with your knee and back to your starting position
- Do half the time on one knee, then change to the other
- Keep your core engaged

HOME WORKOUT 12

1) Skiing Torso Rotation

- Keep your feet wider than shoulder-width apart, toes pointing out
- Keep your chest up and lift your arms straight out at the side, at shoulder height

- Reach down to your left foot with the opposite hand
- Come back to the upright position with arms outstretched and jump up
- Then reach down to your right foot with the opposite hand
- Bend your knee a little when reaching towards your foot and keep your other arm straight at the back

2) Squats Increasing Claps

- Keep your feet shoulder-width apart
- You are going to squat and clap
- Increase the claps by one with each repetition
- This means you are staying in squat-hold position longer each time!

3) Leg Kick, Tap with Opposite Hand

- Stand upright
- Kick with your right foot then lunge back with your left foot and touch the ground with your left hand
- And repeat
- Halfway through, switch sides
- Now kick with your left foot and lunge back with your right foot and touch the ground with your right hand

4) Reverse Crunches with Knee Flexion

- This exercise is on the mat
- Sit on the mat and tuck your knees in close to your chest
- You are going to do reverse crunches very slowly down and then fast on the way up
- As you lower down slowly to the mat, lift your legs up and keep them straight; stretch out your arms over your head
- As you come up, bring your knees in towards your chest, hold them for a split second then lower down to the mat again slowly

5) Side Tap, Side Laterals

- Stand up, feet hip-width apart, knees soft
- Gently lean forward, sidestep with a straight leg and at the same time lift both arms up to shoulder height

- Alternate your feet
- Make sure you keep your moving leg straight and the other one bent from the knee

6) Burpees and Forward Lunges

- You are going to do one burpee followed by a forward lunge on each leg
- Place your hands on your hips during the lunges
- Make sure your toes, knee and hip are in line
- Engage your core and keep your chest up

HOME WORKOUT 13

1) Press-ups/Star Jumps

- Take up a press-up position
- You are going to do one press-up, then touch your knees on the ground
- Bring your knees back up and star jump your feet
- Touching your knees on the ground will work your core more, so make sure you engage your core

2) Low Kick Dance

- This is fun!
- Stand up with your feet hip-width apart
- Kick each foot as if you are passing a football and alternate your feet each time
- Keep your arms bent with your hands by your torso and keep your core engaged

3) Squat Side Jumps

- This is a hard one!
- You are going to squat, touch the ground, jump to the side and squat again
- After each squat, jump to the alternate side

4) Triceps Dips

- You'll need a chair, step or a bench for this one
- Sit on a chair, place your hands next to you on the chair-seat, your legs bent in front of you

- Dip down and push yourself back up
- Make sure you keep the back of your torso close to the chair
- To make this exercise more challenging, keep your legs straight in front of you

5) Single Leg Hops

- Stand up on one foot
- Hop on the spot
- Switch sides halfway through
- Make sure you engage your core

6) Lying Flying

- Lie on your front
- Stretch both arms out to the side, palms facing down
- Raise your chest as much as possible and squeeze your shoulder-blades together by lifting your arms up
- Make sure you breathe in and out during every repetition

HOME WORKOUT 14

1) 5 Split Squats and Jumps to Alternate Foot

- Start with feet apart
- Chest up, core engaged, hands on your hips
- After 5 split squats, jump and swap your feet
- And carry on with the split squats
- If jumping as you swap feet is hard, just step and swap

2) Diagonal Toe Touch Crunches

- Lie on your back, keeping both feet up in the air throughout the exercise
- Reach one hand towards the opposite foot, then come back to the mat, keeping your hands next to your ears
- Change hands and repeat
- Feel those oblique muscles when you curl up and twist
- If it is hard for you to touch your toes, that's OK. Try to reach up as much as possible

3) Clap under Thighs/Squat Jumps

- You are going to jump onto one foot, kick the other foot upwards and clap under that leg
- Then the other leg
- Each time after you have done both legs, touch the ground and do a squat jump

4) Plank

- This is active rest
- You are going to stay in the plank position
- Hold yourself in plank position on your toes and on your forearms
- Keep your core engaged
- Tilt your pelvis forward, which helps you engage your core

5) Press-ups to Sides

- You are going to do one press-up
- Then move your hands 20-30 cm to the right and do another press-up
- Then back to the left and another press-up
- Make sure when moving to the right, you move your left hand to the right first
- And vice versa
- And if this is hard, feel free to do these press-ups on your knees

6) Leg Oblique Side Drops

- Lie on your back
- Feet up, bending from your hips and knees at 90 degrees
- Arms straight out on each side to give you support, palms facing up
- You are going to lower your legs to the left, keeping your right shoulder on the ground
- And then the other side: lower your legs to the right, keeping your left shoulder on the ground
- It is very important to do this exercise slowly in a controlled movement
- You need to use your core and oblique muscles to keep the movement controlled

HOME WORKOUT 15

1) Horizontal Side Jumps

- Get into a press-up position with feet together, either on your hands or on your fists
- Start with your feet to one side of the central line of your body, as you will be jumping to the other side
- Engage your core and side-jump to left and right
- Make sure you are breathing regularly
- Good work: this is a good cardio exercise and also works your core

2) Leg Raises

- Lie on your back
- Place your arms by your sides with your hands under your bum
- Keep your legs bent and rest your head on the ground
- You are going to raise your bum as well as your legs
- Contract your abdominal muscles each time you raise your bum

3) Press-ups and Diagonal Touch

- Take up a press-up position
- You are going to do one press-up followed by a knee touch
- Drop your chest down as much as possible, keep your core engaged and once you push yourself up, touch your knee with your opposite hand
- Feel free to do the press-ups on your knees and again touch your opposite knee each time

4) Heel Touches

- Lie on your back
- Keep your head up, legs bent
- You are going to touch your heels, alternating from side to side
- Squeeze your oblique muscles
- This works your abdominals as well as your obliques

5) Jumping Lunges

- I will be honest, this is a hard one!
- Take up a lunge position, one foot forward with the back knee down, hands on your hips
- You are going to jump and swap your feet
- Make sure you engage your core and try to lower your back knee as much as possible
- If this is hard, you can step back rather than jump

11.3 THE RECIPE COLLECTION: EASY, HEALTHY AND NUTRITIOUS DISHES

Welcome to my recipe collection! I've specially selected each of these dishes as offering the perfect combination of speed, ease and nutritional value.

You'll see with each dish that I have broken down the macro content (those crucial fats, protein and carbohydrates proportions) and the calorie count.

I've divided the recipes into categories as you'll see below:

BREAKFAST/BRUNCHES

1. Banana pancake
2. Melemen
3. Frittata
4. Overnight Oats
5. Homemade Granola with Protein Powder

LUNCHES

1. Green and Minty Soup
2. Turkish Red Lentil Soup
3. Tofu Scrambled Eggs
4. Bulgur Wheat with Halloumi and Peppers
5. Heavenly Salad of Grains and Pulses

DINNERS

1. Lentil and Cauliflower Masaman
2. Minced Beef with Fresh Runner Beans
3. Yoghurt-Marinated Salmon with Lentils
4. Prawn and Mushroom Casserole
5. Quinoa and Black Bean Salad

SALADS/SNACKS

1. Lentil Koftes
2. Piyaz
3. Feta and Beetroot with Lentils
4. Spinach and Strawberry Salad
5. Falafel with Beetroot and Garlic Dip

BREAKFASTS/BRUNCHES

1) BANANA PANCAKES

You can opt to add yoghurt/berries for a delicious breakfast (additional macros they provide are not included below).

SERVES 2 – MAKES 8 SMALL PANCAKES
PREPARATION TIME: 5 MINUTES
COOKING TIME: 10 MINUTES
Per Serving
Calories: 138 cals
Protein: 6.8g
Carbs: 17.5g
Fat: 5.3g

1 banana, mashed with a fork
2 whole eggs
a pinch of ground cinnamon
a pinch of baking soda
coconut oil spray, for cooking

Put the mashed banana, eggs, cinnamon and baking soda into a food processor, and whizz together for 30 seconds. Alternatively you can put the ingredients in a tall jug and use a stick blender to combine them.

Heat a medium, non-stick frying pan, add a few sprays of coconut oil, and cook the pancakes in batches, a few at a time, turning once. Keep the heat low, otherwise they will burn. Serve with optional berries and/or yoghurt.

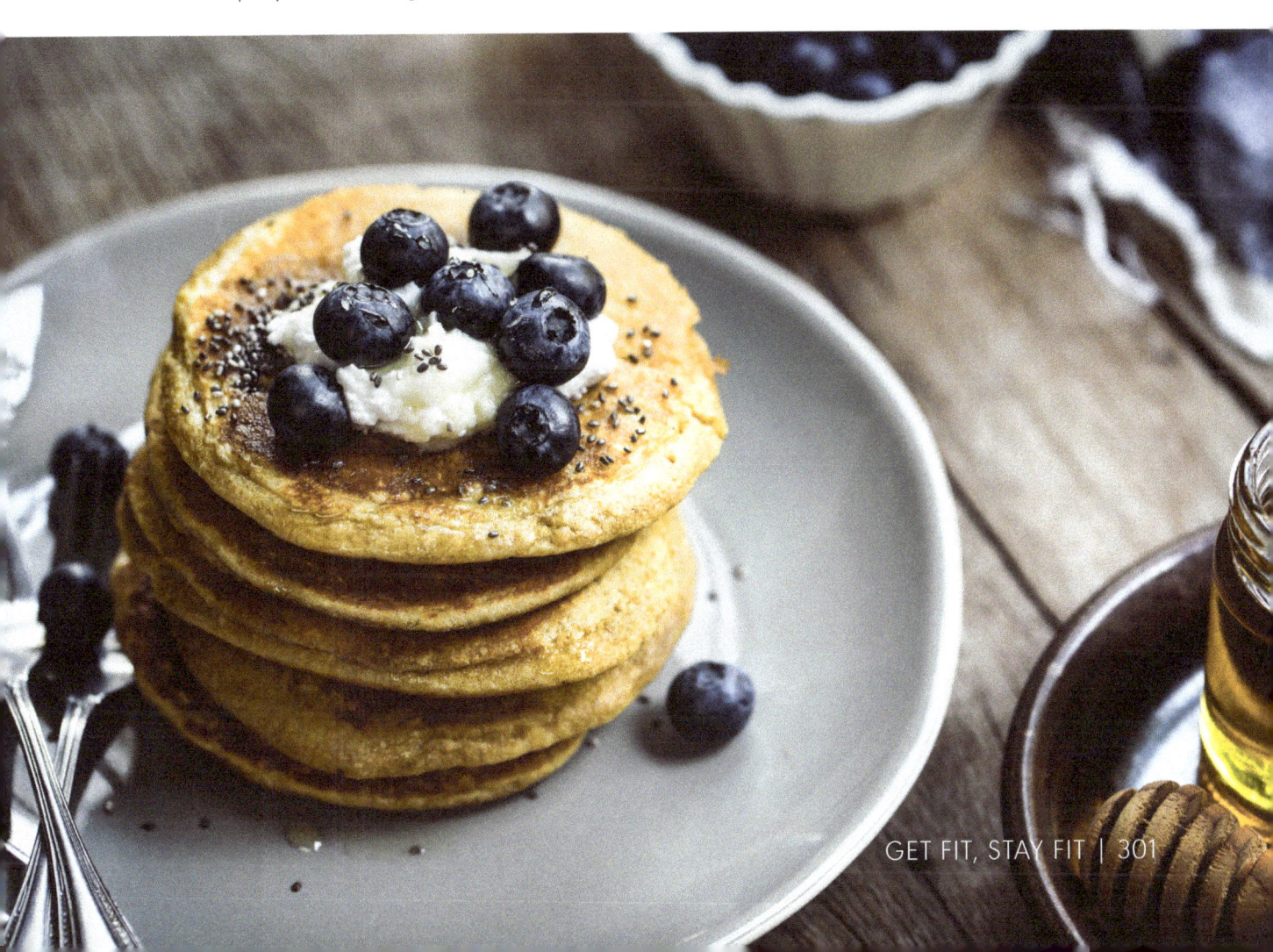

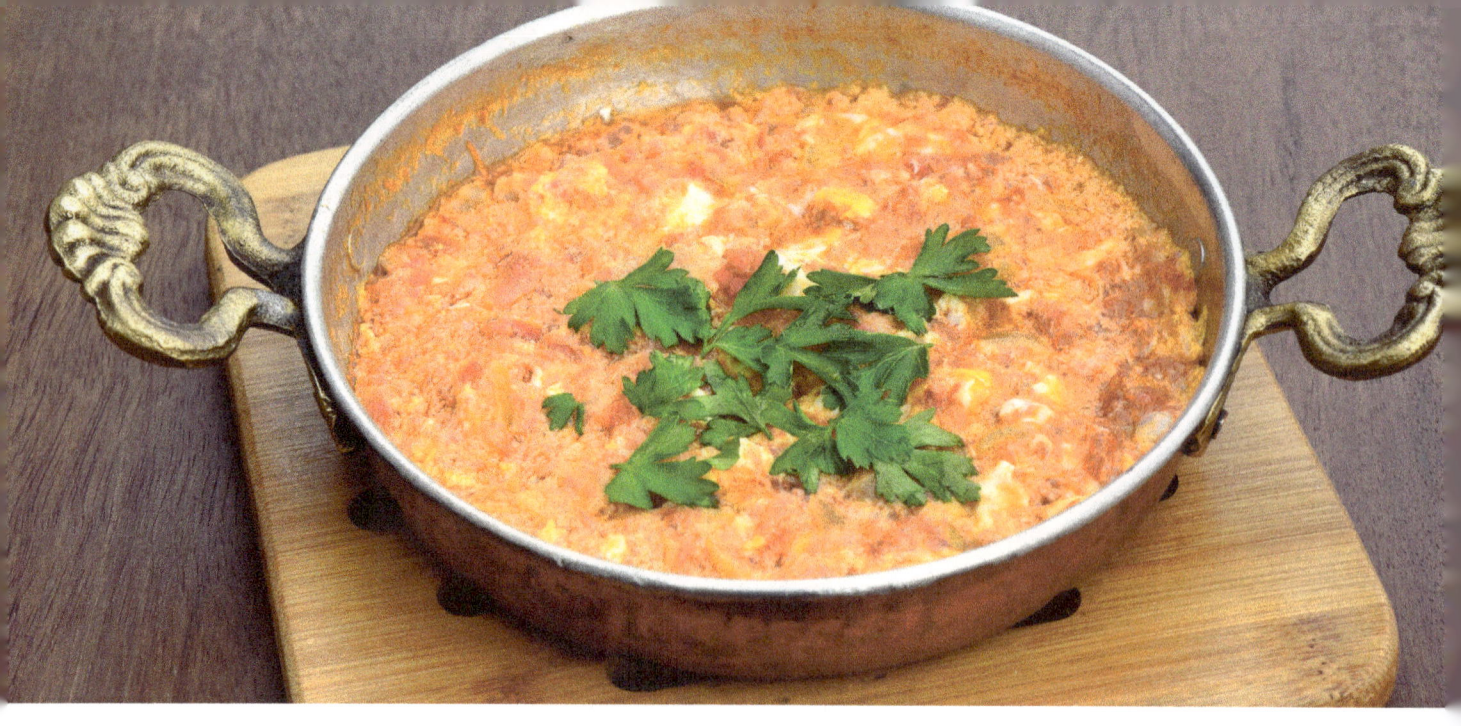

2) MELEMEN

This is a great protein-packed breakfast or brunch. It reminds me of hot summer days in my Turkish home town of Izmir. It is a very popular breakfast dish and almost everyone claims that theirs is the best Melemen!

SERVES 2

PREPARATION TIME: 5 MINUTES

COOKING TIME: 20 MINUTES

Per Serving

Calories: 345 cals

Protein: 20.6g

Carbs: 17g

Fat: 22.3g

1 tbsp olive oil

1 medium onion, diced

1 green pepper, diced

1 garlic clove, crushed (optional)

½ tsp black mustard seeds

½ tsp chilli flakes

2 medium tomatoes, or half a tin of chopped tomatoes (200g)

6 eggs

1 tbsp parsley, chopped

salt and pepper to taste

Heat the oil in a medium-sized saucepan, and when it's hot fry the onion and peppers over a low heat for 5-7 minutes, until soft.

Add the garlic, mustard seeds and chilli flakes, and cook for a further minute.

Add the tomatoes – if you are using fresh then a splash of water in the pan is a good idea. Cook for 5 more minutes and season with a little salt and pepper.

Make 4 pockets in the mixture in the bottom of the pan and crack the eggs in. Cover the pan with a lid, and cook until just set. Sprinkle over the parsley and serve.

3) FRITTATA

This is a very easy recipe. You can cut this into slabs to take with you to work, with a salad. Feel free to add a little chilli if you'd like a bit of heat.

SERVES 4
PREPARATION TIME: 5 MINUTES
COOKING TIME: 30 MINUTES
Per Serving
Calories: 223 cals
Protein: 14.6g
Carbs: 9.9g
Fat: 13.9g

1 tbsp vegetable oil
1 onion, thinly sliced
1 red pepper, thinly sliced
75g button mushrooms, thinly sliced
8 eggs
pinch of dried rosemary
pinch of dried oregano
50ml semi-skimmed milk (optional)
10 cherry tomatoes
salt and black pepper to taste

Pre-heat the oven to 200°C/Fan 180°C/Gas Mark 6

Add the vegetable oil to a large (25cm) oven-proof frying pan, and when the oil is hot add the onions and peppers, cooking over a low heat for 5-7 minutes until soft. If you don't have such a large ovenproof frying pan you could use a medium-sized baking tray instead.

Add the mushrooms and cook for a further 3-4 minutes.

Mix the eggs with the dried herbs, seasoning and milk. Add this to the pan with the vegetables. Halve the cherry tomatoes and dot around the pan. Put the pan into the oven and cook the frittata for around 20-25 minutes, by which time it should be set.

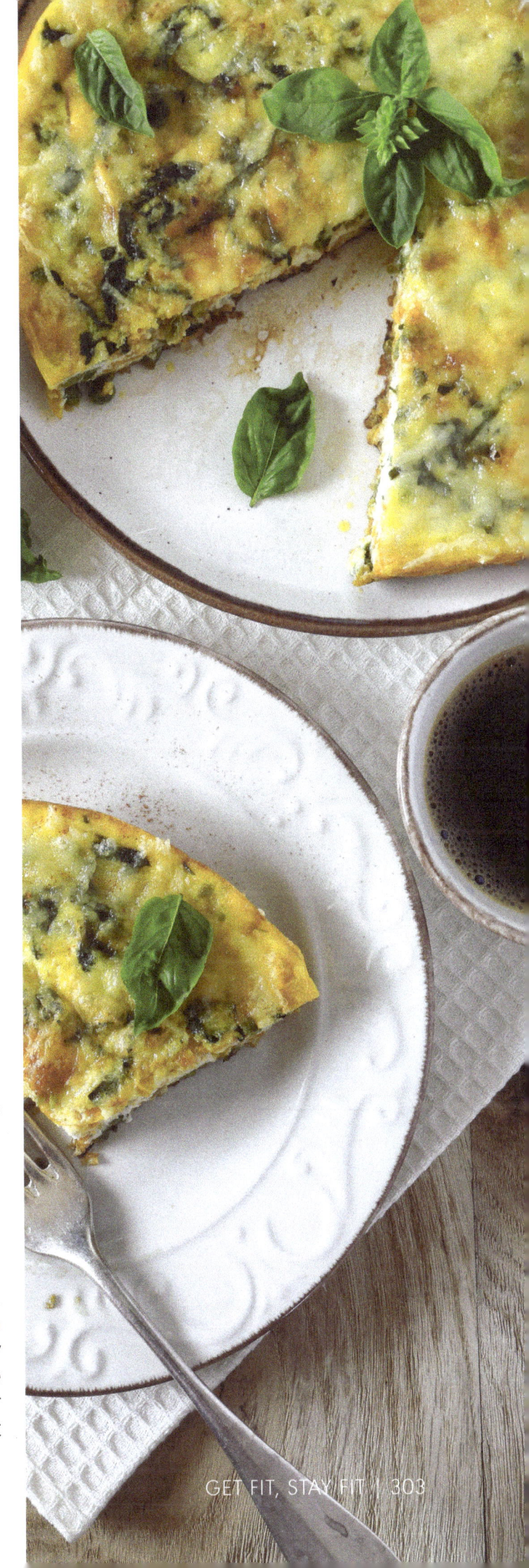

4) OVERNIGHT OATS

Chia seeds are packed with antioxidants, full of fibre and high in protein. They are also a great source of Omega 3, which helps increase your good cholesterol, protecting against heart disease and stroke. Do make sure you measure the seeds, to ensure you don't increase your calorie count too much.

SERVES 2

PREPARATION TIME: 5 MINUTES

COOKING TIME: JUST OVERNIGHT SOAKING FOR THE OATS

Per Serving (with semi-skimmed milk)

Calories: 216 cals

Protein: 16.8g

Carbs: 23.2g

Fat: 5.9g

50g porridge oats

2 tsp chia seeds

200ml semi-skimmed milk (or soya, almond, or coconut milk)

25g protein powder

Mix the porridge oats, chia seeds and milk in an airtight jar or plastic container, and leave in the fridge overnight.

In the morning loosen the mixture with a little more milk, then add your favourite protein powder. If using unflavoured powder, you might like to add a pinch of cinnamon or ¼ tsp vanilla extract. The oats can also be served with berries or a spoonful of nut butter.

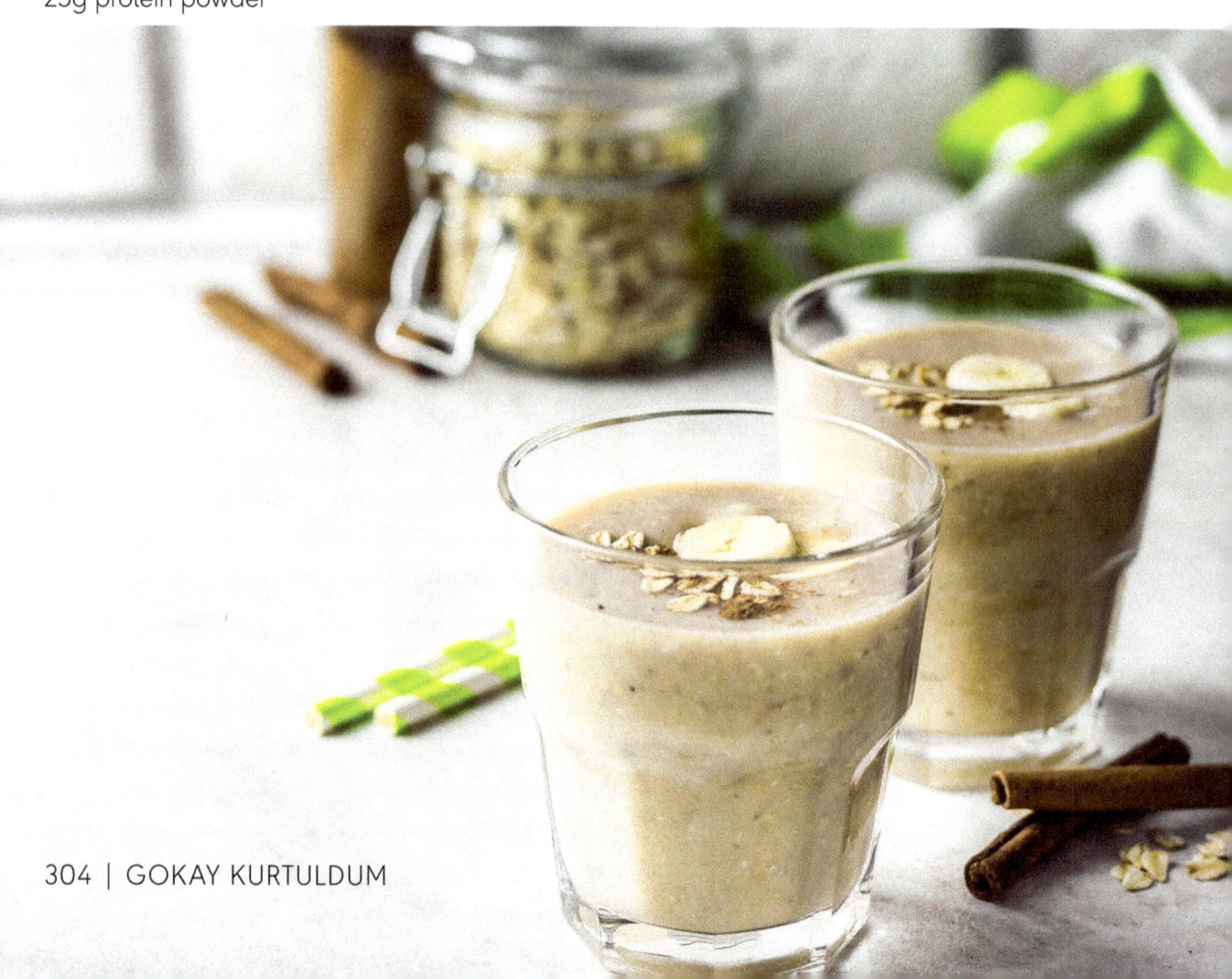

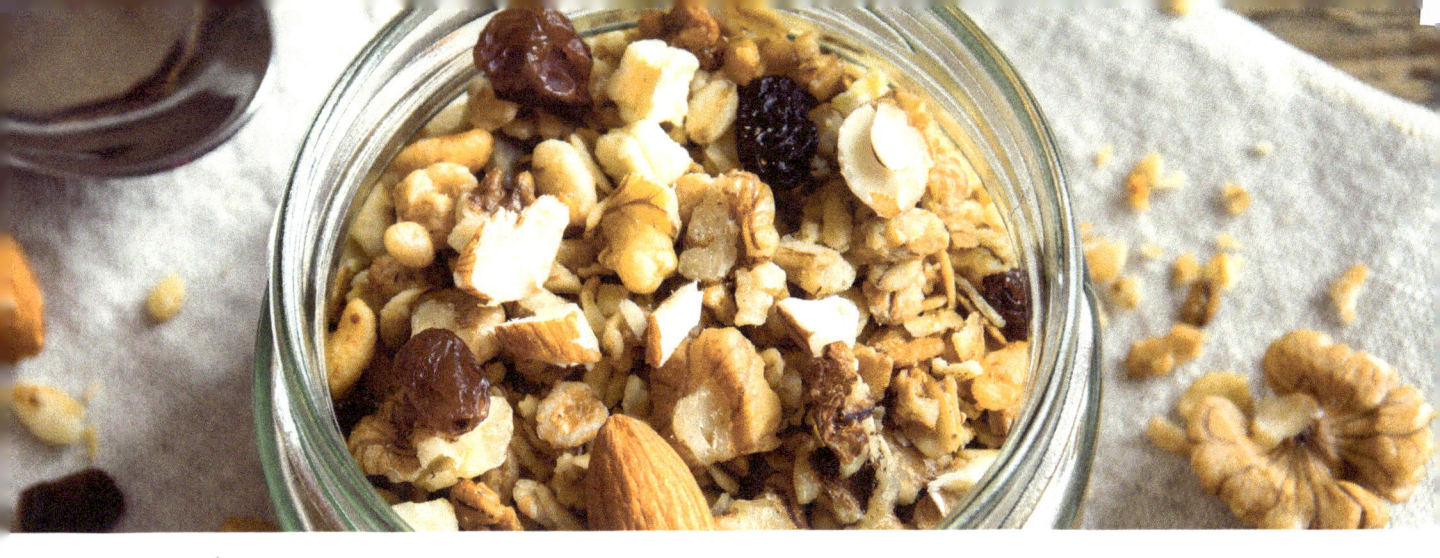

5) HOMEMADE GRANOLA WITH PROTEIN POWDER

I love it when I can make a much better version of a product at home, such as this granola - it's great that it's not full of sugar and I can add my own favourite nuts and berries. I keep mine for at least a month in an airtight container.

MAKES 12 PORTIONS

PREPARATION TIME: 5 MINUTES

COOKING TIME: 20 MINUTES

Per Serving (with one 25g scoop of protein powder included)

Calories: 378 cals

Protein: 25.9g

Carbs: 32.7g

Fat: 16.3g

300g porridge oats

50g sunflower seeds

50g pecan nuts or walnuts

100g flaked almonds

50g raisins

50g dried cranberries

1 tsp ground cinnamon

100g maple syrup or honey

3 tbsp coconut oil, or other natural oil

25g protein powder (per serving)

Preheat the oven to 150°C/130°C Fan/Gas Mark 2

Mix the oats, seeds, nuts, raisins, dried cranberries and cinnamon together in a large bowl.

Put both the maple syrup and coconut oil in a small saucepan and heat gently, stirring until combined. Pour this over the dry ingredients, mixing everything together.

Lay a piece of parchment on a baking tray, tip the mixture in and bake for 20 minutes, turning halfway through. It will be ready when it looks golden brown, and the almonds are toasted. The granola will harden as it cools.

I add milk and a 25g scoop of protein powder to the granola, just before eating.

LUNCHES

1) GREEN AND MINTY SOUP

This makes enough for 6 people, so you could portion the soup and freeze some to eat another day.

SERVES 6
PREPARATION TIME: 10 MINUTES
COOKING TIME: 15 MINUTES
Per Serving
Calories: 226 cals
Protein: 14.4g
Carbs: 36.4g
Fat: 3.4g

1 tbsp olive oil
2 onions, roughly chopped
1 courgette, chopped
200g mangetout, chopped
150g green beans, chopped
2 garlic cloves, sliced
1 litre vegetable stock
500g frozen peas
100g spinach, washed
15g fresh mint leaves
1 tsp sea salt
freshly ground black pepper

Heat the olive oil in a saucepan and fry the onions for 7-8 minutes over a medium to low heat until soft.

Add the courgette, mangetout and green beans, and fry for 2 minutes.

Add the garlic and cook for a further minute. Pour in the stock and bring everything to the boil. Reduce the heat and add the peas and the spinach. Stir and remove the pan from the heat, and add the mint and seasoning.

Using a hand blender or food processor, blitz until smooth. Serve with a few extra mint leaves if you like.

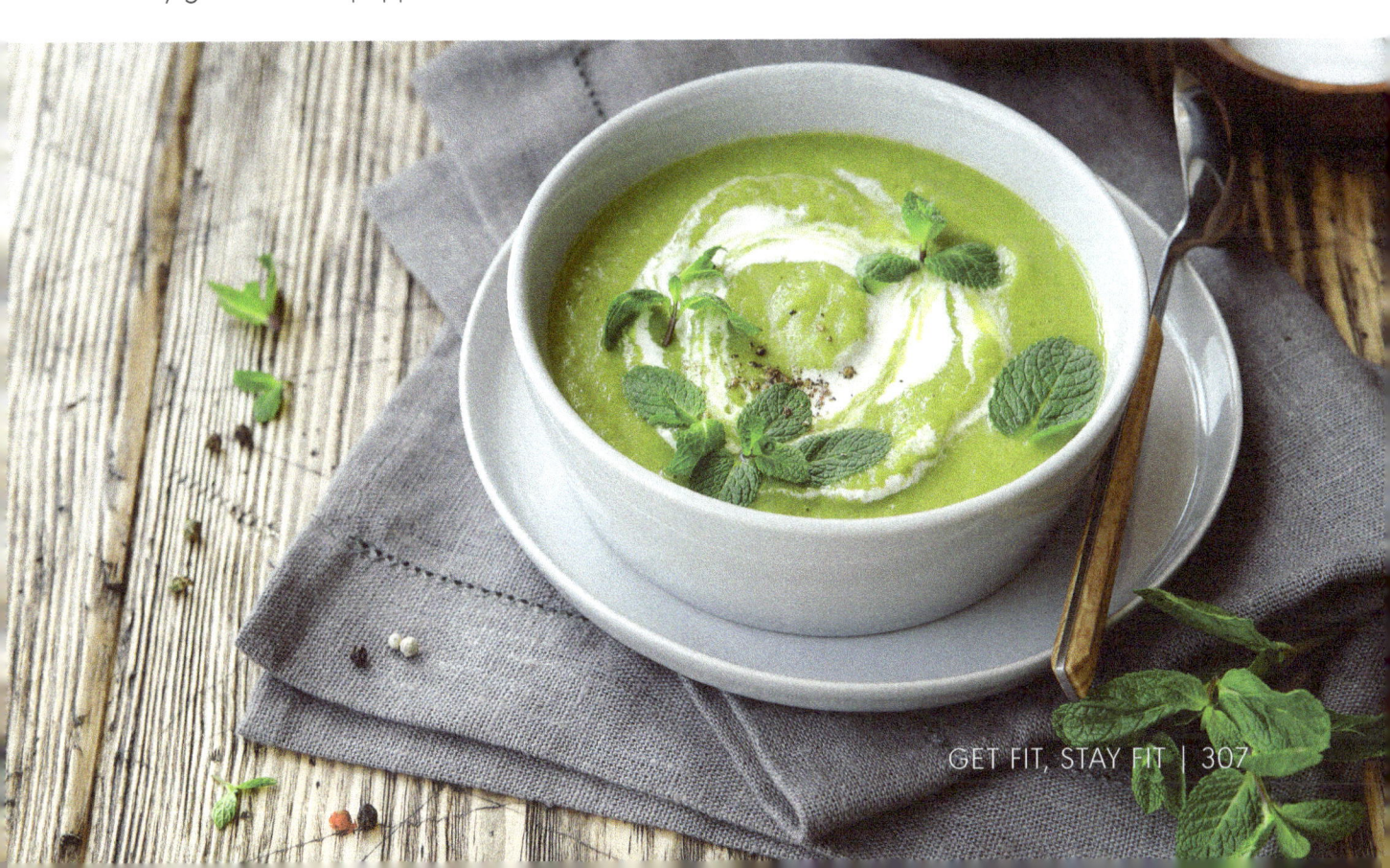

2) TURKISH RED LENTIL SOUP

I simply can't get enough of this soup. When I was a child, I used to have it once a week and just tasting it takes me right back to that time in my life! It's also a very popular winter starter dish in most restaurants in Izmir.

SERVES 6 (SUITABLE FOR BATCH COOKING AND FREEZING)

PREPARATION TIME: 10 MINUTES

COOKING TIME: 30 MINUTES

Per Serving

Calories: 114 cals

Protein: 4.4g

Carbs: 13.6g

Fat: 5g

200g red lentils, rinsed

2 tbsp olive oil

1 large onion, diced

1 large carrot, peeled and diced

2 celery sticks, diced

1 heaped tbsp tomato purée

2 tsp ground cumin

1 tsp paprika

½ tsp dried mint

½ tsp dried oregano

¼ tsp black pepper

¼ tsp crushed red chillies

600ml vegetable stock

600ml water

½ tsp salt

squeeze of lemon juice, to serve

pinch of ground cumin (optional, to serve)

pinch of black pepper (optional, to serve)

Heat the olive oil in a large saucepan and when hot add the onion and fry for 5 minutes. Add the carrots and celery, plus a pinch of salt, and cook for 3 more minutes.

Add the tomato purée and simmer for a minute or two, before adding all of the herbs and spices. Cook for another couple of minutes.

Now add the lentils, stock and water. Bring it all to the boil before reducing the heat and simmering for 15 minutes.

Use a hand blender to achieve a smooth consistency, taste for seasoning and add a big squeeze of lemon juice to taste. You can also add a pinch of ground cumin and black pepper to your bowl if you like.

GET FIT, STAY FIT | 309

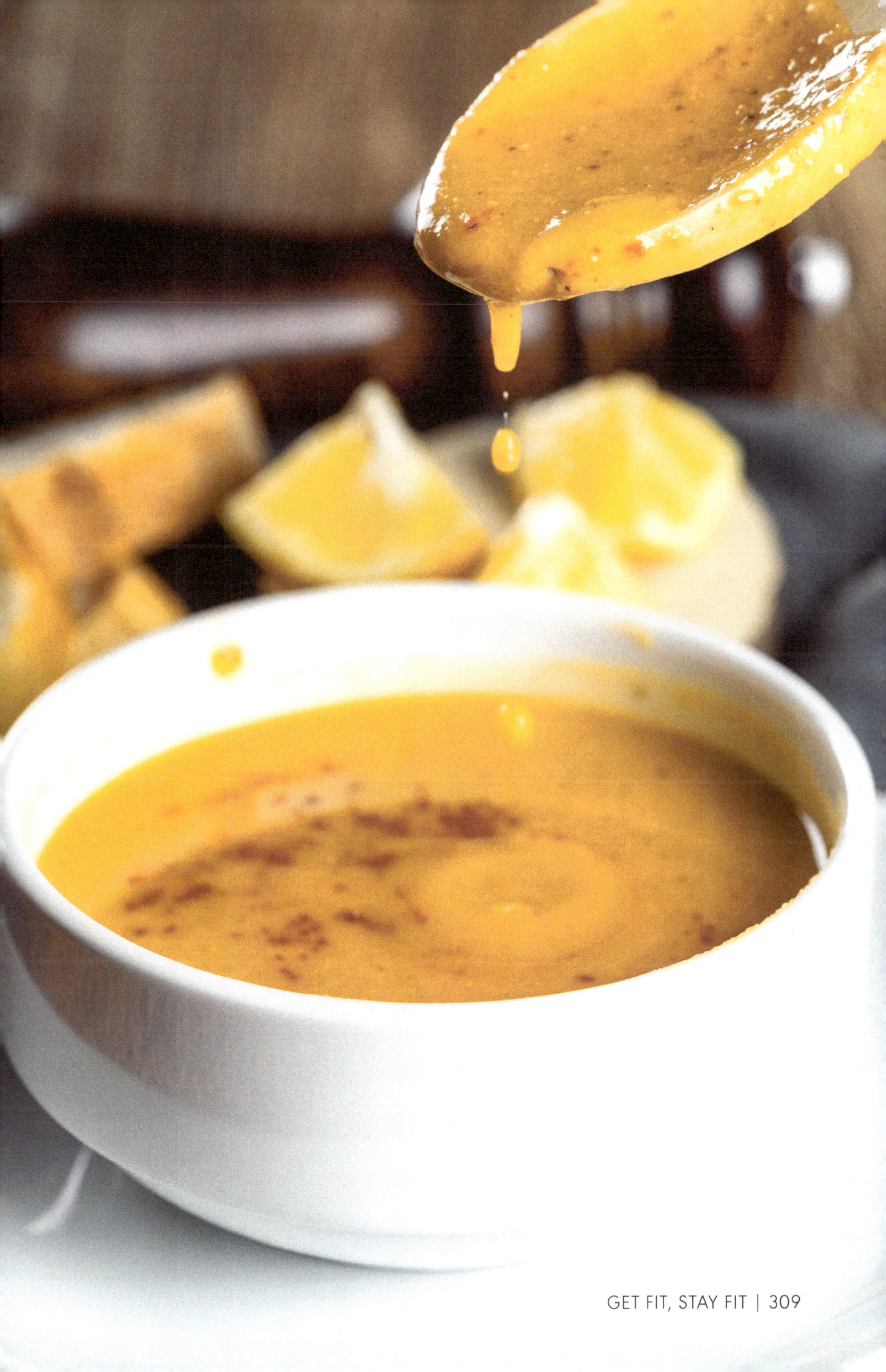

3) TOFU SCRAMBLED EGGS

This dish is super-quick to prepare and super-nutritious too!

SERVES 2

PREPARATION TIME: LESS THAN FIVE MINUTES

COOKING TIME: LESS THAN FIVE MINUTES

Per Serving

Calories: 336 cals

Protein: 19.2g

Carbs: 10.6g

Fat: 24.3g

30g butter

5 button mushrooms, thinly sliced

100g firm tofu, crumbled

30g feta cheese, diced

100g peas, defrosted

3 eggs

salt and black pepper, to taste

Melt the butter over a medium heat in a small, non-stick frying pan. When it froths, add the mushrooms and cook for a couple of minutes.

While the mushrooms are cooking, put the remaining ingredients in a bowl and mix together.

Pour the mixture into the pan with the mushrooms and stir everything gently until the eggs are just set.

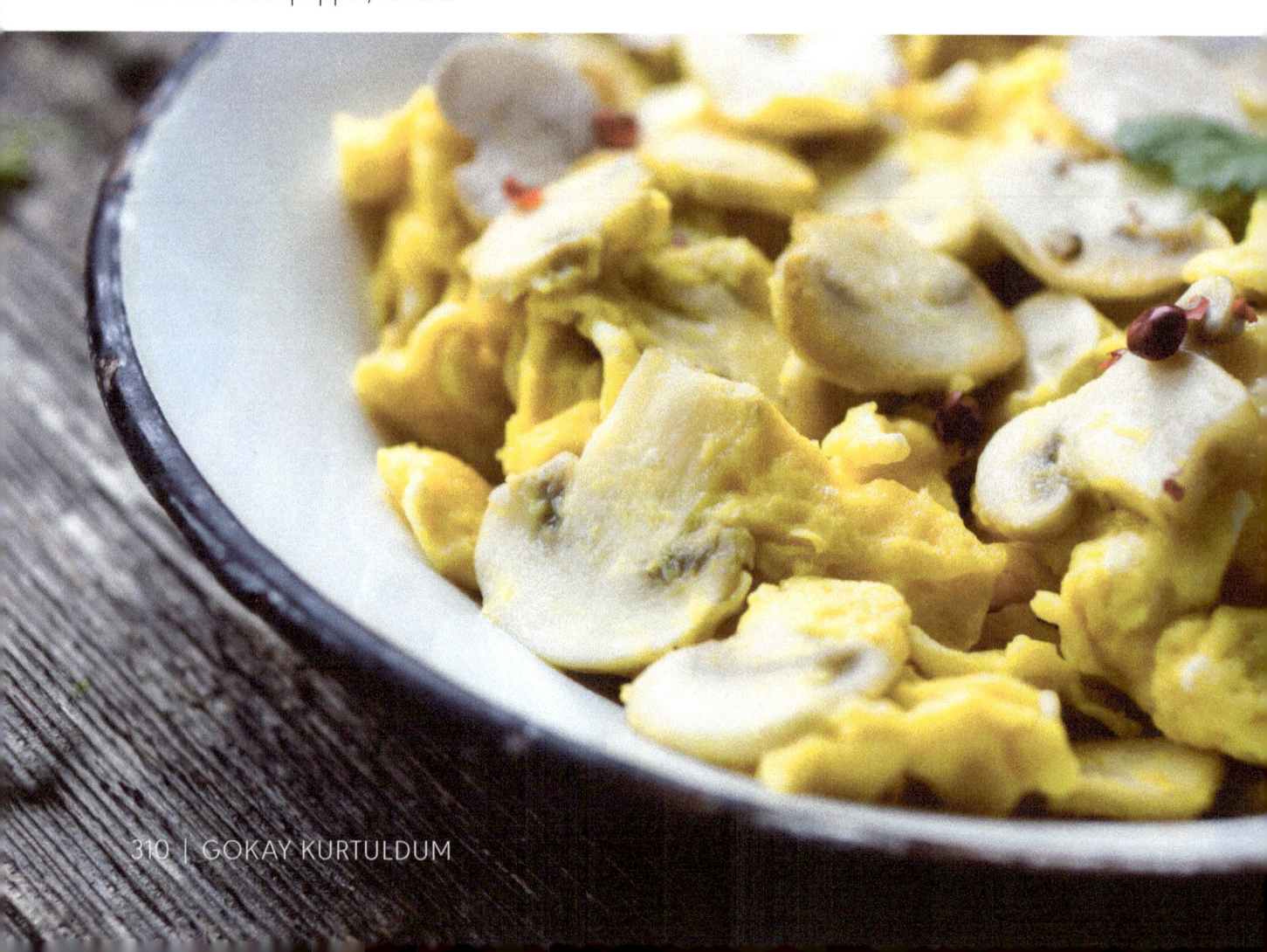

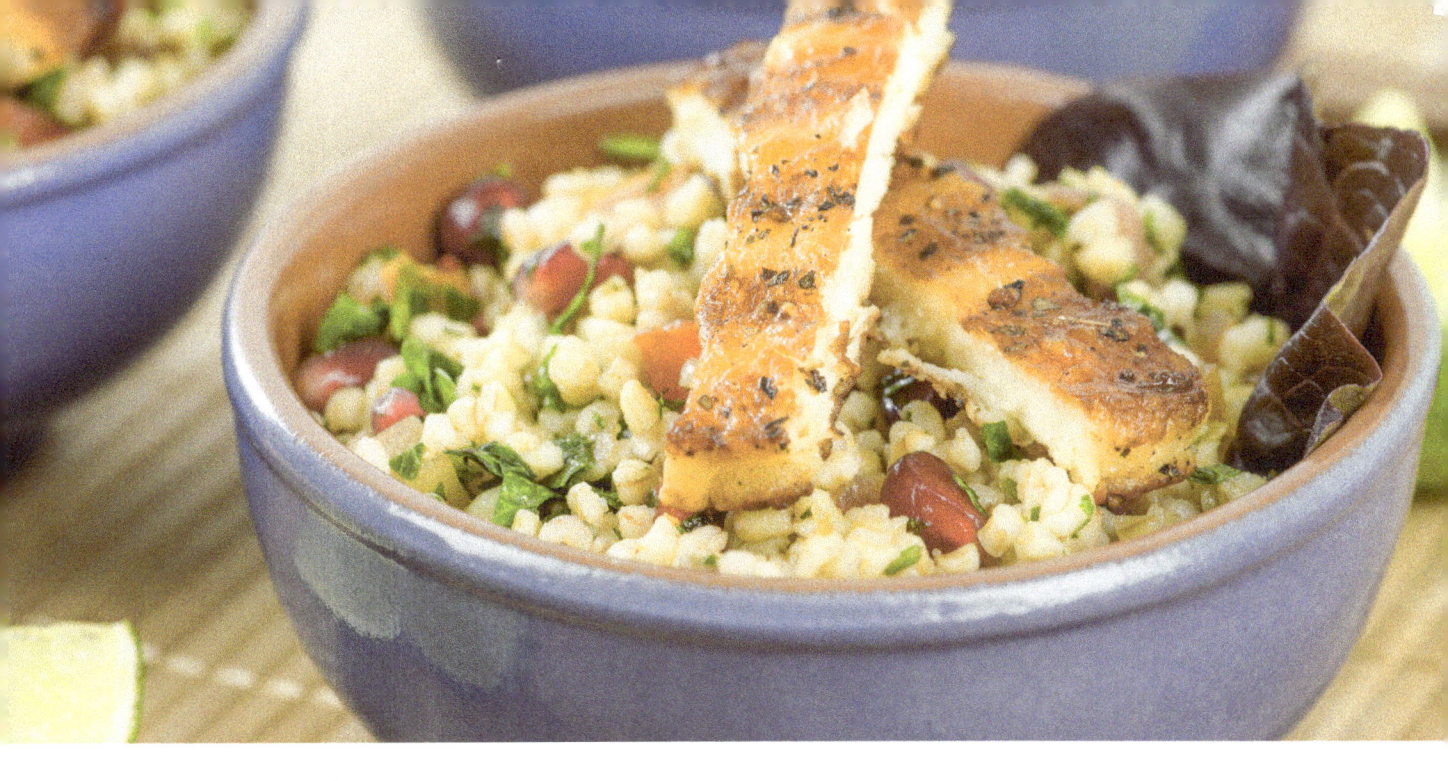

4) BULGUR WHEAT WITH HALLOUMI AND PEPPERS

I find this recipe very satisfying – although it doesn't contain meat, the consistency of halloumi makes it feel as though it does!

SERVES 2
PREPARATION TIME: 10 MINUTES
COOKING TIME: 20 MINUTES

Per Serving

Calories: 657 cals

Protein: 27.6g

Carbs: 18.4g

Fat: 55.2g

100g bulgur wheat

175ml vegetable stock

1-calorie spray vegetable oil

200g halloumi cheese, sliced

100g roasted red peppers, from a jar

50g walnuts, roughly chopped

a small handful of fresh basil

1 tbsp olive oil

2 tbsp freshly squeezed lime juice

salt and black pepper

Put the bulgur wheat in a large bowl, pour in the boiling hot stock and cover the bowl with clingfilm. Set aside for 15-20 minutes, until the stock is absorbed and the grains are tender.

Spray the oil onto a medium, non-stick frying pan and once the oil is hot, fry the halloumi cheese for a couple of minutes on each side, till golden brown.

Slice the peppers, tear the basil, and set aside.

When the bulgur is ready, dress it with the olive oil and lime juice, and season with salt and pepper to taste. Remember the halloumi is salty, so you may not need to add salt.

Add the peppers, basil, walnuts and halloumi to the bowl, combine everything gently and transfer to a dish to serve.

5) HEAVENLY SALAD OF GRAINS AND PULSES

Use a ready-cooked pack of lentils from the supermarket to make this super-easy, colourful salad. It will keep in the fridge for several days.

SERVES 2

PREPARATION TIME: 10 MINUTES

COOKING TIME: 20 MINUTES

Per Serving

Calories: 679 cals

Protein: 49.4g

Carbs: 72.5g

Fat: 19.1g

80g pearled spelt

40g bulgur wheat

85ml vegetable stock

50g green lentils (from a pre-cooked pack)

½ red pepper, diced

½ yellow pepper, diced

200g chickpeas (half a can)

2 tbsp parsley, finely chopped

1 spring onion, finely chopped

salt and pepper

200g grilled chicken, to serve

For the Dressing:

4 tsp pomegranate molasses

2 tbsp olive oil

juice of half a lemon

2 shallots, finely chopped

salt and pepper to taste

Rinse the spelt, put it in a small saucepan and bring to the boil, before reducing the heat to a simmer for 20 minutes. Drain, and set aside to cool.

Put the bulgur wheat in a large bowl, pour in the boiling hot stock and cover the bowl with clingfilm. Leave for 15-20 minutes, until the stock is absorbed and the grains are tender. Set aside to cool.

In a small bowl whisk together the ingredients for the dressing.

Put the spelt, bulgur, chickpeas and lentils together in a large bowl and mix. Add the peppers, parsley, spring onion, and mix together again. Taste and add seasoning.

Pour the dressing over the salad and serve with grilled chicken.

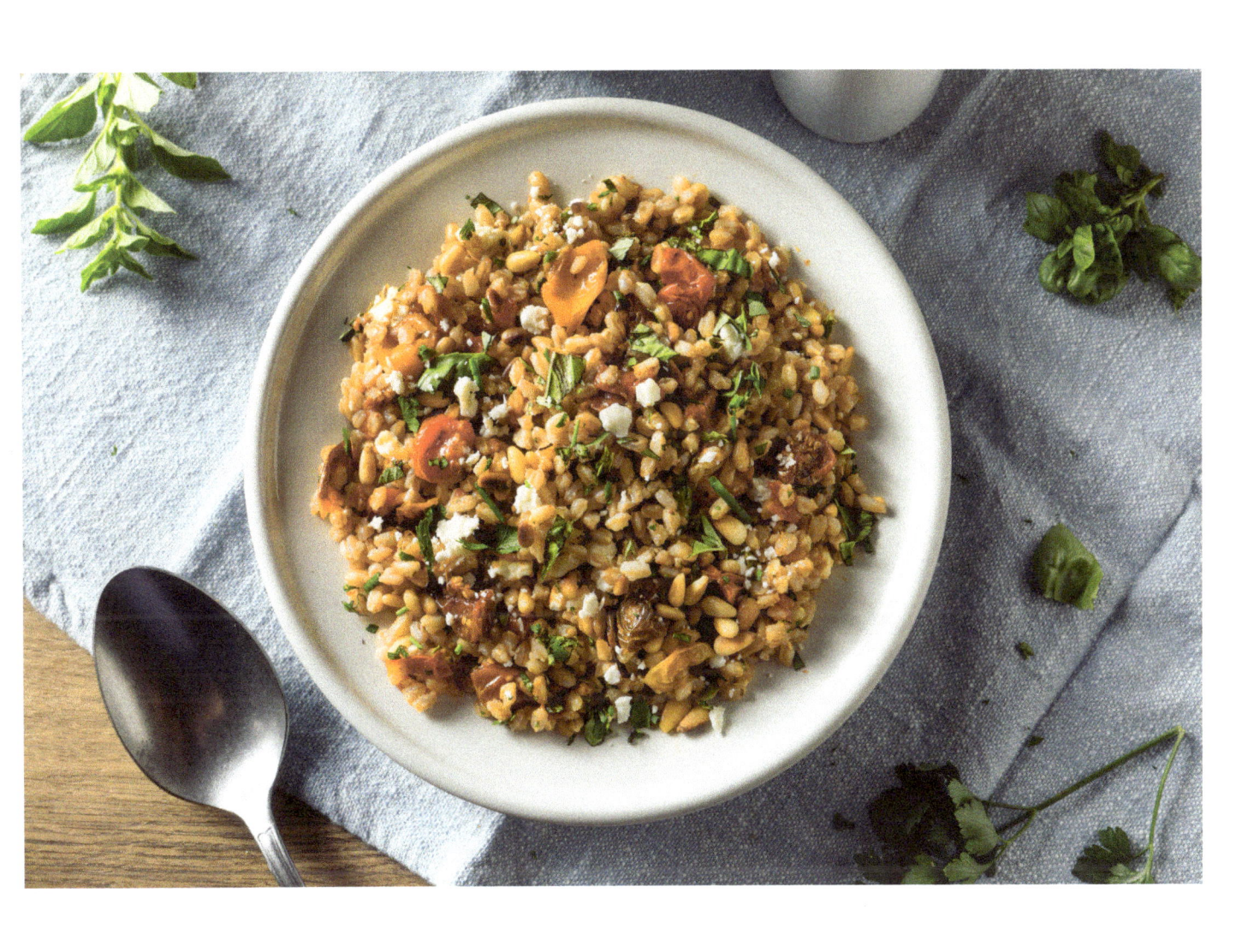

DINNERS

1) LENTIL AND CAULIFLOWER MASAMAN

You can keep this aromatic vegetarian curry in the fridge for a couple of days: the flavour will be even better! Make the Masaman paste if you have time, but supermarket-bought paste does just as well here too.

SERVES 4
PREPARATION TIME: 15 MINUTES
COOKING TIME: 30 MINUTES
Per Serving
Calories: 383 cals
Protein: 16g
Carbs: 47.6g
Fat: 16g

For the Masaman paste:

Add all the ingredients below to a food processor, processing until the mix forms a paste. The quantity will be more than you need for this recipe, but you can keep it in a sterile jar in the fridge, using it within 2 weeks.

65g roasted peanuts
1 tbsp ground coriander
1 tsp ground cumin
½ tsp ground cinnamon
¼ tsp ground cloves
pinch ground white pepper
pinch ground nutmeg
pinch ground cardamom
1 tsp turmeric
5-15 dried red chilli peppers soaked in water for about 10 minutes and deseeded (use gloves!)
1 stalk of lemongrass, minced
5 cm fresh ginger, peeled and sliced
1 shallot
juice of 2 limes, plus 1½ tsp grated lime peel
50ml soy sauce
50ml maple syrup

For the cauliflower and lentils:

200g red lentils, rinsed
2 tbsp vegetable oil
2 onions, diced
1 carrot, diced
1 cauliflower, leaves removed
1 tbsp masaman curry paste
2 cm fresh ginger, grated
400ml vegetable stock
salt and black pepper
10g fresh coriander, chopped, to serve
a few mint leaves, chopped, to serve

Add the lentils to a medium saucepan, cover with cold water, bring to the boil, reduce the heat and cook for 15 minutes. Drain the lentils and set aside.

In a second medium saucepan, heat the oil and when hot add the onions and carrots, cooking over a low heat for 5 minutes.

Separate the cauliflower into small florets and add them to the saucepan, letting them colour a little, which is great for adding flavour.

Add the curry paste, cook for a minute or two, then add the grated ginger and stock.

Pop a lid on the saucepan and simmer everything for around 8 minutes, stirring from time to time.

Add the lentils to heat through, stir everything together and add a sprinkle of coriander and mint leaves before serving.

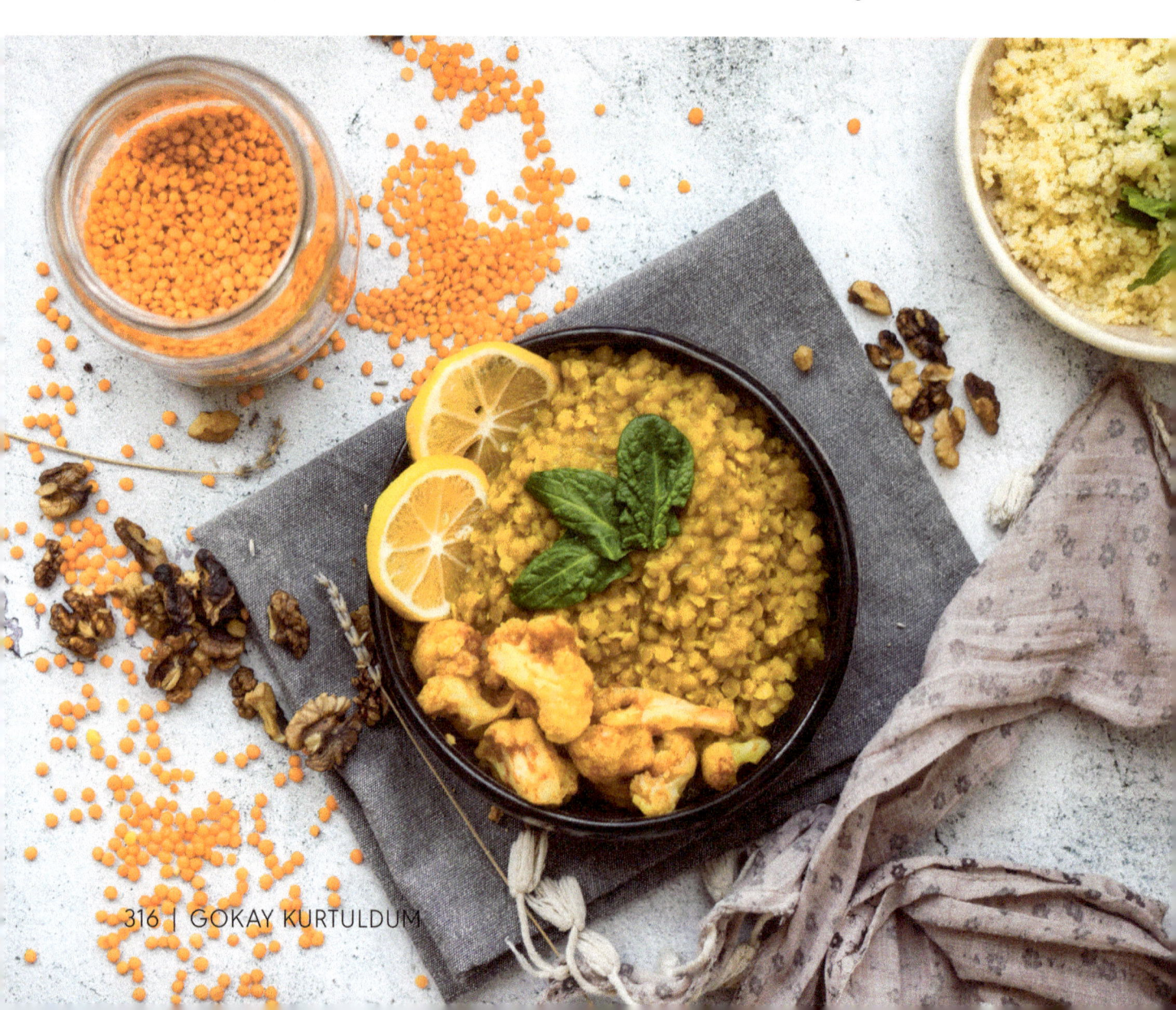

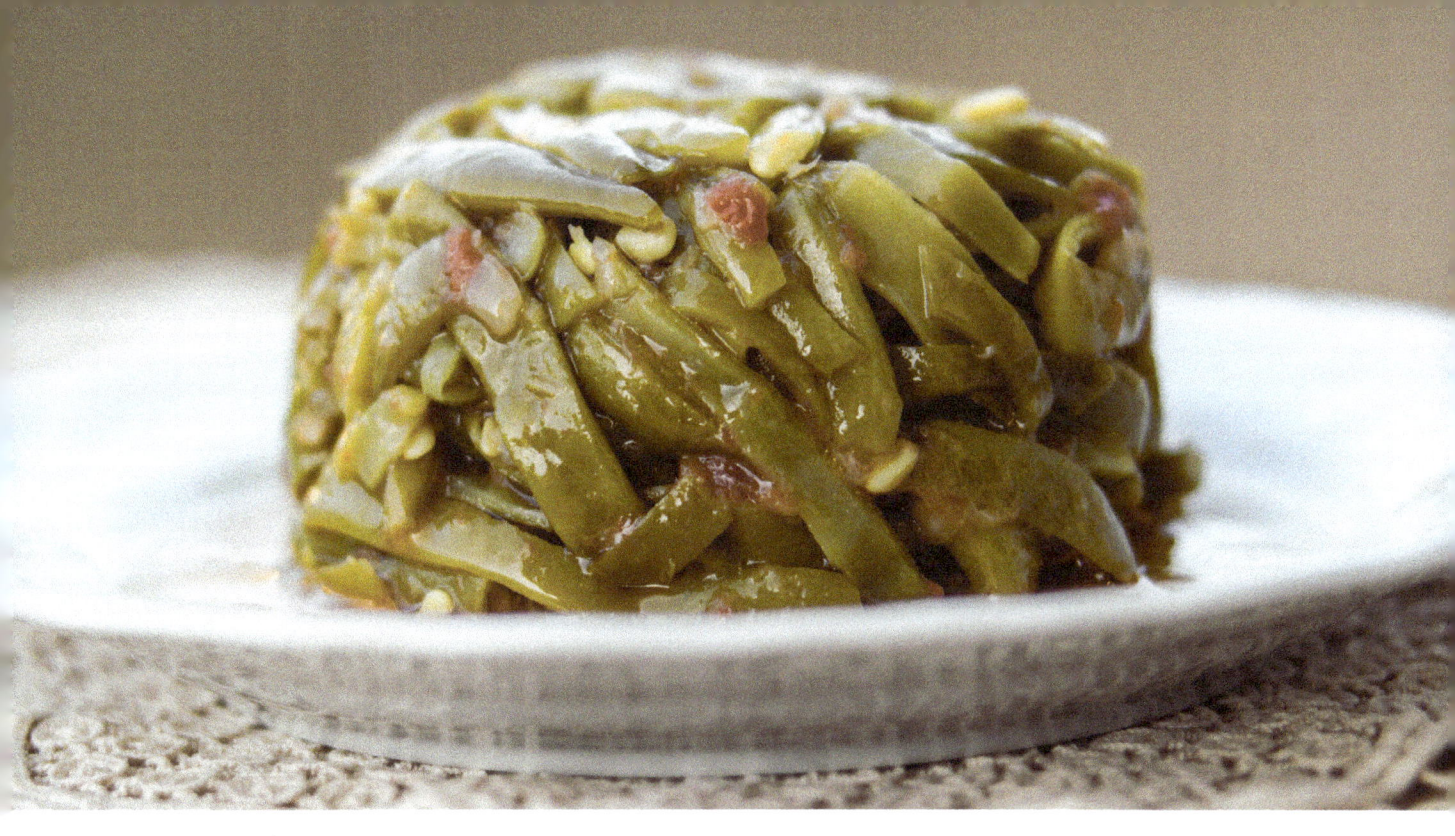

2) MINCED BEEF WITH FRESH RUNNER BEANS

Feel free to cook this without the meat, though if you want to increase protein content in order to build and repair muscle then using mince is good here. For a more filling meal add around 50g of brown rice per person.

SERVES 2 (SUITABLE FOR FREEZING)
PREPARATION TIME: 10 MINUTES
COOKING TIME: 30 MINUTES
Per Serving
Calories: 212 cals
Protein: 11.2g
Carbs: 20.1g
Fat: 10.6g

1 tbsp vegetable oil

1 onion, finely chopped

1 tbsp tomato purée

250g beef mince

400g tin chopped tomatoes

250ml beef stock

250g runner beans, topped, tailed and cut in half

Heat the vegetable oil in a medium saucepan and fry the onion for 5-7 minutes over a low heat, until soft.

Add the tomato purée to the pan, cook for a couple of minutes, then add the minced beef and cook over a medium heat until browned.

Add the stock, tinned tomatoes and runner beans, and bring everything to the boil before reducing the heat to a simmer for 25-30 minutes. The beans are soft when cooked like this, so if you prefer a more crunchy texture add them ten minutes before the end of the cooking time instead.

3) YOGHURT-MARINATED SALMON WITH LENTILS

Feel free to grab ready-cooked lentils from the supermarket for a speedy meal.

SERVES 2

PREPARATION TIME: 5 MINUTES PLUS 20 MINUTES FOR MARINADE

COOKING TIME: UNDER 10 MINUTES

Per Serving

Calories: 683 cals

Protein: 47.6g

Carbs: 60.7g

Fat: 30.1g

2 salmon fillets, without skin

150g natural yoghurt

juice of 1 lemon

pinch of salt

¼ small cucumber

1-calorie olive oil spray

250g pack of ready-cooked lentils

1 tbsp sesame seeds

First place the fish in a bowl. Combine the yoghurt, lemon juice and salt and pour this over the salmon. Cover the bowl and put it in the fridge for 20 minutes to marinate.

Meanwhile cut the cucumber into ribbons with either a potato peeler or a spiraliser.

Remove the fish from the fridge and use some paper towels to remove excess yoghurt. Add a few sprays of olive oil to a medium non-stick frying pan and fry the salmon for 3 minutes on each side.

Put the lentils into a serving dish, add the cucumber and salmon and sprinkle over the sesame seeds.

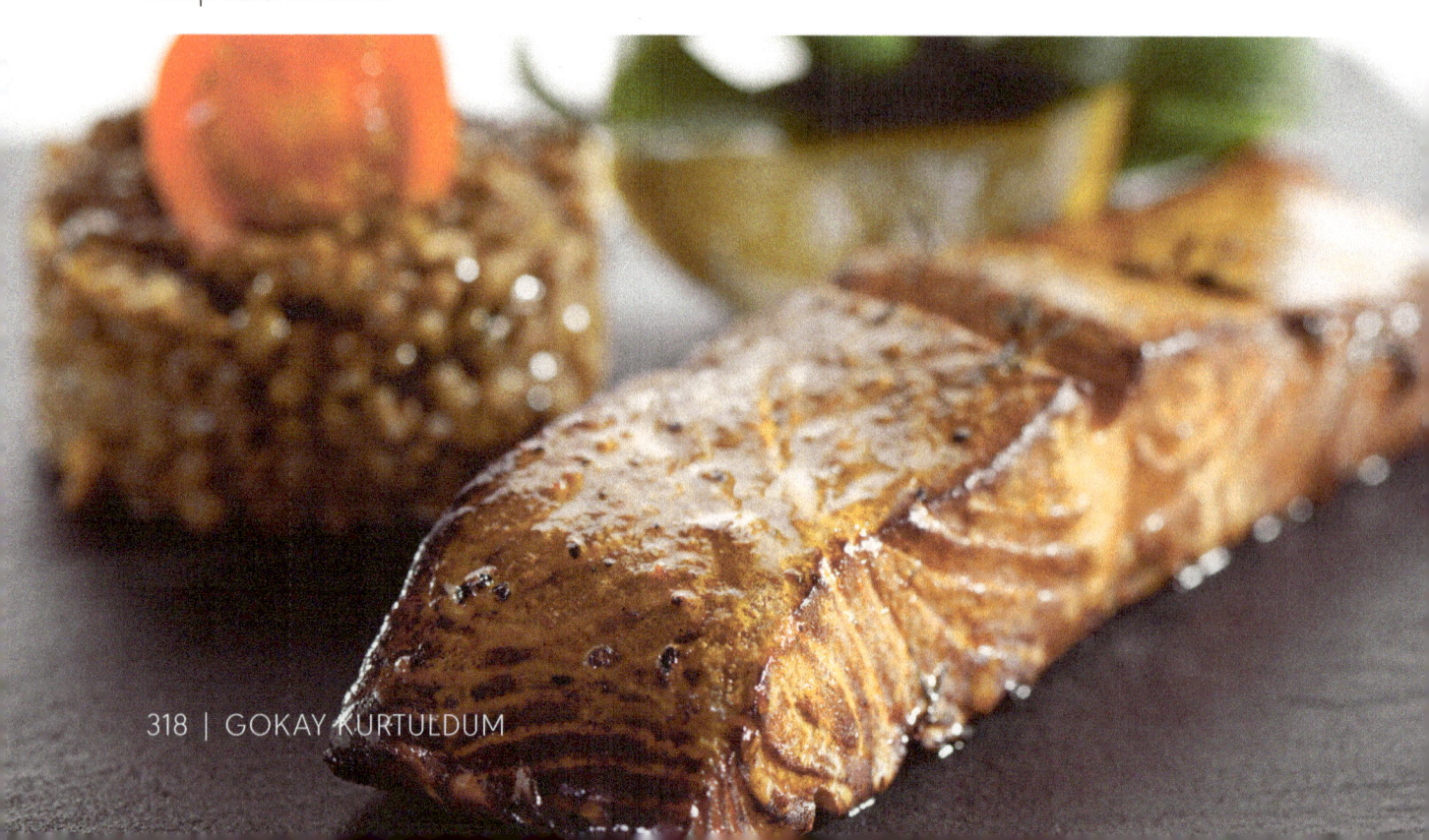

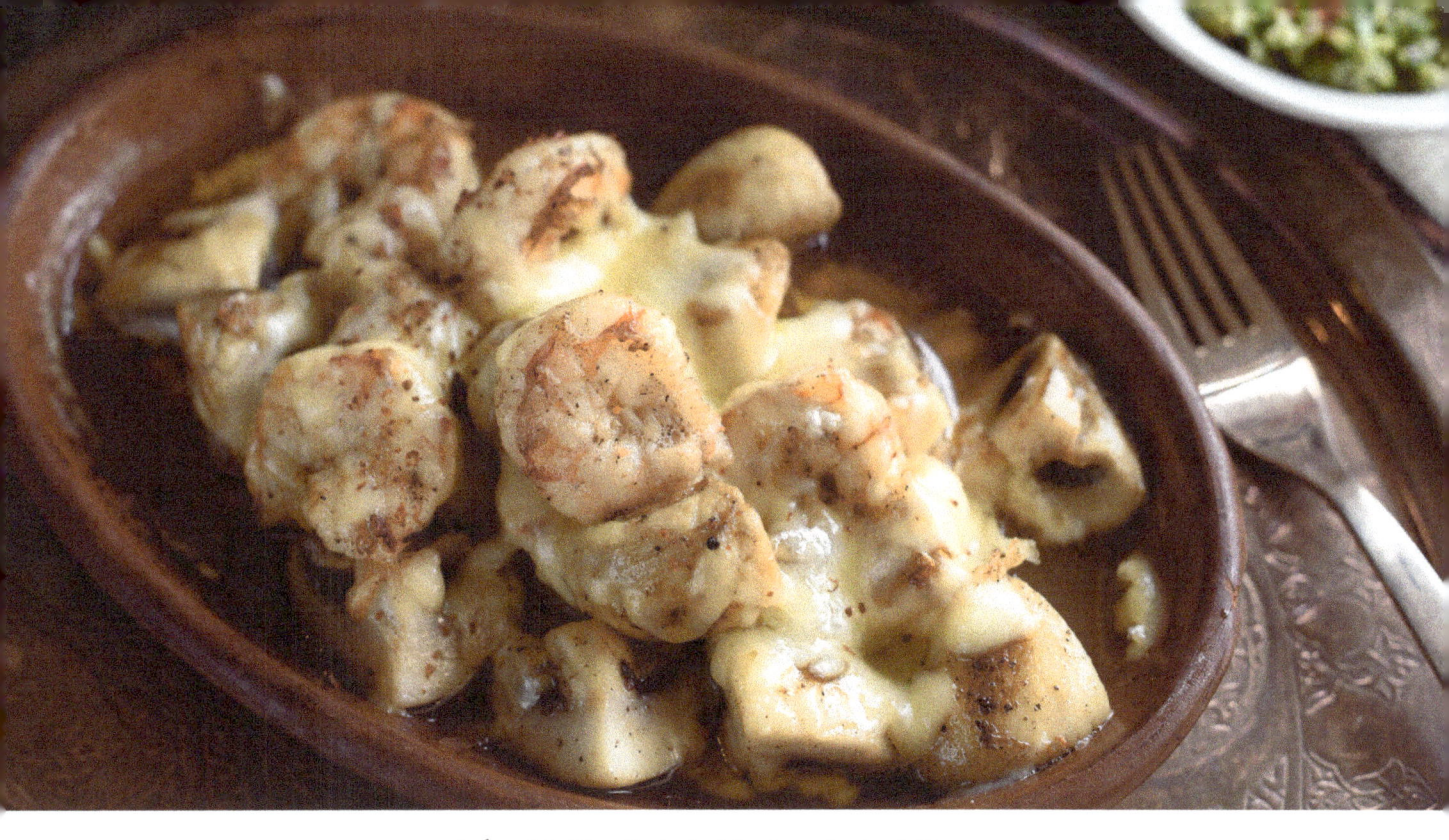

4) PRAWN AND MUSHROOM CASSEROLE

Prawns are a great addition to dishes, as they are full of protein, yet low in calories.

SERVES 2
PREPARATION TIME: 10 MINUTES
COOKING TIME: 30 MINUTES
Per Serving
Calories: 524 cals
Protein: 41.3g
Carbs: 18.7g
Fat: 29.2g

2 tbsp vegetable oil
15g butter
1 medium onion, diced
1 red pepper, diced
1 tsp tomato purée
250g button mushrooms
250g small cooked prawns
45g cheddar cheese, grated
½ tsp chilli flakes
salt and black pepper
250ml water
100g sugar snap peas

Pre-heat the oven to 200°C/180°C Fan/Gas Mark 6

Add the vegetable oil and butter to a small casserole dish, and cook the onion and pepper over a low heat for 5-7 minutes, until soft.

Add the tomato purée, and cook for a couple of minutes.

Add the mushrooms, and stir for a few minutes over a high heat, until any water has evaporated.

Now add the prawns, cheese, chilli flakes, seasoning and water, pop a lid on the pan and put in the oven for 20 minutes.

Once the dish is out of the oven, add the sugar snap peas and stir through before serving.

5) QUINOA AND BLACK BEAN SALAD

Feel free to add tuna or grilled chicken to this tasty salad which is full of different colours and textures.

SERVES 2

PREPARATION TIME: 10 MINUTES

COOKING TIME: 15 MINUTES

Per Serving

Calories: 584 cals

Protein: 19.2g

Carbs: 81.4g

Fat: 20.2g

100g quinoa

1 tbsp vegetable oil

1 onion, finely chopped

1 garlic clove, crushed

300ml chicken stock

1 tsp cumin

½ tsp chilli flakes

200g sweetcorn (1 small tin)

400g tin of black beans

¼ cucumber, diced

100g green olives

10g coriander, chopped

10g mint, chopped

Rinse the quinoa under cold water and set aside to drain.

Add the vegetable oil to a medium saucepan and fry the onion for 5-7 minutes over a low heat until soft. Add the garlic and cook for a further minute.

Add the quinoa and stock, bring to the boil, then reduce the heat and simmer for 15 minutes. The liquid should be fully absorbed by then and the grains swollen, though still with some bite.

Drain both the sweetcorn and the black beans, and add them to the pan.

Add the cucumber, olives, coriander and mint, mix everything well together, and serve.

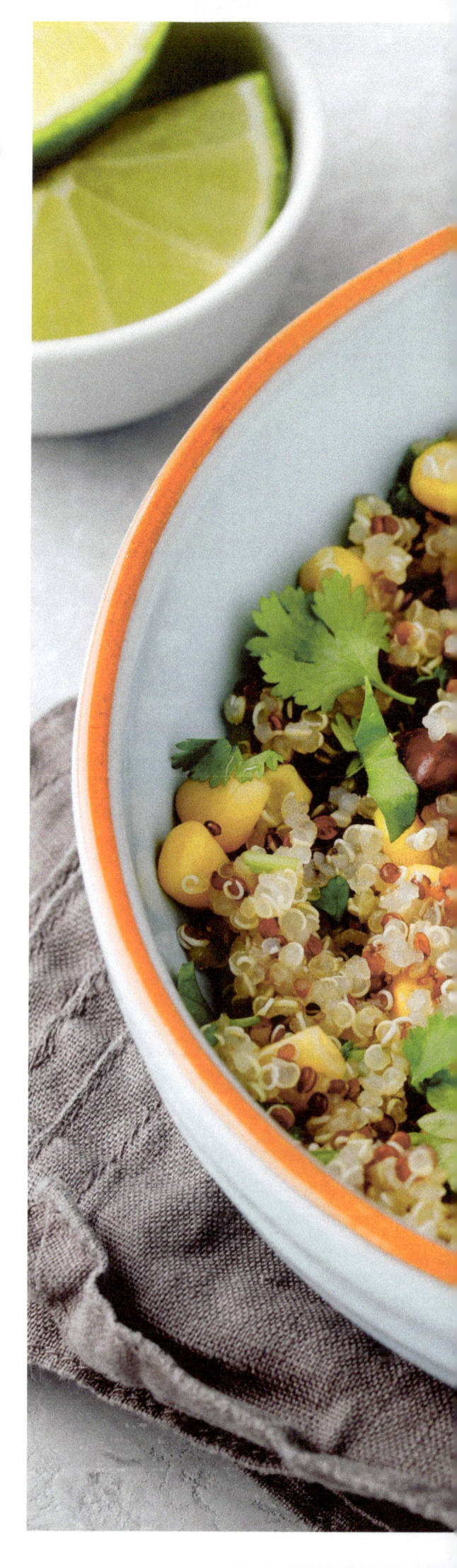

SALADS/SNACKS

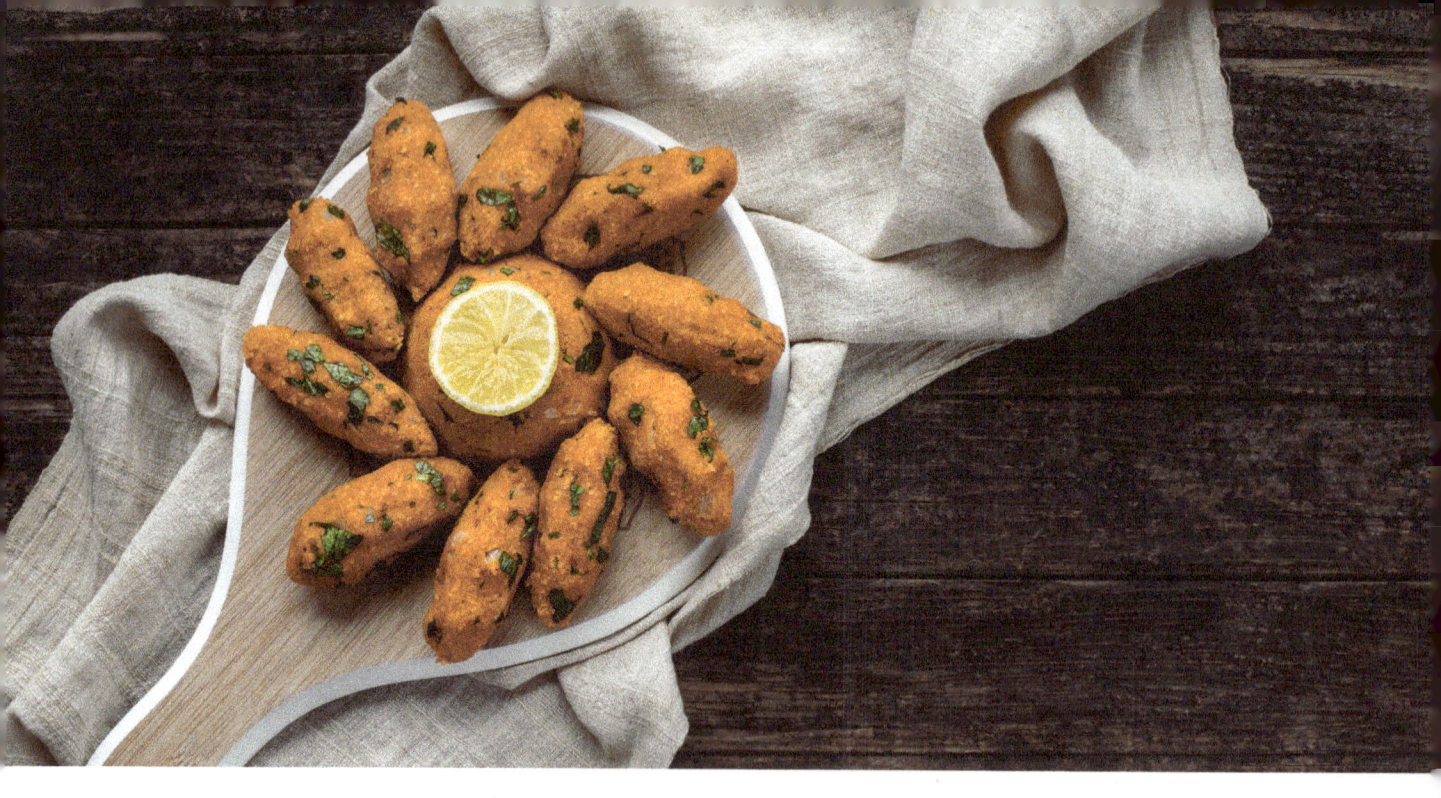

1) LENTIL KOFTES

This recipe makes 24 little patties, perfect for batch cooking. They can then be frozen and used as a quick easy meal when you are short of time.

SERVES 8 (3 patties each) (SUITABLE FOR FREEZING)

PREPARATION TIME: 5 MINUTES

COOKING TIME: 15 MINUTES

Per Serving

Calories: 204 cals

Protein: 7.9g

Carbs: 39.2g

Fat: 2.9g

200g red lentils, rinsed

300g fine bulgur wheat

1 tbsp vegetable oil

1 medium onion, finely chopped

2 tbsp tomato purée

2 tsp ground cumin

2 tsp chilli flakes

2 tsp black pepper

2 spring onions, finely chopped

8 tbsp parsley, finely chopped

salt

Put the rinsed lentils in a saucepan with 750ml of cold water. Bring to the boil, then lower the heat and simmer for 15 minutes, until the lentils are soft. Add the bulgur wheat to the saucepan, cover with a lid and set aside for 30 minutes.

Add the vegetable oil to a small frying pan and fry the onion over a low heat for 5-7 minutes, until soft. Add the tomato purée and cook for a further couple of minutes, stirring frequently.

Tip the lentils and bulgur onto a plate and allow them to cool for a few minutes.

Put the onion mixture into a bowl, then add the cooled lentils and bulgur, as well as the spices, and mix well. If the mixture looks a little dry, add a tablespoon of water.

Add the spring onions and parsley, and mix well together again. Check for seasoning and add a little salt if necessary. Finally shape the mixture into oval-shaped patties and serve. They are usually served with lettuce leaves.

2) PIYAZ

This salad is great as it is or served with meatballs or fish for added protein.

SERVES 2
PREPARATION TIME: 10 MINUTES
COOKING TIME: 7 MINUTES

Per Serving

Calories: 599 cals

Protein: 32.9g

Carbs: 75.3g

Fat: 19.3g

3 eggs

1 red onion

pinch of salt

juice of half a lemon

400g tin cannellini beans

400g tin chickpeas

1 green pepper, diced

1 large tomato, deseeded and chopped

4 lettuce leaves, thinly sliced

2 tbsp parsley, chopped

1 tsp black pepper

1 tsp sumac

1 tbsp olive oil

salt, to taste

First boil the eggs. Bring a small saucepan of water to the boil and gently lower them into the water. Cook the eggs for 1 minute only, then remove the pan from the heat, put a lid on, and allow to sit for 7 minutes before running them under cold water to prevent further cooking. Peel the eggs and set aside.

Cut the onion in half, then slice very thinly, in half-moon shapes. Rub the onion slices with the lemon juice and salt and keep to one side in a small bowl.

Drain both the beans and the chickpeas, and add them to a large bowl. Add the green pepper, tomato, lettuce and parsley.

Chop two of the eggs into cubes, and the remaining one into quarters.

When ready to serve, add the marinated onions to the big bowl, as well as the sumac, cubed eggs, black pepper and olive oil. Mix together gently and taste, as you might like to add a little more lemon juice and some salt.

Transfer to a serving dish and finish with the egg quarters.

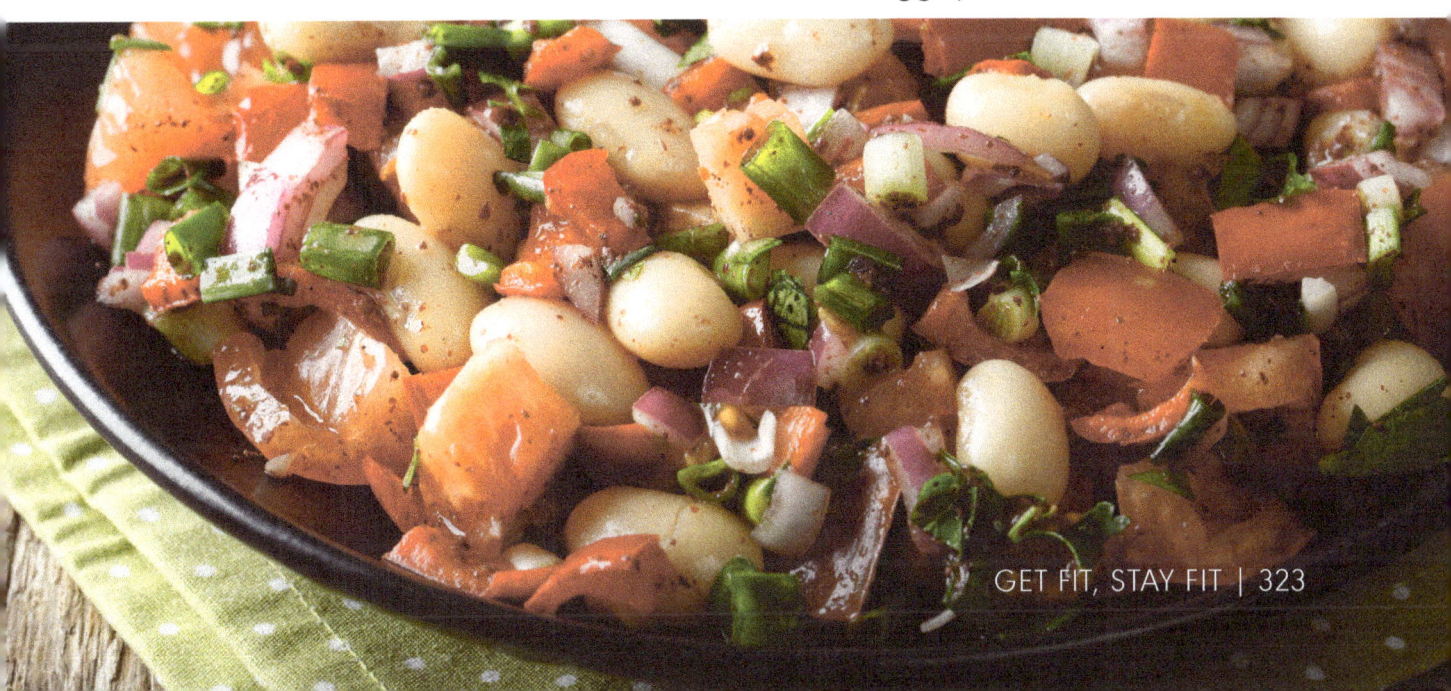

3) FETA AND BEETROOT WITH LENTILS

You may not need to use all of the pecans in the salad, but it's worth making the full amount here as they are a really handy snack.

SERVES 2
PREPARATION TIME: 10 MINUTES
COOKING TIME: 30 MINUTES
Per Serving
Calories: 574 cals
Protein: 21.8g
Carbs: 47.3g
Fat: 32.8g

80g green lentils, rinsed

40g pecans or walnuts

15g butter

2 tbsp light brown sugar

75g feta cheese

150g cooked beetroot (vacuum packed)

mixed salad leaves

1 tbsp sesame oil

salt and pepper

Put the rinsed lentils into a saucepan, add cold water, bring the pan to the boil, then reduce the heat to a low simmer for 25-30 minutes, until soft. Drain, season lightly with salt and pepper, add the sesame oil to combine, and set aside to cool.

For the candied nuts, add the butter and sugar to a small frying pan over a low heat, and add the nuts, stirring to mix, for a couple of minutes. Tip the nuts out onto a lightly oiled baking tray.

Cut the feta into cubes, and the beetroot into small wedges.

When you are ready to assemble the salad, layer a serving dish first with the lentils, then the leaves, beetroot, feta and nuts.

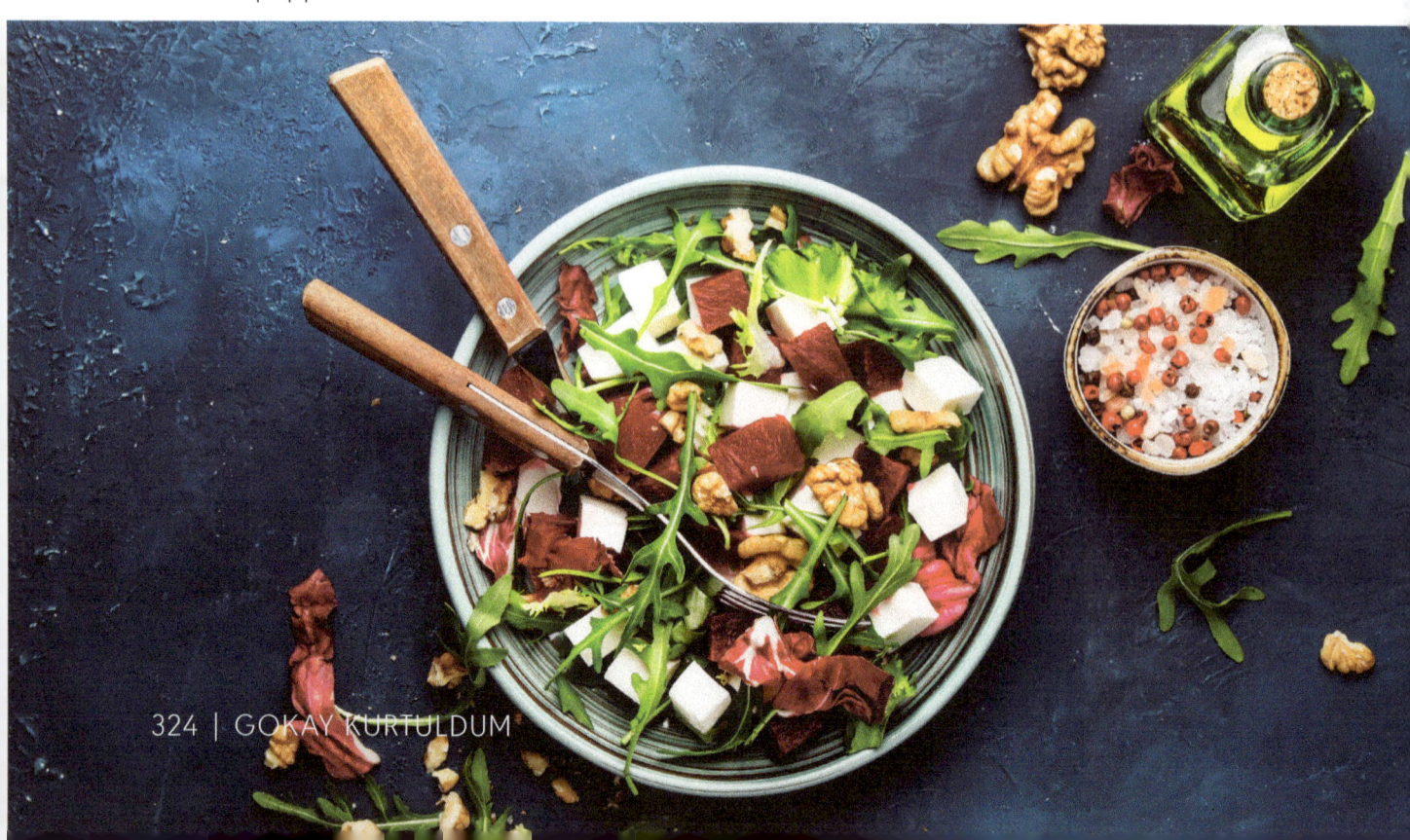

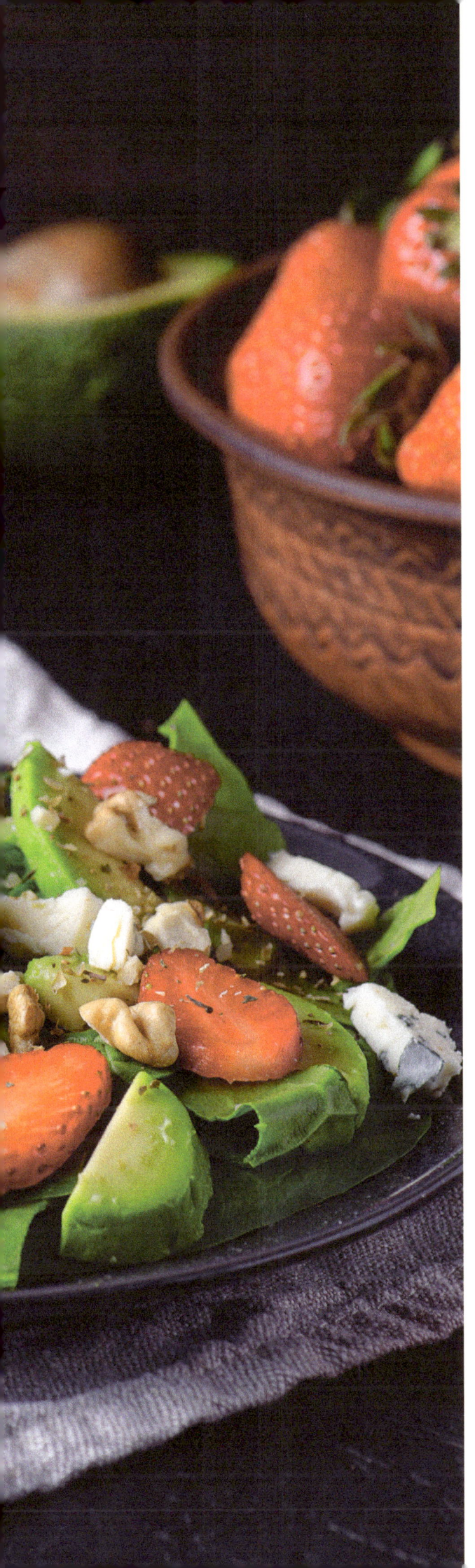

4) SPINACH AND STRAWBERRY SALAD

This colourful, no cook salad is put together in seconds, and the zingy dressing can be used to perk up many other salads too, so it's great to have in the fridge. Add prawns if you like for extra protein.

SERVES 2

PREPARATION TIME: 10 MINUTES

Per Serving

Calories: 582 cals

Protein: 11.7g

Carbs: 22.2g

Fat: 52.1g

80g spinach, washed

½ an avocado

6 strawberries

50g feta cheese, cubed

50g hazelnuts

1 tsp sesame seeds

1 tsp nigella seeds

For the Dressing:

4 tbsp olive oil

1 tbsp lemon juice

1 tbsp vinegar

1 tsp agave syrup (optional)

½ tsp salt

To assemble the salad, cut the strawberries into quarters and slice the avocado.

Whisk together the ingredients for the dressing in a bowl.

Spread the spinach out on a serving plate, and arrange the avocado, strawberries, feta and hazelnuts on top.

Scatter the sesame and nigella seeds over, then add the dressing and it's ready to serve.

5) FALAFEL WITH BEETROOT AND GARLIC DIP

This is great served with pitta and salad, or just as salad alone if you are limiting carbs.

MAKES 24 – SERVES 8 (SUITABLE FOR FREEZING)
PREPARATION TIME: 10 MINUTES
COOKING TIME: 30 MINUTES
Per Serving
Calories: 250 cals
Protein: 9.2g
Carbs: 22g
Fat: 11.9g

For the Falafel:

15g fresh coriander

15g fresh parsley

2 cloves garlic, crushed

juice of 2 lemons

2 tbsp olive oil

half a red onion

1 tbsp ground cumin

1 tbsp turmeric

1 tbsp tahini

pinch of bicarbonate of soda

salt and pepper

800g tinned chickpeas, drained

50g pine nuts

For the beetroot dip:

300g cooked beetroots (vacuum packed)

3 tbsp natural yoghurt

1 clove garlic, crushed

1 tsp sea salt

Pre-heat the oven to 200°C/180°C Fan/Gas Mark 6

For the falafel:

Put all of the ingredients, except the chickpeas and pine nuts, into a food processor, and blend until smooth.

Add the chickpeas and pine nuts, and mix for 15 seconds only, as you want the patties to have some texture.

Divide the mixture into 24 golf ball-sized balls, then flatten lightly into patty shapes.

Put the patties on a flat baking tray, covered with a piece of baking parchment, and bake them in the oven for 30 minutes, turning them halfway through.

For the beetroot dip: cut the beetroot into quarters and add these and all the other ingredients to a food processor. Whizz to a purée, and transfer to a serving bowl.

Serve the falafel with the beetroot dip on the side.

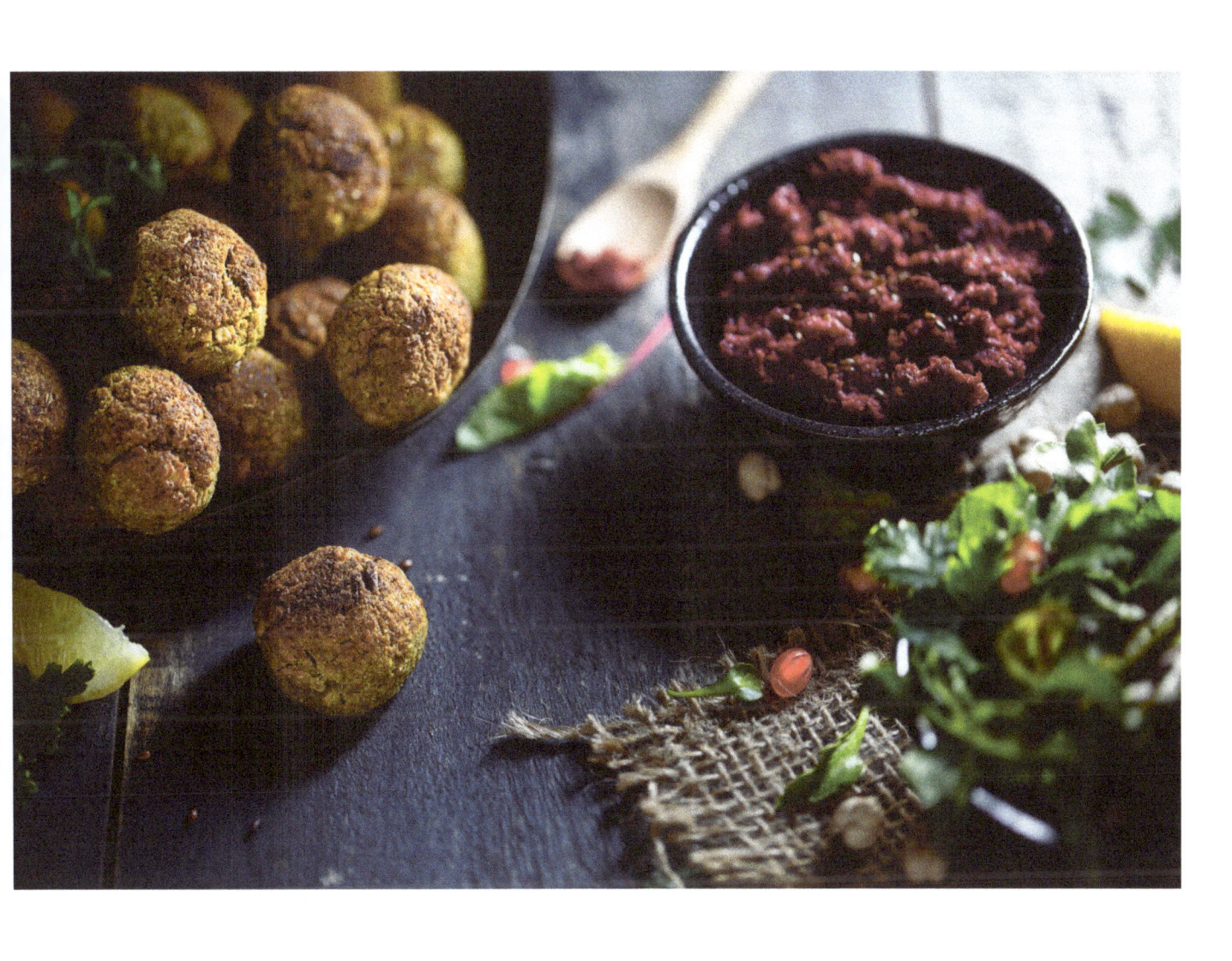

ACKNOWLEDGEMENTS

Firstly I'd like to thank my sister, who raised me after our mum died when I was a child, for being so thoughtful, supportive and for playing multiple roles in my life. I'd like to thank my parents for giving me life too.

Special thanks to my editor Lorna Fergusson of Fictionfire Literary Consultancy, who has been absolutely amazing, working on my book with so much patience and care. This book would have never have come alive without her!

I'd like to thank:

Clare Josa, my Author Mastermind Coach, who in just a two minute conversation during a coffee break inspired me to change my idea of writing a basic recipe book into a much more detailed fitness guide book for men. And all my peers in Clare's Mastermind Programme for being very supportive.

Liz Appleton, my proofreader whose attention to detail is brilliant and her error finding sensors probably 100 times better than any normal person!

Vicki Howard, who named OCADO, for helping me to come up with the acronym AIMBEST.

All my clients for having an amazing connection with me; it almost feels like I have a second family.

In particular, (not in any specific order):

Richard Housley, who is a great example of someone who is very successful in his career, plus a very good family man, who makes fitness, working out and healthy eating his priorities, seeing all this as forming his new lifestyle.

Emma Davidson, who has been a loyal and dedicated client since 2010, and my most long-standing female client.

Sue Riches, who always supports me and who is my star pupil, achieving so much in such a short period of time in terms of fitness and wellbeing, and also for being my brainstorming buddy.

Christopher Barret, who has changed his lifestyle, got fit and healthy and is one of the clients whose story I share with other clients for inspiration.

Finally, I'd like to thank Daniel Priestley for being an amazing coach and an inspirational entrepreneur. His coaching programmes are priceless and he has changed the way I see the world. I'd also like to thank my peers who have been on the same journey with me in Daniel's coaching programmes.